WORLD HEALTH ORGANIZATION

INTERNATIONAL AGENCY FOR RESEARCH ON CANCER

IARC MONOGRAPHS
ON THE
EVALUATION OF THE
CARCINOGENIC RISK
OF CHEMICALS TO HUMANS

Some Antineoplastic and Immunosuppressive Agents

VOLUME 26

This publication represents the views and expert opinions
of an IARC Working Group on the
Evaluation of the Carcinogenic Risk of Chemicals to Humans
which met in Lyon,
14-21 October 1980

May 1981

INTERNATIONAL AGENCY FOR RESEARCH ON CANCER

IARC MONOGRAPHS

In 1971, the International Agency for Research on Cancer (IARC) initiated a programme on the evaluation of the carcinogenic risk of chemicals to humans involving the production of critically evaluated monographs on individual chemicals. In 1980, the programme was expanded to include the evaluation of the carcinogenic risk associated with employment in specific occupations.

The objective of the programme is to elaborate and publish in the form of monographs critical reviews of data on carcinogenicity for chemicals and complex mixtures to which humans are known to be exposed, and on specific occupational exposures, to evaluate these data in terms of human risk with the help of international working groups of experts in chemical carcinogenesis and related fields, and to indicate where additional research efforts are needed.

International Agency for Research on Cancer 1981

ISBN 92 8 321226 6

PRINTED IN SWITZERLAND

CONTENTS 3

RISK OF CHEMICALS TO HUMANS:

SOME ANTINEOPLASTIC AND IMMUNOSUPPRESSIVE AGENTS

Lyon, 14-21 October 1980

Members[1]

R. Althouse, University of Oxford, Clinical Medical School, Radcliffe Hospital, Oxford OX2 6HE, UK

W.F. Benedict, Division of Hematology-Oncology, University of Southern California School of Medicine, 4650 Sunset Boulevard, Los Angeles CA 90054, USA *(Co-rapporteur section 3.2)*

H. Calvert, Institute of Cancer Research, Department of Biochemical Pharmacology, Block E, Clifton Avenue, Belmont, Sutton, Surrey SM2 5PX, UK

M. Clavel, Centre Léon Berard, 28 rue Laënnec, 69008 Lyon, France

T.A. Connors, Director, MRC Toxicology Unit, Medical Research Council Laboratories, Woodmansterne Road, Carshalton, Surrey SM5 4EF, UK *(Co-rapporteur section 3.2)*

J.F. Cordero, Birth Defects Branch, Chronic Diseases Division, Bureau of Epidemiology, Human Services, Center for Disease Control, Atlanta, GA 30333, USA

L. Fiore-Donati, Director, Istituto di Anatomia e Istologie Patologica, Policlinico 'Borgo Roma', 37100 Verona, Italy

M.H. Greene, Environmental Epidemiology Branch, Division of Cancer Cause and Prevention, National Cancer Institute, Landow Building, 3C07, Bethesda, MD 20205, USA

R.A. Griesemer, Director, Biology Division, Oak Ridge National Laboratory, PO Box Y, Oak Ridge, TN 37830, USA *(Co-rapporteur section 3.1)*

---

[1] Unable to attend: C. Schlatter, Institut für Toxikologie der Eidgenössischen Technischen Hochschule und der Universität Zürich, Schorenstrasse 16, 8603 Schwerzenbach bei Zürich, Switzerland

M. Habs, Institut für Toxikologie und Chemotherapie, Deutsches Krebsforschungszentrum, Im Neuenheimer Feld 280, Postfach 101949, D 6900 Heidelberg 1, Federal Republic of Germany

L. Kinlen, University of Oxford, Radcliffe Infirmary, Oxford OX2 6HE, UK

T.M. Mack, University of Southern California School of Medicine, Department of Pathology, 2225 Zonal Avenue, Los Angeles, CA 90033, USA *(Co-rapporteur section 3.3)*

H. Marquardt, Pharmakologisches Institut, Universitäts-Krankenhaus Eppendorf, Grindelallee 117, 2000 Hamburg 13, Federal Republic of Germany

J.G. McVie, Netherlands Cancer Institute, Antoni van Leeuwenhoekhuis, Plesmanlaan 121, 1066 CX Amsterdam, The Netherlands

D. Neubert, Institut für Toxikologie und Embryonal-Pharmakologie der Freien Universitat Berlin, Garystrasse 9, 1000 Berlin 33, Federal Republic of Germany *(Co-rapporteur section 3.2)*

I. Penn, Department of Surgery, Health Sciences Center, University of Colorado, 4200 East Ninth Avenue, Denver, CO 80262, USA *(Vice-chairman; co-rapporteur section 3.2)*

D. Schmähl, Director, Institut für Toxikologie und Chemotherapie, Deutsches Krebsforschungszentrum, Im Neuenheimer Feld 280, Postfach 101949, D 6900 Heidelberg 1, Federal Republic of Germany *(Chairman)*

J.-L. Touraine, INSERM - Unité 80, Unité de Recherche sur la Pathologie métabolique et rénale, Hôpital Edouard Herriot, Pavillon P, 5 place d'Arsonval, 69374 Lyon Cédex 2, France

R. Truhaut, Faculté des Sciences pharmaceutiques et biologiques de Paris-Luxembourg, Laboratoire de Toxicologie et d'Hygiène industrielle, 4 avenue de l'Observatoire, 75006 Paris, France

V. Turusov, Cancer Research Centre, USSR Academy of Medical Sciences, Kashirskoye Shosse, 115478 Moscow, USSR

G.M. Williams, Associate Director, Naylor Dana Institute for Disease Prevention, American Health Foundation, 1 Dana Road, Valhalla, NY 10595, USA

Representative from the National Cancer Institute

M.I. Kelsey, Division of Cancer Cause and Prevention, National Cancer Institute, Landow Building, 3C37, 9000 Rockville Pike, Bethesda, MD 20205, USA

Representative from SRI International

J. Johansson, Bio-organic Chemistry Department, SRI International, 333 Ravenswood, Menlo Park, CA 94025, USA *(Co-rapporteur sections 1 and 2)*

Representative from the Pharmaceutical Manufacturers' Association

G.M. Lyon, Director, Drug Regulatory Affairs, Burroughs Wellcome Co., 3030 Cornwallis Road, Research Triangle Park, NC 27709, USA

Secretariat

C. Agthe, Division of Epidemiology and Biostatistics

H. Bartsch, Division of Environmental Carcinogenesis *(Co-rapporteur section 3.2)*

J.R.P. Cabral, Division of Environmental Carcinogenesis *(Co-rapporteur section 3.1)*

M. Friesen, Division of Environmental Carcinogenesis *(Co-rapporteur sections 1 and 2)*

L. Haroun, Division of Environmental Carcinogenesis *(Co-secretary)*

E. Heseltine *(Editor)*

A. Likhachev, Division of Environmental Carcinogenesis

D. Mietton, Division of Environmental Carcinogenesis *(Library assistant)*

H. Ohshima, Division of Environmental Carcinogenesis

C. Partensky, Division of Environmental Carcinogenesis *(Technical officer)*

I. Peterschmitt, Division of Environmental Carcinogenesis *(Bibliographic researcher)*

R. Saracci, Division of Epidemiology and Biostatics *(Co-rapporteur section 3.3)*

L. Simonato, Division of Epidemiology and Biostatistics

L. Tomatis, Director, Division of Environmental Carcinogenesis *(Head of the Programme)*

J. Wahrendorf, Division of Epidemiology and Biostatistics

J. Wilbourn, Division of Environmental Carcinogenesis *(Co-secretary)*

Secretarial assistance
- A. Beevers
- M.-J. Ghess
- S. Reynaud
- J. Smith

NOTE TO THE READER

The term 'carcinogenic risk' in the *IARC Monograph* series is taken to mean the probability that exposure to a chemical or complex mixture or employment in a particular occupation will lead to cancer in humans.

The fact that a monograph has been prepared on a chemical, complex mixture or occupation does not imply that a carcinogenic hazard is associated with the exposure, only that the published data have been examined. Equally, the fact that a chemical, complex mixture or occupation has not yet been evaluated in a monograph does not mean that it does not represent a carcinogenic hazard.

Anyone who is aware of published data that may alter an evaluation of the carcinogenic risk of a chemical, complex mixture or employment in an occupation is encouraged to make this information available to the Division of Environmental Carcinogenesis, International Agency for Research on Cancer, Lyon, France, in order that the chemical, complex mixture or occupation may be considered for re-evaluation by a future Working Group.

Although every effort is made to prepare the monographs as accurately as possible, mistakes may occur. Readers are requested to communicate any errors to the Division of Environmental Carcinogenesis, so that corrections can be reported in future volumes.

IARC MONOGRAPH PROGRAMME ON THE EVALUATION OF THE CARCINOGENIC RISK OF CHEMICALS TO HUMANS

PREAMBLE

BACKGROUND

In 1971, the International Agency for Research on Cancer (IARC) initiated a programme on the evaluation of the carcinogenic risk of chemicals to humans with the object of producing monographs on individual chemicals[1]. The criteria established at that time to evaluate carcinogenic risk to humans were adopted by all the working groups whose deliberations resulted in the first 16 volumes of the *IARC Monograph* series. In October 1977, a joint IARC/WHO *ad hoc* Working Group met to re-evaluate these guiding criteria; this preamble reflects the results of their deliberations(1) and those of a subsequent IARC *ad hoc* Working Group which met in April 1978(2).

A further *ad hoc* Working Group, which met in Lyon in April 1979 to prepare criteria to select chemicals for *IARC Monographs*(3), recommended that the *Monograph* programme be expanded to include consideration of human exposures in selected occupations. The Working Group which met in June 1980 therefore considered occupational exposures in wood, leather and some associated industries; their deliberations resulted in Volume 25 of the *Monograph* series.

OBJECTIVE AND SCOPE

The objective of the programme is to elaborate and publish in the form of monographs critical reviews of data on carcinogenicity for groups of chemicals to which humans are known to be exposed, to evaluate those data in terms of human risk with the help of international working groups of experts in chemical carcinogenesis and related fields, and to indicate where additional research efforts are needed.

The critical analyses of the data are intended to assist national and international authorities in formulating decisions concerning preventitive measures. No recommendations are given concerning legislation, since this depends on risk-benefit evaluations, which seem best made by individual governments and/or other international agencies. In this connection, WHO recommendations on food additives(4), drugs(5), pesticides and contaminants(6) and occupational carcinogens(7) are particularly informative.

---

[1] Since 1972, the programme has undergone considerable expansion, primarily with the scientific collaboration and financial support of the US National Cancer Institute, Bethesda, MD.

Up to May 1981, 26 volumes of the *Monographs* had been published or were in press(8). A total of 553 compounds, industrial processes or occupational exposures had been evaluated or re-evaluated. For 41 chemicals, groups of chemicals, industrial processes or industrial exposures, a positive association or a strong suspicion of an association with human cancer has been found. For 22 of the individual chemicals, exposures are predominantly in occupational settings, although the general population may be exposed through environmental contamination. For 12 chemicals, human exposure was related to therapeutic uses; for one compound exposure occurs *via* the diet. The preponderance of experimental data over epidemiological data on the 553 compounds or processes is striking: data on humans were available for only 70 of the chemicals, and 134 of them were evaluated for human carcinogenicity solely on the basis of *sufficient evidence* of carcinogenicity in experimental animals. The remainder could not be evaluated for carcinogenicity to humans.

The *IARC Monographs* are recognized as an authoritative source of information on the carcinogenicity of environmental chemicals. The first users' survey, made in 1976, indicates that the monographs are consulted routinely by various agencies in 24 countries. Each volume is printed in 4000 copies and distributed *via* the WHO publications service. (See last page for a listing of IARC publications and back outside cover for distribution and sales services.)

SELECTION OF CHEMICALS FOR MONOGRAPHS

The chemicals (natural and synthetic, including those which occur as mixtures and in manufacturing processes) are selected for evaluation on the basis of two main criteria: (a) there is evidence of human exposure, and (b) there is some experimental evidence of carcinogenicity and/or there is some evidence or suspicion of a risk to humans. In certain instances, chemical analogues are also considered. The scientific literature is surveyed for published data relevant to the monograph programme. In addition, the IARC *Survey of Chemicals Being Tested for Carcinogenicity*(9) often indicates those chemicals that may be scheduled for future meetings.

Inclusion of a chemical in a volume does not imply that it is carcinogenic, only that the published data have been examined. The evaluations must be consulted to ascertain the conclusions of the Working Group. Equally, the fact that a chemical has not appeared in a monograph does not mean that it is without carcinogenic hazard.

As new data on chemicals for which monographs have already been prepared and new principles for evaluating carcinogenic risk receive acceptance, re-evaluations will be made at subsequent meetings, and revised monographs will be published as necessary.

WORKING PROCEDURES

Approximately one year in advance of a meeting of a working group, a list of the substances to be considered is prepared by IARC staff in consultation with other experts. Subsequently, all relevant biological data are collected by IARC; in addition to the published literature, US Public Health Service Publication No. 149(10) has been particularly valuable and has been used in conjunction with other recognized sources of information on chemical carcinogenesis and systems such as CANCERLINE, MEDLINE and TOXLINE. The major collection of data and the preparation of first drafts for the sections on chemical and physical properties, on production, use, occurrence and on analysis are carried out by SRI International, Stanford, CA, USA under a separate contract with the US National Cancer Institute. Most of the data so obtained on production, use and occurrence refer to the United States and Japan; SRI International and IARC supplement this information with that from other sources in Europe. Bibliographical sources for data on mutagenicity and teratogenicity are the Environmental Mutagen Information Center and the Environmental Teratology Information Center, both located at the Oak Ridge National Laboratory, TN, USA.

Six to nine months before the meeting, reprints of articles containing relevant biological data are sent to an expert(s), or are used by the IARC staff, for the preparation of first draft monographs. These drafts are edited by IARC staff and are sent prior to the meeting to all participants of the Working Group for their comments. The Working Group then meets in Lyon for seven to eight days to discuss and finalize the texts of the monographs and to formulate the evaluations. After the meeting, the master copy of each monograph is verified by consulting the original literature, then edited and prepared for reproduction. The monographs are usually published within six months after the Working Group meeting.

DATA FOR EVALUATIONS

With regard to biological data, only reports that have been published or accepted for publication are reviewed by the working groups, although a few exceptions have been made. The monographs do not cite all of the literature on a particular chemical: only those data considered by the Working Group to be relevant to the evaluation of the carcinogenic risk of the chemical to humans are included.

Anyone who is aware of data that have been published or are in press which are relevant to the evaluations of the carcinogenic risk to humans of chemicals for which monographs have appeared is urged to make them available to the Division of Environmental Carcinogenesis, International Agency for Research on Cancer, Lyon, France.

THE WORKING GROUP

The tasks of the Working Group are five-fold: (a) to ascertain that all data have been collected;   (b) to select the data relevant for the evaluation;   (c) to ensure that the summaries of the data enable the reader to follow the reasoning of the committee;   (d) to judge the significance of the results of experimental and epidemiological studies;   and (e) to make an evaluation of the carcinogenic risk of the chemical.

Working Group participants who contributed to the consideration and evaluation of chemicals within a particular volume are listed, with their addresses, at the beginning of each publication (see p. 5).   Each member serves as an individual scientist and not as a representative of any organization or government. In addition, observers are often invited from national and international agencies, organizations and industries.

GENERAL PRINCIPLES FOR EVALUATING THE CARCINOGENIC
RISK OF CHEMICALS

The widely accepted meaning of the term 'chemical carcinogenesis', and that used in these monographs, is the induction by chemicals of neoplasms that are not usually observed, the earlier induction by chemicals of neoplasms that are usually observed, and/or the induction by chemicals of more neoplasms than are usually found - although fundamentally different mechanisms may be involved in these three situations. Etymologically, the term 'carcinogenesis' means the induction of cancer, that is, of malignant neoplasms; however, the commonly accepted meaning is the induction of various types of neoplasms or of a combination of malignant and benign tumours. In the monographs, the words 'tumour' and 'neoplasm' are used interchangeably. (In scientific literature the terms 'tumourigen', 'oncogen' and 'blastomogen' have all been used synonymously with 'carcinogen', although occasionally 'tumourigen' has been used specifically to denote a substance that induces benign tumours.)

Experimental Evidence

Qualitative aspects

Both the interpretation and evaluation of a particular study as well as the overall assessment of the carcinogenic activity of a chemical involve several qualitatively important considerations, including: (a) the experimental parameters under which the chemical was tested, including route of administration and exposure, species, strain, sex, age, etc.;   (b) the consistency with which the chemical has been shown to be carcinogenic, e.g., in how many species and at which target organ(s);   (c) the spectrum of neoplastic response, from benign neoplasm to multiple malignant tumours;   (d) the stage of tumour formation in which a chemical may be involved: some chemicals act as complete carcinogens and have initiating and promoting activity, while others are promoters only; and (e) the possible role of modifying factors.

There are problems not only of differential survival but of differential toxicity, which may be manifested by unequal growth and weight gain in treated and control animals. These complexities are also considered in the interpretation of data.

Many chemicals induce both benign and malignant tumours. Few instances are recorded in which only benign neoplasms are induced by chemicals that have been studied extensively. Benign tumours may represent a stage in the evolution of a malignant neoplasm or they may be 'end-points' that do not readily undergo transition to malignancy. If a substance is found to induce only benign tumours in experimental animals, it should be suspected of being a carcinogen and requires further investigation.

Hormonal carcinogenesis

Hormonal carcinogenesis presents certain distinctive features: the chemicals involved occur both endogenously and exogenously; in many instances, long exposure is required; tumours occur in the target tissue in association with a stimulation of non-neoplastic growth, but in some cases, hormones promote the proliferation of tumour cells in a target organ. Hormones that occur in excessive amounts, hormone-mimetic agents and agents that cause hyperactivity or imbalance in the endocrine system may require evaluative methods comparable with those used to identify chemical carcinogens; particular emphasis must be laid on quantitative aspects and duration of exposure. Some chemical carcinogens have significant side effects on the endocrine system, which may also result in hormonal carcinogenesis. Synthetic hormones and anti-hormones can be expected to possess other pharmacological and toxicological actions in addition to those on the endocrine system, and in this respect they must be treated like any other chemical with regard to intrinsic carcinogenic potential.

Quantitative aspects

Dose-response studies are important in the evaluation of carcinogenesis: the confidence with which a carcinogenic effect can be established is strengthened by the observation of an increasing incidence of neoplasms with increasing exposure.

The assessment of carcinogenicity in animals is frequently complicated by recognized differences among the test animals (species, strain, sex, age), route(s) of administration and in dose/duration of exposure; often, target organs at which a cancer occurs and its histological type may vary with these parameters. Nevertheless, indices of carcinogenic potency in particular experimental systems [for instance, the dose-rate required under continuous exposure to halve the probability of the animals remaining tumourless(11)] have been formulated in the hope that, at least among categories of fairly similar agents, such indices may be of some predictive value in other systems, including humans.

Chemical carcinogens differ widely in the dose required to produce a given level of tumour induction, although many of them share common biological properties, which include metabolism to reactive [electrophilic(12-14)] intermediates capable of interacting with DNA. The reason for this variation in dose-response is not understood, but it may be due either to differences within a common metabolic process or to the operation of qualitatively distinct mechanisms.

Statistical analysis of animal studies

Tumours which would have arisen had an animal lived longer may not be observed because of the death of the animal from unrelated causes, and this possibility must be allowed for. Various analytical techniques have been developed which use the assumption of independence of competing risks to allow for the effects of intercurrent mortality on the final numbers of tumour-bearing animals in particular treatment groups.

For externally visible tumours and for neoplasms that cause death, methods such as Kaplan-Meier (i.e., 'life-table', 'product-limit', or 'actuarial') estimates(11), with associated significance tests(15, 16), have been recommended.

For internal neoplasms which are discovered 'incidentally'(15) at autopsy but which did not cause the death of the host, different estimates(17) and significance tests(15,16) may be necessary for the unbiased study of the numbers of tumour-bearing animals.

All of these methods(11, 15-17) can be used to analyse the numbers of animals bearing particular tumour types, but they do not distinguish between animals with one or many such tumours. In experiments which end at a particular fixed time, with the simultaneous sacrifice of many animals, analysis of the total numbers of internal neoplasms per animal found at autopsy at the end of the experiment is straightforward. However, there are no adequate statistical methods for analysing the numbers of particular neoplasms that kill an animal. The design and statistical analysis of long-term carcinogenicity experiments were recently reviewed, in Supplement 2 to the *Monograph* series(18).

Evidence of Carcinogenicity in Humans

Evidence of carcinogenicity in humans can be derived from three types of study, the first two of which usually provide only suggestive evidence: (1) reports concerning individual cancer patients (case reports), including a history of exposure to the supposed carcinogenic agent; (2) descriptive epidemiological studies in which the incidence of cancer in human populations is found to vary (spatially or temporally) with exposure to the agent; and (3) analytical epidemiological studies (e.g., case-control or cohort studies) in which individual exposure to the agent is found to be associated with an increased risk of cancer.

An analytical study that shows a positive association between an agent and a cancer may be interpreted as implying causality to a greater or lesser extent, on the basis of the following criteria: (a) There is no identifiable positive bias. [By 'positive bias' is meant the operation of factors in study design or execution which lead erroneously to a more strongly positive association between an agent and disease than in fact exists. Examples of positive bias include, in case-control studies, better documentation of exposure to the agent for cases than for controls, and, in cohort studies, the use of better means of detecting cancer in individuals exposed to the agent than in individuals not exposed.]   (b) The possibility of positive confounding has been considered. [By 'positive confounding' is meant a situation in which the relationship between an agent and a disease is rendered more strongly positive than it truly is as a result of an association between that agent and another agent which either causes or prevents the disease. An example of positive confounding is the association between coffee consumption and lung cancer, which results from their joint association with cigarette smoking.]   (c) The association is unlikely to be due to chance alone.   (d) The association is strong.   (e) There is a dose-response relationship.

In some instances, a single epidemiological study may be strongly indicative of a cause-effect relationship; however, the most convincing evidence of causality comes when several independent studies done under different circumstances result in 'positive' findings.

Analytical epidemiological studies that show no association between an agent and a cancer ('negative' studies) should be interpreted according to criteria analogous to those listed above: (a) there is no identifiable negative bias;   (b) the possibility of negative confounding has been considered;   and (c) the possible effects of misclassification of exposure or outcome have been weighed.   In addition, it must be recognized that in any study there are confidence limits around the estimate of association or relative risk.   In a study regarded as 'negative', the upper confidence limit may indicate a relative risk substantially greater than unity;   in that case, the study excludes only relative risks that are above this upper limit.   This usually means that a 'negative' study must be large to be convincing.   Confidence in a 'negative' result is increased when several independent studies carried out under different circumstances are in agreement.   Finally, a 'negative' study may be considered to be relevant only to dose levels within or below the range of those observed in the study and is pertinent only if sufficient time has elapsed since first human exposure to the agent.   Experience with human cancers of known etiology suggests that the period from first exposure to a chemical carcinogen to development of clinically observed cancer is usually measured in decades and may be in excess of 30 years.

The Working Group whose deliberations resulted in Supplement 1 to the *Monographs* (IARC, 1979) defined *sufficient evidence* of the carcinogenicity of a chemical to humans as that which provides a causal association between exposure and cancer; *limited evidence* was defined as that which indicates a possible carcinogenic effect in humans.

Relevance of Experimental Data to the Evaluation of Carcinogenic Risk to Humans

No adequate criteria are presently available to interpret experimental carcinogenicity data directly in terms of carcinogenic potential for humans. Nonetheless, utilizing data collected from appropriate tests in animals, positive extrapolations to possible human risk can be approximated.

Information compiled from the first 26 volumes of the *IARC Monographs* (19-21) shows that of the 41 chemicals, groups of chemicals, manufacturing processes or occupational exposures now generally accepted to cause or probably to cause cancer in humans, all but possibly two (arsenic and benzene) of those which have been tested appropriately produce cancer in at least one animal species. For several of the chemicals that are carcinogenic for humans (aflatoxins, 4-aminobiphenyl, diethylstilboestrol, melphalan, mustard gas and vinyl chloride), evidence of carcinogenicity in experimental animals preceded evidence obtained from epidemiological studies or case reports.

In general, the evidence that a chemical produces tumours in experimental animals is of two degrees: (a) *sufficient evidence* of carcinogenicity is provided by the production of malignant tumours; and (b) *limited evidence* of carcinogenicity reflects qualitative and/or quantitative limitations of the experimental results.

Sufficient evidence of carcinogenicity is provided by experimental studies that show an increased incidence of malignant tumours: (i) in multiple species or strains, and/or (ii) in multiple experiments (routes and/or doses), and/or (iii) to an unusual degree (with regard to incidence, site, type and/or precocity of onset). Additional evidence may be provided by data concerning dose-response, mutagenicity or structure.

For many of the chemicals evaluated in the first 26 volumes of the *IARC Monographs* for which there is *sufficient evidence* of carcinogenicity in animals, data relating to carcinogenicity for humans are either insufficient or nonexistent. In the absence of adequate data on humans, it is reasonable, for practical purposes, to regard such chemicals as if they presented a carcinogenic risk to humans.

In the present state of knowledge, it would be difficult to define a predictable relationship between the dose (mg/kg bw/day) of a particular chemical required to produce cancer in test animals and the dose which would produce a similar incidence of cancer in humans. The available data suggest, however, that such a relationship may exist(22, 23), at least for certain classes of carcinogenic chemicals. Data that provide sufficient evidence of carcinogenicity in test animals may therefore be used in an approximate quantitative evaluation of the human risk at some given exposure level, provided that the nature of the chemical concerned and the physiological, pharmacological and toxicological differences between the test animals and humans are taken into account. However, no acceptable methods are currently available for quantifying the possible errors in such a procedure, whether it is used to generalize between species or to extrapolate from high to low doses. The methodology for such quantitative extrapolation to humans requires further development.

Evidence for the carcinogenicity of some chemicals in experimental animals may be *limited* for two reasons. Firstly, experimental data may be restricted to such a point that it is not possible to determine a causal relationship between administration of a chemical and the development of a particular lesion in the animals. Secondly, there are certain neoplasms, including lung tumours and hepatomas in mice, which have been considered of lesser significance than neoplasms occurring at other sites for the purpose of evaluating the carcinogenicity of chemicals. Such tumours occur spontaneously in high incidence in these animals, and their malignancy is often difficult to establish. An evaluation of the significance of these tumours following administration of a chemical is the responsibility of particular Working Groups preparing individual monographs, and it has not been possible to set down rigid guidelines; the relevance of these tumours must be determined by considerations which include experimental design and completeness of reporting.

Some chemicals for which there is *limited evidence* of carcinogenicity in animals have also been studied in humans with, in general, inconclusive results. While such chemicals may indeed be carcinogenic to humans, more experimental and epidemiological investigation is required.

Hence, *'sufficient evidence'* of carcinogenicity and *'limited evidence'* of carcinogenicity do not indicate categories of chemicals: the inherent definitions of those terms indicate varying degrees of experimental evidence, which may change if and when new data on the chemicals become available. The main drawback to any rigid classification of chemicals with regard to their carcinogenic capacity is the as yet incomplete knowledge of the mechanism(s) of carcinogenesis.

In recent years, several short-term tests for the detection of potential carcinogens have been developed. When only inadequate experimental data are available, positive results in validated short-term tests (see p.23) are an indication that the compound is a potential carcinogen and that it should be tested in animals for an assessment of its carcinogenicity. Negative results from short-term tests cannot be considered sufficient evidence to rule out carcinogenicity. Whether short-term tests will eventually be as reliable as long-term tests in predicting carcinogenicity in humans will depend on further demonstrations of consistency with long-term experiments and with data from humans. Available screening assays are evaluated in Supplement 2 to the *Monographs*(18).

EXPLANATORY NOTES ON THE MONOGRAPH CONTENTS

Chemical and Physical Data (Section 1)

The Chemical Abstracts Services Registry Number, the latest Chemical Abstracts Primary Name (9th Collective Index)(24) and the IUPAC Systematic Name(25) are recorded in section 1. Other synonyms and trade names are given, but no comprehensive list is provided. Further, some of the trade names are those of mixtures in which the compound being evaluated is only one of the ingredients.

The structural and molecular formulae, molecular weight and chemical and physical properties are given. The properties listed refer to the pure substance, unless otherwise specified, and include, in particular, data that might be relevant to carcinogenicity (e.g., lipid solubility) and those that concern identification.

A separate description of the composition of technical products includes available information on impurities and formulated products.

Production, Use, Occurrence and Analysis (Section 2)

The purpose of section 2 is to provide indications of the extent of past and present human exposure to the chemical.

Synthesis

Since cancer is a delayed toxic effect, the dates of first synthesis and of first commercial production of the chemical are provided. In addition, methods of synthesis used in past and present commercial production are described. This information allows a reasonable estimate to be made of the date before which no human exposure could have occurred.

Production

Since Europe, Japan and the United States are reasonably representative industrialized areas of the world, most data on production, foreign trade and uses are obtained from those countries. It should not, however, be inferred that those nations are the sole or even the major sources or users of any individual chemical.

Production and foreign trade data are obtained from both governmental and trade publications by chemical economists in the three geographical areas. In some cases, separate production data on organic chemicals manufactured in the United States are not available because their publication could disclose confidential information. In such cases, an indication of the minimum quantity produced can be inferred from the number of companies reporting commercial production. Each company is required to report on individual chemicals if the sales value or the weight of the annual production exceeds a specified minimum level. These levels vary for chemicals classified for different uses, e.g., medicinals and plastics; in fact, the minimal annual sales value is between $1000 and $50,000 and the minimal annual weight of production is between 450 and 22, 700 kg. Data on production in some European countries are obtained by means of general questionnaires sent to companies thought to produce the compounds being evaluated. Information from the completed questionnaires is compiled by country, and the resulting estimates of production are included in the individual monographs.

Use

Information on uses is meant to serve as a guide only and is not complete. It is usually obtained from published data but is often complemented by direct contact with manufacturers of the chemical. In the case of drugs, mention of their therapeutic uses does not necessarily represent current practice nor does it imply judgement as to their clinical efficacy.

Statements concerning regulations and standards (e.g., pesticide registrations, maximum levels permitted in foods, occupational standards and allowable limits) in specific countries are mentioned as examples only. They may not reflect the most recent situation, since such legislation is in a constant state of change; nor should it be taken to imply that other countries do not have similar regulations.

Occurrence

Information on the occurrence of a chemical in the environment is obtained from published data, including that derived from the monitoring and surveillance of levels of the chemical in occupational environments, air, water, soil, foods and tissues of animals and humans. When available, data on the generation, persistence and bioaccumulation of a chemical are also included.

Analysis

The purpose of the section on analysis is to give the reader an indication, rather than a complete review, of methods cited in the literature. No attempt is made to evaluate critically or to recommend any of the methods.

Biological Data Relevant to the Evaluation of Carcinogenic Risk to Humans (Section 3)

In general, the data recorded in section 3 are summarized as given by the author; however, comments made by the Working Group on certain shortcomings of reporting, of statistical analysis or of experimental design are given in square brackets. The nature and extent of impurities/contaminants in the chemicals being tested are given when available.

Carcinogenicity studies in animals

The monographs are not intended to cover all reported studies. Some studies are purposely omitted (a) because they are inadequate, as judged from previously described criteria(26-29) (e.g., too short a duration, too few animals, poor survival); (b) because they only confirm findings that have already been fully described; or (c) because they are judged irrelevant for the purpose of the evaluation. In certain cases, however, such studies are mentioned briefly, particularly when the information is considered to be a useful supplement to other reports or when it is the only data available. Their inclusion does not, however, imply acceptance of the adequacy of their experimental design and/or of the analysis and interpretation of their results.

Mention is made of all routes of administration by which the compound has been adequately tested and of all species in which relevant tests have been done(6, 28). In most cases, animal strains are given. [General characteristics of mouse strains have been reviewed (30).] Quantitative data are given to indicate the order of magnitude of the effective carcinogenic doses. In general, the doses and schedules are indicated as they appear in the paper; sometimes units have been converted for easier comparison. Experiments in which the compound was administered in conjunction with known carcinogens and experiments on factors that modify the carcinogenic effect are also reported. Experiments on the carcinogenicity of known metabolites, chemical precursors, analogues and derivatives are also included.

Other relevant biological data

Lethality data are given when available, and other data on toxicity are included when considered relevant. The metabolic data are restricted to studies that show the metabolic fate of the chemical in animals and humans, and comparisons of data from animals and humans are made when possible. Information is also given on absorption, distribution, excretion and placental transfer.

Prenatal toxicity

Data on effects on reproduction, teratogenicity and feto- and embryotoxicity from studies in experimental animals and from observations in humans are also included. There appears to be no causal relationship between teratogenicity (31) and carcinogenicity, but chemicals often have both properties. Evidence of prenatal toxicity suggests transplacental transfer, which is a prerequisite for transplacental carcinogenesis.

Indirect tests (mutagenicity and other short-term tests)

Data from indirect tests are also included. Since most of these tests have the advantage of taking less time and being less expensive than mammalian carcinogenicity studies, they are generally known as 'short-term' tests. They comprise assay procedures which rely on the induction of biological and biochemical effects in *in vivo* and/or *in vitro* systems. The end-point of the majority of these tests is the production not of neoplasms in animals but of changes at the molecular, cellular or multicellular level: these include the induction of DNA damage and repair, mutagenesis in bacteria and other organisms, transformation of mammalian cells in culture, and other systems.

The short-term tests may be useful (a) in predicting potential carcinogenicity in the absence of carcinogenicity data in animals, (b) as a contribution in deciding which chemicals should be tested in animals, (c) in identifying active fractions of complex mixtures containing carcinogens, (d) for recognizing active metabolites of known carcinogens in human and/or animal body fluids and (e) in helping to elucidate mechanisms of carcinogenesis. [See Supplement 2 to the *Monographs*(18) and references 48-56.]

Although the theory that cancer is induced as a result of somatic mutation suggests that agents which damage DNA *in vivo* may be carcinogens, the precise relevance of short-term tests to the mechanism by which cancer is induced is not known. Predictions of potential carcinogenicity are currently based on correlations between responses in short-term tests and data from animal carcinogenicity and/or human epidemiological studies. This approach is limited because the number of chemicals known to be carcinogenic in humans is insufficient to provide a basis for validation, and most validation studies involve chemicals that have been evaluated for carcinogenicity only in animals. The selection of chemicals is in turn limited to those classes for which data on carcinogenicity are available. The results of validation studies could be strongly influenced by such selection of chemicals and by the proportion of carcinogens in the series of chemicals tested; this should be kept in mind when evaluating the predictivity of a particular test. The usefulness of any test is reflected by its ability to classify carcinogens and noncarcinogens, using the animal data as a standard; however, animal tests may not always provide a perfect standard. The attainable level of correlation between short-term tests and animal bioassays is still under investigation.

Since many chemicals require metabolism to an active form, tests that do not take this into account may fail to detect certain potential carcinogens. The metabolic activation systems used in short-term tests (e.g., the cell-free systems used in bacterial tests) are meant to approximate the metabolic capacity of the whole organism. Each test has its advantages and limitations; thus, more confidence can be placed in the conclusions when negative or positive results for a chemical are confirmed in several such test systems. Deficiencies in metabolic competence may lead to misclassification of chemicals, which means that not all tests are suitable for assessing the potential carcinogenicity of all classes of compounds.

The present state of knowledge does not permit the selection of a specific test(s) as the most appropriate for identifying potential carcinogenicity. Before the results of a particular test can be considered to be fully acceptable for predicting potential carcinogenicity, certain criteria should be met: (a) the test should have been validated with respect to known animal carcinogens and found to have a high capacity for discriminating between carcinogens and noncarcinogens, and (b), when possible, a structurally related carcinogen(s) and noncarcinogen(s) should have been tested simultaneously with the chemical in question. The results should have been reproduced in different laboratories, and a prediction of carcinogenicity should have been confirmed in additional test systems. Confidence in positive results is increased if a mechanism of action can be deduced and if appropriate dose-response data are available. For optimum usefulness, data on purity must be given.

The short-term tests in current use that have been the most extensively validated are the *Salmonella typhimurium* plate-incorporation assay(32-36), the X-linked recessive lethal test in *Drosophila melanogaster*(37), unscheduled DNA synthesis(38) and *in vitro* transformation(36,39). Each is compatible with current concepts of the possible mechanism(s) of carcinogenesis.

An adequate assessment of the genetic activity of a chemical depends on data from a wide range of test systems. The monographs include, therefore, data not only from those already mentioned, but also on the induction of point mutations in other systems(40-45), on structural(46) and numerical chromosome aberrations, including dominant lethal effects (47), on mitotic recombination in fungi(40) and on sister chromatid exchanges (48-50).

The existence of a correlation between quantitative aspects of mutagenic and carcinogenic activity has been suggested (6,47-53), but it is not sufficiently well established to allow general use.

Further information about mutagenicity and other short-term tests is given in references 48-56 .

Case reports and epidemiological studies

Observations in humans are summarized in this section. The criteria for including a study in this section are described above (pp. 16-17).

Summary of Data Reported and Evaluation (Section 4)

Section 4 summarizes the relevant data from animals and humans and gives the critical views of the Working Group on those data.

Experimental data

Data relevant to the evaluation of the carcinogenicity of the chemical in animals are summarized in this section. The animal species mentioned are those in which the carcinogenicity of the substance was clearly demonstrated. Tumour sites are also indicated. If the substance has produced tumours after prenatal exposure or in single-dose experiments, this is indicated. Dose-response data are given when available.

Results from validated mutagenicity and other short-term tests and from tests for prenatal toxicity are reported if the Working Group considered the data to be relevant.

Human data

Human exposure to the chemical is summarized on the basis of data on production. use and occurrence. Case reports and epidemiological studies that are considered to be pertinent to an assessment of human carcinogenicity are described. Other biological data which are considered to be relevant are also mentioned.

Evaluation

This section comprises the overall evaluation by the Working Group of the carcinogenic risk of the chemical, complex mixture or occupational exposure to humans. All of the data in the monograph, and particularly the summarized experimental and human data, are considered in order to make this evaluation.

References

1. IARC (1977) IARC Monograph Programme on the Evaluation of the Carcinogenic Risk of Chemicals to Humans. Preamble. *IARC intern. tech. Rep. No. 77/002*

2. IARC (1978) Chemicals with *sufficient evidence* of carcinogenicity in experimental animals - *IARC Monographs* volumes 1-17. *IARC intern. tech. Rep. No. 78/003*

3. IARC (1979) Criteria to select chemicals for *IARC Monographs. IARC intern. tech. Rep. No. 79/003*

4. WHO (1961) Fifth Report of the Joint FAO/WHO Expert Committee on Food Additives. Evaluation of carcinogenic hazard of food additives. *WHO tech. Rep. Ser., No. 220,* pp. 5, 18, 19

5. WHO (1969) Report of a WHO Scientific Group. Principles for the testing and evaluation of drugs for carcinogenicity. *WHO tech. Rep. Ser., No. 426,* pp. 19, 21, 22

6. WHO (1974) Report of a WHO Scientific Group. Assessment of the carcinogenicity and mutagenicity of chemicals. *WHO tech. Rep. Ser.,* No. 546

7. WHO (1964) Report of a WHO Expert Committee. Prevention of cancer. *WHO tech. Rep. Ser., No. 276,* pp. 29, 30

8. IARC (1972-1980) *IARC Monographs on the Evaluation of the Carcinogenic Risk of Chemicals to Humans,* Volumes 1-24, Lyon, France

    Volume 1 (1972) Some Inorganic Substances, Chlorinated Hydrocarbons, Aromatic Amines, *N*-Nitroso Compounds and Natural Products (19 monographs), 184 pages

    Volume 2 (1973) Some Inorganic and Organometallic Compounds (7 monographs), 181 pages

    Volume 3 (1973) Certain Polycyclic Aromatic Hydrocarbons and Heterocyclic Compounds (17 monographs), 271 pages

    Volume 4 (1974) Some Aromatic Amines, Hydrazine and Related Substances, *N*-Nitroso Compounds and Miscellaneous Alkylating Agents (28 monographs), 286 pages

    Volume 5 (1974) Some Organochlorine Pesticides (12 monographs), 241 pages

    Volume 6 (1974) Sex Hormones (15 monographs), 243 pages

    Volume 7 (1974) Some Anti-thyroid and Related Substances, Nitrofurans and Industrial Chemicals (23 monographs), 326 pages

    Volume 8 (1975) Some Aromatic Azo Compounds (32 monographs), 357 pages

    Volume 9 (1975) Some Aziridines, *N-, S-* and *O*-Mustards and Selenium (24 monographs), 268 pages

    Volume 10 (1976) Some Naturally Occurring Substances (32 monographs), 353 pages

Volume 11 (1976) Cadmium, Nickel, Some Epoxides, Miscellaneous Industrial Chemicals and General Considerations on Volatile Anaesthetics (24 monographs), 306 pages

Volume 12 (1976) Some Carbamates, Thiocarbamates and Carbazides (24 monographs), 282 pages

Volume 13 (1977) Some Miscellaneous Pharmaceutical Substances (17 monographs), 255 pages

Volume 14 (1977) Asbestos (1 monograph), 106 pages

Volume 15 (1977) Some Fumigants, the Herbicides, 2,4-D and 2,4,5-T, Chlorinated Dibenzodioxins and Miscellaneous Industrial Chemicals (18 monographs), 354 pages

Volume 16 (1978) Some Aromatic Amines and Related Nitro Compounds - Hair Dyes, Colouring Agents, and Miscellaneous Industrial Chemicals (32 monographs), 400 pages

Volume 17 (1978) Some *N*-Nitroso Compounds (17 monographs), 365 pages

Volume 18 (1978) Polychlorinated Biphenyls and Polybrominated Biphenyls (2 monographs), 140 pages

Volume 19 (1979) Some Monomers, Plastics and Synthetic Elastomers, and Acrolein (17 monographs), 513 pages

Volume 20 (1979) Some Halogenated Hydrocarbons (25 monographs), 609 pages

Volume 21 (1979) Sex Hormones (II) (22 monographs), 583 pages

Volume 22 (1980) Some Non-Nutritive Sweetening Agents (2 monographs), 208 pages

Volume 23 (1980) Some Metals and Metallic Compounds (4 monographs), 438 pages

Volume 24 (1980) Some Pharmaceutical Drugs (16 monographs), 337 pages

Volume 25 (1981) Wood, Leather and Some Associated Industries (7 monographs), 412 pages

Volume 26 (1981) Some Antineoplastic and Immunosuppressive Agents (18 monographs), 411 pages

9. IARC (1973-1979) *Information Bulletin on the Survey of Chemicals Being Tested for Carcinogenicity, Numbers 1-8*, Lyon, France

Number 1 (1973) 52 pages
Number 2 (1973) 77 pages
Number 3 (1974) 67 pages
Number 4 (1974) 97 pages
Number 5 (1975) 88 pages
Number 6 (1976) 360 pages
Number 7 (1978) 460 pages
Number 8 (1979) 604 pages

10. PHS 149 (1951-1976) Public Health Service Publication No. 149, *Survey of Compounds which have been Tested for Carcinogenic Activity,* Washington DC, US Government Printing Office

    1951 Hartwell, J.L., 2nd ed., Literature up to 1947 on 1329 compounds, 583 pages

    1957 Shubik, P. & Hartwell, J.L., Supplement 1, Literature for the years 1948-1953 on 981 compounds, 388 pages

    1969 Shubik, P. & Hartwell, J.L., edited by Peters, J.A., Supplement 2, Literature for the years 1954-1960 on 1048 compounds, 655 pages

    1971 National Cancer Institute, Literature for the years 1968-1969 on 882 compounds, 653 pages

    1973 National Cancer Institute, Literature for the years 1961-1967 on 1632 compounds, 2343 pages

    1974 National Cancer Institute, Literature for the years 1970-1971 on 750 compounds, 1667 pages

    1976 National Cancer Institute, Literature for the years 1972-1973 on 966 compounds, 1638 pages

11. Pike, M.C. & Roe, F.J.C. (1963) An actuarial method of analysis of an experiment in two-stage carcinogenesis. *Br. J. Cancer, 17,* 605-610

12. Miller, E.C. & Miller, J.A. (1966) Mechanisms of chemical carcinogenesis: nature of proximate carcinogens and interactions with macromolecules. *Pharmacol. Rev., 18,* 805-838

13. Miller, J.A. (1970) Carcinogenesis by chemicals: an overview - G.H.A. Clowes Memorial Lecture. *Cancer Res., 30,* 559-576

14. Miller, J.A. & Miller, E.C. (1976) *The metabolic activation of chemical carcinogens to reactive electrophiles.* In: Yuhas, J.M., Tennant, R.W. & Reagon, J.D., eds, *Biology of Radiation Carcinogenesis,* New York, Raven Press

15. Peto, R. (1974) Guidelines on the analysis of tumour rates and death rates in experimental animals. *Br. J. Cancer, 29,* 101-105

16. Peto, R. (1975) Letter to the editor. *Br. J. Cancer, 31,* 697-699

17. Hoel, D.G. & Walburg, H.E., Jr (1972) Statistical analysis of survival experiments. *J. natl Cancer Inst., 49,* 361-372

18. IARC (1980) *IARC Monographs on the Evaluation of the Carcinogenic Risk of Chemicals to Humans,* Supplement 2, *Long-term and Short-term Screening Assays for Carcinogens: A Critical Appraisal,* Lyon

19. IARC Working Group (1980) An evaluation of chemicals and industrial processes associated with cancer in humans based on human and animal data: *IARC Monographs* Volumes 1 to 20. *Cancer Res., 40,* 1-12

20. IARC (1979) *IARC Monographs on the Evaluation of the Carcinogenic Risk of Chemicals to Humans, Supplement 1, Chemicals and Industrial Processes Associated with Cancer in Humans,* Lyon

21. IARC (1979) *Annual Report, 1979,* Lyon, pp. 89-99

22. Rall, D.P. (1977) *Species differences in carcinogenesis testing.* In: Hiatt, H.H., Watson, J.D. & Winsten, J.A., eds, *Origins of Human Cancer,* Book C, Cold Spring Harbor, NY, Cold Spring Harbor Laboratory, pp. 1383-1390

23. National Academy of Sciences (NAS) (1975) *Contemporary Pest Control Practices and Prospects: the Report of the Executive Committee,* Washington DC

24. Chemical Abstracts Services (1978) *Chemical Abstracts Ninth Collective Index (9CI), 1972-1976,* Vols 76-85, Columbus, OH

25. International Union of Pure & Applied Chemistry (1965) *Nomenclature of Organic Chemistry,* Section C, London, Butterworths

26. WHO (1958) Second Report of the Joint FAO/WHO Expert Committee on Food Additives. Procedures for the testing of intentional food additives to establish their safety and use. *WHO tech. Rep. Ser., No. 144*

27. WHO (1967) Scientific Group. Procedures for investigating intentional and unintentional food additives. *WHO tech. Rep. Ser., No. 348*

28. Berenblum, I., ed. (1969) Carcinogenicity testing. *UICC tech. Rep. Ser., 2*

29. Sontag, J.M., Page, N.P. & Saffiotti, U. (1976) Guidelines for carcinogen bioassay in small rodents. *Natl Cancer Inst. Carcinog. tech. Rep. Ser., No. 1*

30. Committee on Standardized Genetic Nomenclature for Mice (1972) Standardized nomenclature for inbred strains of mice. Fifth listing. *Cancer Res., 32,* 1609-1646

31. Wilson, J.G. & Fraser, F.C. (1977) *Handbook of Teratology,* New York, Plenum Press

32. Ames, B.N., Durston, W.E., Yamasaki, E. & Lee, F.D. (1973) Carcinogens are mutagens: a simple test system combining liver homogenates for activation and bacteria for detection. *Proc. natl Acad. Sci., USA, 70,* 2281-2285

33. McCann, J., Choi, E., Yamasaki, E. & Ames, B.N. (1975) Detection of carcinogens as mutagens in the *Salmonella*/microsome test: assay of 300 chemicals. *Proc. natl Acad. Sci. USA, 72,* 5135-5139

34. McCann, J. & Ames, B.N. (1976) Detection of carcinogens as mutagens in the *Salmonella*/microsome test: assay of 300 chemicals: discussion. *Proc. natl Acad. Sci. USA, 73,* 950-954

35. Sugimura, T., Sato, S., Nagao, M., Yahagi, T., Matsushima, T., Seino, Y., Takeuchi, M. & Kawachi, T. (1977) *Overlapping of carcinogens and mutagens.* In: Magee, P.N., Takayama, S., Sugimura, T. & Matsushima, T., eds, *Fundamentals in Cancer Prevention,* Baltimore, University Park Press, pp. 191-215

36. Purchase, I.F.M., Longstaff, E., Ashby, J., Styles, J.A., Anderson, D., Lefevre, P.A. & Westwood, F.R. (1976) Evaluation of six short-term tests for detecting organic chemical carcinogens and recommendations for their use. *Nature, 264,* 624-627

37. Vogel, E. & Sobels, F.H. (1976) *The function of* Drosophila *in genetic toxicology testing.* In: Hollaender, A., ed., *Chemical Mutagens: Principles and Methods for Their Detection,* Vol. 4, New York, Plenum Press, pp. 93-142

38. San, R.H.C. & Stich, H.F. (1975) DNA repair synthesis of cultured human cells as a rapid bioassay for chemical carcinogens. *Int. J. Cancer, 16,* 284-291

39. Pienta, R.J., Poiley, J.A. & Lebherz, W.B. (1977) Morphological transformation of early passage golden Syrian hamster embryo cells derived from cryopreserved primary cultures as a reliable *in vitro* bio-assay for identifying diverse carcinogens. *Int. J. Cancer, 19,* 642-655

40. Zimmermann, F.K. (1975) Procedures used in the induction of mitotic recombination and mutation in the yeast *Saccharomyces cerevisiae. Mutat. Res., 31,* 71-86

41. Ong, T.-M. & de Serres, F.J. (1972) Mutagenicity of chemical carcinogens in *Neurospora crassa. Cancer Res., 32,* 1890-1893

42. Huberman, E. & Sachs, L. (1976) Mutability of different genetic loci in mammalian cells by metabolically activated carcinogenic polycyclic hydrocarbons. *Proc. natl Acad. Sci. USA, 73,* 188-192

43. Krahn, D.F. & Heidelburger, C. (1977) Liver homogenate-mediated mutagenesis in Chinese hamster V79 cells by polycyclic aromatic hydrocarbons and aflatoxins. *Mutat. Res., 46,* 27-44

44. Kuroki, T., Drevon, C. & Montesano, R. (1977) Microsome-mediated mutagenesis in V79 Chinese hamster cells by various nitrosamines. *Cancer Res., 37,* 1044-1050

45. Searle, A.G. (1975) The specific locus test in the mouse. *Mutat. Res., 31,* 277-290

46. Evans, H.J. & O'Riordan, M.L. (1975) Human peripheral blood lymphocytes for the analysis of chromosome aberrations in mutagen tests. *Mutat. Res., 31,* 135-148

47. Epstein, S.S., Arnold, E., Andrea, J., Bass, W. & Bishop, Y. (1972) Detection of chemical mutagens by the dominant lethal assay in the mouse. *Toxicol. appl. Pharmacol., 23,* 288-325

48. Perry, P. & Evans, H.J. (1975) Cytological detection of mutagen-carcinogen exposure by sister chromatid exchanges. *Nature, 258,* 121-125

49. Stetka, D.G. & Wolff, S. (1976) Sister chromatid exchanges as an assay for genetic damage induced by mutagen-carcinogens. I. *In vivo* test for compounds requiring metabolic activation. *Mutat. Res., 41,* 333-342

50. Bartsch, H. & Grover, P.L. (1976) *Chemical carcinogenesis and mutagenesis.* In: Symington, T. & Carter, R.L., eds, *Scientific Foundations of Oncology,* Vol IX, *Chemical Carcinogenesis,* London, Heinemann Medical Books Ltd, pp. 334-342

51. Hollaender, A., ed. (1971a,b, 1973, 1976) *Chemical Mutagens: Principles and Methods for Their Detection,* Vols 1-4, New York, Plenum Press

52. Montesano, R. & Tomatis, L., eds (1974) *Chemical Carcinogenesis Essays (IARC Scientific Publications No. 10),* Lyon, International Agency for Research on Cancer

53. Ramel, C., ed. (1973) Evaluation of genetic risk of environmental chemicals: report of a symposium held at Skokloster, Sweden, 1972. *Ambio Spec. Rep., No. 3*

54. Stoltz, D.R., Poirier, L.A., Irving, C.C., Stich, H.F., Weisburger, J.H. & Grice, H.C. (1974) Evaluation of short-term tests for carcinogenicity. *Toxicol. appl. Pharmacol., 29,* 157-180

55. Montesano, R., Bartsch, H. & Tomatis, L., eds (1976) *Screening Tests in Chemical Carcinogenesis (IARC Scientific Publications No. 12),* Lyon, International Agency for Research on Cancer

56. Committee 17 (1976) Environmental mutagenic hazards. *Science, 187,* 503-514

This 26th volume of the *IARC Monographs* comprises 18 monographs on some anti-neoplastic and immunosuppressive drugs.   Two compounds, chlorambucil and cyclo-phosphamide, had been evaluated by a previous Working Group (IARC, 1975); new data that had become available on those compounds have been included in the present monographs and taken into consideration in the re-evaluations. Two other immunosuppressive agents that can be used in humans, cyclosporin A and antilymphocyte globin (ALG), were not considered in this volume.

The Working Group considered that any assessment of the carcinogenicity in experi-mental animals of compounds of this group was complicated by the fact that many of them are used as anticancer agents and could thus inhibit tumour growth at the same time as causing it.   A further complication in testing these drugs was posed by their immuno-suppressive effects, which make it difficult to test the compounds at sufficiently high doses throughout the normal lifespan of experimental animals.

An area of major concern to the Working Group was that of combination effects among the chemicals, particularly since many of the compounds considered are used clinically in various combinations.   Unfortunately, the experimental data on this subject that were available to the Working Group were limited and did not permit an evaluation of their significance in assessing the carcinogenicity of the individual compounds and/or of the combinations of compounds. Such information has therefore not always been included.

The compounds considered in this volume include alkylating agents, antimetabolites, mitotic inhibitors and/or immunosuppressants. Alkylating agents were generally found to be carcinogenic and mutagenic and to produce neoplasms at multiple organ sites. For other agents the results were often less clear cut.

For several of the drugs, no epidemiological study was available that compared the observed numbers of cancers in patients who had received the drug in question with expected numbers of cancers.   In certain studies in which the total number of patients treated was specified, it was possible to infer that there had been an increased frequency of cancer, even in the absence of calculated expected numbers and a precise estimate of risk. For the majority of the drugs considered here, however, only case reports were available. Case reports of cancer associated with exposure to particular drugs reflect the interests of those who report them and the preferences of the editors who publish them; the factors that influence clinicians and editors cannot be known, although it is evident that reports of a particular association tend to encourage other reports of a similar type.   Moreover, the number of patients who have received the drug of interest is usually also unknown. For example, the use of prednisone has been so extensive that a large number of case reports of subsequent cancer would be expected by chance alone. At the other extreme, the paucity of case reports of cancer in patients who received dacarbazine may simply reflect the fact that dacarbazine is most widely used in the treatment of patients with terminal neoplastic disease; it cannot be used as evidence for lack of carcinogenic risk of this agent. Case reports cannot, therefore, prove that a particular drug increases the incidence of a neoplasm, although they can certainly be valuable in indicating areas in which epidemiological studies should be made. Exceptions to the limited usefulness of case reports are rare, but the case reports of non-Hodgkin's lymphoma in transplant recipients, most of whom would have received azathioprine and prednisone, were sufficiently numerous in 1970 to deduce that the incidence must be greatly increased, even with very conservative assumptions (Doll & Kinlen, 1970).

The use of any medication that is associated with an adverse effect must be considered in relation to its therapeutic efficacy and to the natural history of the disorder under treatment. When they were first introduced, most of the drugs considered in this volume were used mainly in patients with advanced neoplastic disease, who rarely survived without therapy; thus, concern about late complications associated with the use of these agents was a minor consideration. However, successful treatment of advanced malignancy in some patients, administration of adjuvant chemotherapy to increasing numbers of patients with early-stage cancers (an unknown but substantial fraction of whom do not develop recurrent cancer), and the use of some of these agents in the treatment of non-neoplastic diseases require a different assessment of risks and benefits. Of particular concern in this regard is the routine use of cytotoxic drugs for the treatment of nonmalignant disorders such as juvenile rheumatoid arthritis or the nephrotic syndrome in children and young adults. Some such patients with a very bad prognosis may have much to gain from therapy, but others may go into remission without therapy.

A theoretical possibility in evaluating risk associated with exposure to a drug is that any observation may reflect a known or suspected effect of the disease for which the drug was administered. This is especially true when the initial disease was also a neoplasm. With regard to the drugs considered here, the available evidence weighs against such a possibility, but co-therapy with radiation and with drugs of recognized carcinogenicity has made evaluation of some of them, such as the vinca alkaloids, difficult or impossible.

Most of the epidemiological evidence cited in this volume is based on restricted periods of follow-up, sometimes because of short survival of the patients. Important additional effects of these drugs, such as increases in the frequency of solid tumours (known often to have a long latent interval), might have appeared.

References

Doll, R. & Kinlen, L. (1970) Immunosurveillance and cancer: epidemiological evidence. *Br. med. J., iv,* 420-422

IARC (1975) *IARC Monographs on the Evaluation of Carcinogenic Risk of Chemicals to Man,* Vol. 9, *Some aziridines, N, S & O-mustards and selenium,* Lyon, pp. 125-156

THE MONOGRAPHS

5-AZACYTIDINE

1. CHEMICAL AND PHYSICAL DATA

1.1 Synonyms and trade names

Chem. Abstr. Services Reg. No.: 320-67-2

Chem. Abstr. Name: 1,3,5-Triazin-2(1*H*)-one, 4-amino-1-β-D-ribofuranosyl-

IUPAC Systematic Name: 4-Amino-1-β-D-ribofuranosyl-*s*-triazin-2(1*H*)-one

Trade names: Antibiotic U 18496; Azacitidine; NSC 102816; U 18496

1.2 Structural and molecular formulae and molecular weight

$C_8H_{12}N_4O_5$ Mol. wt: 244.2

1.3 Chemical and physical properties of the pure substance

From Winkley & Robins (1970) or Von Hoff *et al.* (1975), unless otherwise specified

(a) *Description:* White crystalline powder

(b) *Melting-point:* 235-237°C (dec.)

(c) *Optical rotation:* $[\alpha]_D^{26} = +22.4°$ (c = 1.00; in water)

(d) *Spectroscopy data:* λ_{max} 241 nm, $A_1^1 = 359$ (in water)

(e) *Solubility:* Soluble in warm water (40 mg/ml); and at 1 mg/ml in ethanol, acetone, chloroform, hexane and dimethyl sulphoxide

(f) *Stability:* Sensitive to oxidation. Most stable at pH 7, when its half-life is about 5 days (Chan *et al.*, 1979). In aqueous solution, it undergoes deamination, ring-opening and loss of C-6 (Notari & DeYoung, 1975).

1.4 Technical products and impurities

5-Azacytidine is available as a lyophilized powder in 20 ml vials containing 100 mg of the compound with 100 mg mannitol for injection (Von Hoff *et al.*, 1975).

2. PRODUCTION, USE, OCCURRENCE AND ANALYSIS

2.1 Production and use

(a) Production

5-Azacytidine was first isolated from a culture of the bacterium *Streptoverticillium ladakanus*, but has been prepared subsequently by synthetic methods. One reported method involved treatment of the trimethylsilyl derivative of 4-amino-1,3,5-triazin-2-one with 2,3,5-tri-*O*-acetyl-D-ribofuranosyl bromide, followed by deacetylation to give 5-azacytidine (Winkley & Robins, 1970).

A company in the Federal Republic of Germany is believed to be the only manufacturer of this chemical. No data were available on the quantity produced.

(b) Use

5-Azacytidine has been used to treat patients with acute myeloblastic and acute lympho-blastic leukaemias. The reported dose was 150 - 200 mg/m^2 body surface (approximately 3.7 - 4.9 mg/kg bw) given intramuscularly or intravenously, daily for 5 days in 14 (Škoda, 1975; Von Hoff *et al.*, 1975; Wade, 1977).

2.2 Occurrence

5-Azacytidine is produced by the bacterium *Streptoverticillium ladakanus* (Winkley & Robins, 1970).

2.3 Analysis

No information on analytical methods for the determination of 5-azacytidine was available to the Working Group.

3. BIOLOGICAL DATA RELEVANT TO THE EVALUATION
OF CARCINOGENIC RISK TO HUMANS

3.1 Carcinogenicity studies in animals

(a)   Intraperitoneal administration

Mouse: Groups of 10 male and 10 female A/He mice, 6 - 8 weeks of age (18 - 20 g), received i.p. injections of 5-azacytidine three times weekly for 8 weeks at total dose levels of 90, 62 and 33 mg/kg bw. Treated animals received the chemical as 0.1 ml of solution in steroid-suspending vehicle (SSV)[1] . Control groups received 24 i.p. injections of 0.1 ml SSV or were untreated. Mice given two dose levels of urethane served as positive controls. All animals were killed 24 weeks after the first injection. The numbers of survivors were 11/20, 15/20 and 19/20 at the high, middle and low dose levels, respectively. The number of lung tumours per mouse in animals of both sexes treated with the highest dose was 0.73, which was significantly higher (P $<$ 0.05) than that in untreated (0.22 in males, 0.17 in females) or vehicle-treated (0.25 in males, 0.23 in females) control mice. With lower doses, the increase in lung tumours per mouse was not statistically significant. The numbers of mice with lung tumours, calculated on the basis of survivors of both sexes, were 6/11 (54%), 5/15 (33%) and 8/19 (42%) in the groups receiving the high, middle and low doses, respectively. In untreated and vehicle-treated groups, results were expressed only as % tumour incidence: 22% (males) and 17% (females) in untreated controls, and 26% (males) and 23% (females) in vehicle-treated controls.   In the positive control groups treated with urethane, there was a 100% tumour incidence at both dose levels used: a single i.p. injection of 5 or 20 mg/mouse (Stoner *et al.*, 1973).

Groups of 35 male and 35 female B6C3F1 mice, 38 days of age, received i.p. injections of 2.2 or 4.4 mg/kg bw 5-azacytidine in 10 ml/kg bw buffered saline 3 times a week for 52 weeks. Groups of 15 male and 15 female mice were untreated or received the vehicle only. Surviving mice were killed at 81 or 82 weeks. All high-dose female mice died before the end of the study; of the low-dose female mice, 17/35 survived until termination of the experiment at week 82. Of the male mice, 7/35 of the high-dose group and 13/35 of the low-dose group lived to the end of the study. The numbers of survivors of both sexes in untreated and vehicle-treated groups were 25/30 and 20/30, respectively. In female mice of the low-dose group, lymphocytic and granulocytic tumours were observed in 17/29 animals at a highly significant   incidence (P $<$ 0.001) compared with the vehicle-control group (0/14); 10 of the 17 animals had granulocytic tumours (9 granulocytic sarcomas, 1 granulocytic leukaemia).

---

[1]
    An aqueous solution of NaC l, polysorbate-80, carboxymethyl cellulose and benzyl alcohol

In 265 female vehicle-control mice of this colony, the incidence of haematopoietic tumours was reported to be 49/265, compared with 17/29 observed in the low-dose female mice in this study; and 1/265 granulocytic sarcoma was reported, compared with 9/29 in the treated animals in this study. No significant incidence of tumours was observed in male mice; tumours of the haematopoietic system occurred in 4/31 low-dose and 3/32 high-dose animals, compared with 0/13 in the vehicle-treated group (National Cancer Institute, 1978).

3.2 Other relevant biological data

(a) Experimental systems

Toxic effects

The LD_{50} in mice administered a single dose of 5-azacytidine intraperitoneally or orally was 116 or 572 mg/kg bw, respectively; the values were 2.5 and 4.4 mg/kg bw after 5 daily doses (Palm & Kensler, 1971).

In hamsters, i.v. injection of 15.6 - 250 mg/kg bw produced a moderate-to-severe but transient reduction in arteriole and venule blood flow with some haemostasis. An i.v. dose of 13.3 mg/kg bw administered to a dog produced no immediate response, but by day 2 the animal appeared dehydrated and semiresponsive. Bradypnoea with bilateral rales, hypotension, hypothermia, tremors and markedly elevated levels of blood urea nitrogen and serum glutamic-pyruvic transaminase were noted. One of 4 dogs died after receiving 2 courses of 5 daily i.v. injections of 1.1 mg/kg bw separated by an interval of 9 days; daily i.v. doses of 4.4 mg/kg bw administered for 3 days were lethal (Palm & Kensler, 1971). Toxic symptoms were observed with 2.5 and 0.55 mg/kg bw but not with 0.28 mg/kg bw (Von Hoff et al., 1975).

Following 5 daily i.v. doses to dogs of 0.55 mg/kg bw 5-azacytidine, bone-marrow depression was indicated by a marked but reversible depression in circulating leucocytes and a slight-to-moderate, transient depression in erythrocyte, haemoglobin and platelet values. Liver degeneration was confirmed by microscopic observation of focal liver necrosis and fatty metamorphosis in animals which received repeated dosages of more than 1.1 mg/kg bw. These lesions were often more pronounced in dogs that had received a second 5-day treatment (Von Hoff et al., 1975).

Effects on reproduction and prenatal toxicity

Random-bred (H strain) mice received 1.5 mg/kg bw 5-azacytidine intraperitoneally on 3 consecutive days, starting either on day 7 or day 14 of pregnancy; the fetuses were evaluated histologically 24 hours after the last injection. This dose regime resulted in 100%

(day 7) or 20% (day 14) embryomortality. When treatment was started on day 14 of pregnancy, histological examination revealed largely destroyed nervous and liver tissues with only a few remaining pyknotic cells and no dividing cells. Following a single injection of 4 mg/kg bw on day 12 of pregnancy, a pronounced effect, again on the developing brain, was seen. The authors concluded that 5-azacytidine, at doses nontoxic to the mother, seriously affects cell proliferation and differentiation, especially in brain and liver but also in placental tissues (Seifertová et al., 1968).

It was reported in an abstract that when pregnant mice were injected with 1 mg/kg bw 5-azacytidine on day 12 of gestation, hindlimb defects and/or kinky tails occurred in about half of the treated offspring but in none of the controls. Furthermore, after prenatal treatment, the brain weights of adult mouse offspring were lower in animals both with and without abnormalities (Rodier, 1979).

It was reported in another abstract that administration of 2 injections of 4 mg/kg bw 5-azacytidine 6 hours apart on day 15 or 19 of pregnancy, or to young mice on postnatal day 3, delayed postnatal growth and physical development. Degenerating cells were seen in the neuroepithelial layer within 16 hours after treatment. The effect was especially pronounced when the drug was given on day 15 of gestation; it was much smaller after postnatal treatment. The offspring treated on day 15 showed tremors and were hyperactive even as adults (Rodier et al., 1973). A closer analysis of the effects of this prenatal treatment with 5-azacytidine on postnatal development revealed extreme reduction of the cerebral cortex in those treated on day 15 and an abnormal layering of the pyramidal cells in the hippocampus; regions of the brain which had completed proliferation prior to the treatment were completely normal. Offspring treated on day 19 showed damage in more restricted areas of the developing brain (Langman et al., 1975).

Absorption, distribution, excretion and metabolism

Studies with $[^{14}C\text{-}4]$- and $[^{14}C\text{-}6]$-5-azacytidine in rabbits revealed that the triazine ring is cleaved hydrolytically, with subsequent loss of C-6 as formate. Most of the radioactivity (25-40%) was excreted in the urine within 8 hours; only 1% was excreted in bile (Chan et al., 1977). Another possible pathway consists in deamination to 5-azauridine with subsequent ring cleavage and loss of C-6. Thus, when 5-azacytidine was given orally to mice together with tetrahydrouridine (a pyrimidine nucleoside deaminase inhibitor), blood levels of 5-azacytidine were about 3 times higher than after administration of 5-azacytidine alone. However, no effect of the deaminase inhibitor was seen when the compounds were administered intraperitoneally (Neil et al., 1975).

5-Azacytidine is also phosphorylated to the mono-, di- and triphosphates. It has been shown to be incorporated into DNA and RNA; and it is an inhibitor of uridine kinase and of orotidylic acid decarboxylase. These reactions may contribute to its cytotoxicity (Von Hoff *et al.*, 1975, 1976).

Mutagenicity and other short-term tests

5-Azacytidine was weakly mutagenic in *Salmonella typhimurium* tester strain TA100 without microsomal activation, and in V79 Chinese hamster cells at the hypoxanthine-guanine phosphoribosyltransferase locus (Marquardt & Marquardt, 1977).

It induced chromosomal aberrations in hamster cells (Karon & Benedict, 1972; Benedict *et al.*, 1977) and in human lymphocytes (Viegas-Péquignot & Dutrillaux, 1976) in culture. Increases in sister chromatid exchanges were observed in hamster cells (Banerjee & Benedict, 1979).

5-Azacytidine also induced morphological transformation of mouse C3H/10T½ clone 8 cells in culture (Benedict *et al.*, 1977).

(b) Humans

Toxic effects

Dose-related leucopenia is reported to be the toxic effect which limits the therapeutic dose that can be given in 30% of patients. The lowest point occurs 18 - 30 days after daily i.v. injections. Thrombocytopenia is less common (17%), with a low point at 14 - 18 days (Von Hoff *et al.*, 1976). S.c. injection or i.v. infusion leads to later myelosuppression. Prolonged infusion is difficult practically, due to rapid breakdown of 5-azacytidine in most infusion fluids; 4 hourly infusions in Ringer's lactate produced lowering of myelotoxicity and gastrointestinal upset (Von Hoff *et al.*, 1975). Nausea and vomiting occur in 70% and diarrhoea in 50% of patients given large, single i.v. injections of 150 - 400 mg/m^2 (approximately 3.7 - 9.9 mg/kg bw). Alterations in hepatic function tests were seen in 7% of patients (Von Hoff *et al.*, 1976), and fatal hepatic coma was reported in 4 patients who had had abnormal liver function prior to receiving 5-azacytidine (Bellet *et al.*, 1973).

Myalgia was common in patients receiving large, single i.v. doses of 200 mg/m^2 (approximately 4.9 mg/kg bw) daily for 5 days (Levi *et al.*, 1975); rhabdomyolysis was also noted (Koeffler & Haskell, 1978); however, with lower doses, infusion or s.c. administration, this complication is uncommon (1%). Other effects that have been observed infrequently are rash, stomatitis (Saiki *et al.*, 1978), fever, hypotension (McCredie *et al.*, 1973) and reversible renal impairment (Greenberg, 1979).

Effects on reproduction and prenatal toxicity

No data were available to the Working Group.

Absorption, distribution, excretion and metabolism

After administration of radiolabelled 5-azacytidine, plasma radioactivity declined, with a half-life of 3.5 hours after single i.v. injection and of 4.2 hours after s.c. injection; 85% and 50% of the radioactivity was excreted in the urine within 48 hours (Troetel *et al.*, 1972).

Mutagenicity and chromosomal effects

No data were available to the Working Group.

3.3 Case reports and epidemiological studies of carcinogenicity in humans

No data were available to the Working Group.

4. SUMMARY OF DATA REPORTED AND EVALUATION

4.1 Experimental data

5-Azacytidine was tested by intraperitoneal administration in two experiments in mice. An increased incidence of lung tumours was observed in mice of both sexes in one experiment. In the other experiment, an increased incidence of granulocytic tumours was observed in females.

5-Azacytidine is embryolethal and can induce teratogenic effects in mice at doses non-toxic to the mother. It is weakly mutagenic in bacteria and in mammalian cells in culture. It also induces morphological transformation in mouse cells.

4.2 Human data

5-Azacytidine has had limited use in the treatment of acute leukaemias in Europe and North America since before 1970.

No data were available to evaluate the teratogenic potential, mutagenicity or chromosomal effects of 5-azacytidine in humans.

No case report or epidemiological study was available to the Working Group.

4.3 Evaluation

There is *limited evidence*[1] for the carcinogenicity of 5-azacytidine in mice. No data from studies in humans were available.

There were insufficient data for the Working Group to evaluate the carcinogenicity of 5-azacytidine to humans.

---

[1] See preamble, p. 19.

5. REFERENCES

Banerjee, A. & Benedict, W.F. (1979) Production of sister chromatid exchanges by various cancer chemotherapeutic agents. *Cancer Res., 39,* 797-799

Bellet, R.E., Mastrangelo, M.J., Engstrom, P.F. & Custer, R.P. (1973) Hepatotoxicity of 5-azacytidine (NSC-102816). (A clinical and pathologic study). *Neoplasma, 20,* 303-309

Benedict, W.F., Banerjee, A., Gardner, A. & Jones, P.A. (1977) Induction of morphological transformation in mouse C3H10T½ clone 8 cells and chromosomal damage in hamster A(T$_1$)C1-3 cells by cancer chemotherapeutic agents. *Cancer Res., 37,* 2202-2208

Chan, K.K., Staroscik, J.A. & Sadée, W. (1977) Synthesis of 5-azacytidine-6-^{13}C and -6-^{14}C. *J. med. Chem., 20,* 598-600

Chan, K.K., Giannini, D.D., Staroscik, J.A. & Sadée, W. (1979) 5-Azacytidine hydrolysis kinetics measured by high-pressure liquid chromatography and ^{13}C-NMR spectroscopy. *J. pharm. Sci., 68,* 807-812

Greenberg, M.S. (1979) Reversible renal dysfunction due to 5-azacytidine. *Cancer Treat. Rep., 63,* 806

Karon, M. & Benedict, W.F. (1972) Chromatid breakage: differential effect of inhibitors of DNA synthesis during G2 phase. *Science, 178,* 62

Koeffler, H.P. & Haskell, C.M. (1978) Rhabdomyolysis as a complication of 5-azacytidine. *Cancer Treat. Rep., 62,* 573-574

Langman, J., Rodier, P., Webster, W., Crowley, K., Cardell, E.L. & Pool, R. (1975) *The influence of teratogens on cellular and tissue behavior during the second half of pregnancy and their effect on postnatal behavior.* In: Neubert, D. & Merker, H.-J., eds, *New Approaches to the Evaluation of Abnormal Embryonic Development,* Stuttgart, Georg Thieme, pp. 439-468

Levi, J.A., Wiernik, P.H., Egan, J.J. & Sutherland, J.C. (1975) A comparative study of 5-azacytidine (Aza-C) and guanazole (GNZ) in previously treated adult acute non-lymphocytic leukemia (ANLL) (Abstract no. 329). *Proc. Am. Assoc. Cancer Res., 16,* 83

Marquardt, H. & Marquardt, H. (1977) Induction of malignant transformation and mutagenesis in cell cultures by cancer chemotherapeutic agents. *Cancer, 40,* 1930-1934

McCredie, K.B., Bodey, C.P., Burgess, M.A., Gutterman, J.U., Rodriguez, V., Sullivan, M.P. & Freireich, E.Y. (1973) Treatment of acute leukemia with 5-azacytidine (NSC-102816). *Cancer Chemother. Rep., 57,* 319-323

National Cancer Institute (1978) *Bioassay of 5-Azacytidine for Possible Carcinogenicity (Technical Report Series No. 42, DHEW Publ. No. (NIH) 78-842),* Washington DC, US Government Printing Office

Neil, G.L., Moxley, T.E., Kuentzel, S.L., Manak, R.C. & Haňka, L.J. (1975) Enhancement by tetrahydrouridine (NSH-112907) of the oral activity of 5-azacytidine (NSC-102816) in L1210 leukemic mice. *Cancer Chemother. Rep., Part 1, 59,* 459-465

Notari, R.E. & DeYoung, J.L. (1975) Kinetics and mechanisms of degradation of the antileukemic agent 5-azacytidine in aqueous solutions. *J. pharm. Sci., 64,* 1148-1157

Palm, P.E. & Kensler, C.J. (1971) Toxicology of a new pyrimidine antimetabolite, 5-azacytidine, in mice, hamsters and dogs (Abstract no. 55). *Toxicol. appl. Pharmacol., 19,* 382-383

Rodier, P.M. (1979) A comparison of gross malformations and quantitative measures as indicants of teratogenicity (Abstract). *Anat. Rec., 193,* 665

Rodier, P., Webster, W. & Langman, J. (1973) Morphological and behavioral anomalies after 5-azacytidine treatment of fetal and neonatal mice (Abstract). *Teratology, 7,* A-25 - A 26

Saiki, J.H., McCredie, K.B., Vietti, T.J., Hewlett, J.S., Morrison, F.S., Costanzi, J.J., Stuckey, W.J., Whitecar, J. & Hoogstraten, B. (1978) 5-Azacytidine in acute leukemia. *Cancer, 42,* 2111-2114

Seifertová, M., Veselý, J. & Šorm, F. (1968) Effect of 5-azacytidine on developing mouse embryo. *Experientia, 24,* 487-488

Škoda, J. (1975) *Azapyrimidine nucleosides.* In: Sartorelli, A.C. & Johns, D.G., eds, *Antineoplastic and Immunosuppressive Agents,* Part II, New York, Springer, pp. 361-372

Stoner, G.D., Shimkin, M.B., Kniazeff, A.J., Weisburger, J.H., Weisburger, E.K. & Gori, G.B. (1973) Test for carcinogenicity of food additives and chemotherapeutic agents by the pulmonary tumor response in strain A mice. *Cancer Res., 33,* 3069-3085

Troetel, W.M., Weiss, A.J., Stambaugh, J.E., Laucius, J.F. & Manthei, R.W. (1972) Absorption, distribution and excretion of 5-azacytidine (NSC-102816) in man. *Cancer Chemother. Rep., 56,* 405-411

Viegas-Péquignot, E. & Dutrillaux, B. (1976) Segmentation of human chromosomes induced by 5-ACR(5-azacytidine). *Hum. Genet., 34,* 247-254

Von Hoff, D.D., Handelsman, H. & Slavik, M. (1975) *5-Azacytidine (NSC 102816), Clinical Brochure,* Bethesda, MD, Division of Cancer Treatment, National Cancer Institute

Von Hoff, D.D., Slavik, M. & Muggia, F.M. (1976) 5-Azacytidine. A new anticancer drug with effectiveness in acute myelogenous leukemia. *Ann. intern. Med., 85,* 237-245

Wade, A., ed. (1977) *Martindale, The Extra Pharmacopoeia,* 27th ed., London, The Pharmaceutical Press, p. 1724

Winkley, M.W. & Robins, R.K. (1970) Direct glycosylation of 1,3,5-triazinones. A new approach to the synthesis of the nucleoside antibiotic 5-azacytidine (4-amino-1-β-D-ribofuranosyl-1,3,5-triazin-2-one) and related derivatives. *J. org. Chem., 35,* 491-495

AZATHIOPRINE

1. CHEMICAL AND PHYSICAL DATA

1.1 Synonyms and trade names

Chem. Abstr. Services Reg. No.: 446-86-6

Chem. Abstr. Name: 1*H*-Purine, 6-[(1-methyl-4-nitro-1*H*-imidazol-5-yl)thio] -

IUPAC Systematic Name: 6-[(1-Methyl-4-nitroimidazol-5-yl)thio] purine

Synonyms: Azathioprin; azatioprin; azothiaprine; azothioprene; azothioprine; methyl-nitroimidazolylmercaptopurine; 6-(1-methyl-4-nitro-imidazole-5-yl)thio-purine; 6-(1-methyl-4-nitro-5-imidazolyl)mercaptopurine; 6-[(1-methyl-4-nitro-imidazol-5-yl)thio] purine

Trade names: Amuran; Azamun; BW 57322; Imuran; Imurek; Imurel; Muran; NSC 39084

1.2 Structural and molecular formulae and molecular weight

$C_9H_7N_7O_2S$ Mol. wt: 277.3

1.3 Chemical and physical properties of the pure substance

From Wade (1977) or Windholz (1976)

(a) *Description:* Crystals from 50% aqueous acetone
(b) *Melting-point:* 243-244°C (dec.)
(c) *Spectroscopy data:* λ_{max} 280 nm (at pH 1); 285 nm (at pH 11)

(d) *Solubility:* Insoluble in water; very slightly soluble in ethanol and chloroform; sparingly soluble in dilute mineral acids; soluble in dilute alkali solutions

(e) *Stability:* Sensitive to oxidation; decomposes in strong alkali solutions

1.4 Technical products and impurities

Various national and international pharmacopoeias give specifications for the purity of azathioprine in pharmaceutical products. For example, azathioprine is available in the US as a USP grade measured as containing 98.0 - 101.5% active ingredient on a dried basis, with 1.0% max. mercaptopurine content and 0.1% max. residue on ignition. It is also available in injections as the sodium salt (trade names, Amuran, Imurek) and in tablets measured as containing 93.0 - 107.0% of the stated amount of azathioprine (US Pharmacopeial Convention, Inc., 1980). In the UK, azathioprine is available in tablets containing 50 mg; as azathioprine sodium, available in a powder for preparing injections; and in vials containing the equivalent of 50 mg azathioprine (Wade, 1977). Azathioprine is available in Japan in tablets containing 125 mg.

2. PRODUCTION, USE, OCCURRENCE AND ANALYSIS

2.1 Production and use

(a) *Production*

Synthesis of azathioprine was first reported (Hitchings & Elion, 1962) by the following steps: reaction of *N,N'*-dimethyloxaldiamide with phosphorus pentachloride produced 5-chloro-2-methylimidazole, which was nitrated to 5-chloro-1-methyl-4-nitro-imidazole.   Condensation of this with purine-6-thiol under appropriate dehydrohalo-genating conditions produced azathioprine (Harvey, 1975). This route is believed to be used for commercial production presently.

Commercial production of azathioprine in the US was first reported in 1970 (US Tariff Commission, 1972). Only one US company currently manufactures it (US International Trade Commission, 1979) in an undisclosed amount (see preamble, p. 20-21). Azathioprine is believed to be produced by one company each in the UK and Finland.

This drug was first marketed in Japan in 1965. In 1978, approximately 30 kg were used, all of which were imported from the UK.

(b) Use

Azathioprine is an immunosuppressive agent used, usually in combination with a corticosteroid, to prevent rejection following renal homotransplantation. It is also used following the transplantation of other organs. Other uses of azathioprine are in the treatment of a variety of presumed autoimmune diseases, including rheumatoid arthritis, ankylosing spondylitis, systemic lupus erythematosus, dermatomyositis, periarteritis nodosa, scleroderma, refractory thrombocytopenic purpura, autoimmune haemolytic anaemia, chronic active liver disease, regional enteritis, ulcerative colitis, various autoimmune diseases of the eye, acute and chronic glomerulonephritis, the nephrotic syndrome, Wegener's granulomatosis and multiple sclerosis (Harvey, 1975; Wade, 1977).

Dosage depends upon clinical and haematological responses of individual patients. Therapy is usually initiated at a level of 2 - 5 mg/kg bw per day, orally, with a long-term maintenance dose of 1 - 3 mg/kg bw per day (Goodman & Gilman, 1970, 1975; Harvey, 1975; Wade, 1977; Baker, 1980).

2.2 Occurrence

Azathioprine is not known to be produced in Nature.

2.3 Analysis

Typical methods for the analysis of azathioprine are summarized in Table 1.

3. BIOLOGICAL DATA RELEVANT TO THE EVALUATION
OF CARCINOGENIC RISK TO HUMANS

3.1 Carcinogenicity studies in animals

(a) Oral administration

Rat: A group of 50 male (6-week-old) and 50 female (8-week-old) Fischer 344 strain rats were fed *ad libitum* a diet containing 150 mg/kg azathioprine for 52 weeks. Ten males and 10 females fed a normal diet served as controls. Male rats tolerated the treatment; females rapidly showed weight loss, diarrhoea and tachypnoea after 5 - 6 weeks on the diet, and more than 40% died within the first 12 weeks of the study. All surviving animals were killed after 52 weeks. Squamous-cell ear-duct carcinomas developed in 3/25 female and 3/17 male treated rats and in none of 20 controls animals. There was no difference in the incidence of other tumour types (Frankel *et al.*, 1970).

Table 1. Methods for the analysis of azathioprine

Sample matrix	Sample preparation	Assay procedure[a]	Limit of detection	Reference
Formulations	Dissolve in dimethyl formamide; titrate with tetrabutylammonium hydroxide	T	not given	US Pharmaco-peial Convention, Inc. (1980)
Tablets	Powder sample; add aqueous sodium hydroxide; dilute with water; add sulphuric acid; transfer to polarographic cell; de-aerate by bubbling nitrogen through	P	not given	US Pharmaco-peial Convention, Inc. (1980)
Aqueous solutions	Add to folic acid assay medium; inoculate with *Lactobacillus casei*; incubate	MA	not given	Harber & Maddocks (1973)
Blood plasma	Add 6-methylmercaptopurine as internal standard, and hydro-chloric acid; extract with ethyl acetate; evaporate; add aceto-nitrile	HPLC-UV	40 ng/ml	Ding & Benet (1979)
Urine	Add gluthathione; allow to stand; add hydrochloric acid; elute through cation exchange resin with water; add ammo-nium hydroxide; evaporate; redissolve in perchloric acid	S	not given	Chalmers (1975)

[a]Abbreviations: T, titrimetric analysis; P, polarography; MA, microbiological assay; HPLC-UV, high-performance liquid chromatography with ultra-violet detection; S, spectrophotometry

(b)   Subcutaneous and/or intramuscular administration

Mouse: A 1% solution of azathioprine was prepared by dissolving 100 mg azathioprine in 2.4 ml 0.1N NaOH and diluting the solution with physiological saline to 10 ml.   A group of 25 male and 21 female C57BL mice, 7 weeks old, received s.c. injections of 100 mg/kg bw azathioprine twice weekly for 2 weeks and then once a week for 7 further months.   A group of 10 males and 6 females remained untreated as controls. The animals were observed for an additional 33 weeks.   No leukaemia occurred in the 16 controls evaluated.   After a latent period of 182-377 days, 11/38 (29%) treated animals developed haematopoietic tumours described as thymic lymphomas (8), a reticulum-cell neoplasm (1) and non-thymic lymphomas (2) (Imamura *et al.*, 1973). [No data on survival were provided.]

Four groups of female New Zealand Black/New Zealand White (NZB/NZW) hybrid mice, which develop antinuclear antibodies and immune complex glomerulonephritis and thus serve as models of systemic lupus erythematosus, were given s.c. injections 5 times per week of azathioprine, which was first lyophilized and dissolved in distilled water then redissolved in a solution of propanediol, dimethylacetamide and K_2HPO_4. Twenty-five mice, 120 days old, and 23 mice, 180 days old, were treated with 0.2 mg/mouse; 24 mice, 120 days old, and 24 mice, 180 days old, were treated with 0.4 mg/mouse. The latter dose induced leucopenia in some animals, which necessitated interruption of treatment. Additionally, 15 mice, 120 days old, and 12 mice, 180 days old, received 2.0 mg/mouse azathioprine every 7 days. Controls were 96 untreated or saline- or solvent-treated mice [proportion and age at start of experiment unspecified]. The study was terminated at the beginning of the 21st month of age for each group. In the control group, the median survival time after start of administration was 292 days: 1/96 (1%) animals died with malignant lymphomas, and uraemia was thought to be the cause of death of 94 mice. The median survival time in the experimental groups was essentially independent of the age at the beginning of administration: for animals treated with 0.2 mg and with 0.4 mg the median survival was 435 and 393 days, respectively; animals that received 2 mg once a week had a median survival of 390 days. Total tumour incidences are summarized in Table 2:

Table 2. Tumour incidences in female NZB/NZW mice treated with azathioprine

Treatment	Tumour incidence		
	All mice	According to age at start of treatment	
		120 days	180 days
Azathioprine 0.2 mg 5 times/week	10/48 (21.0%)	5/25 (20.0%)	5/23 (22.5%)
Azathioprine 0.4 mg 5 times/week	29/48 (60.5%)	17/24 (71.0%)	12/24 (50.0%)
Azathioprine 2 mg/week	4/27 (15.0%)	4/15 (16.5%)	0/12 (0%)
Controls	3/96 (3.0%)	-	-

The experimental groups treated both with low and high doses of azathioprine displayed a statistically higher incidence of neoplasia than the controls (P < 0.05). Daily high doses of azathioprine led to a greater tumour frequency than did low doses (P < 0.05). There was no significant difference in tumour frequency between animals treated with weekly doses of 2 mg azathioprine and controls. However, since the 4 animals observed to have tumours were all in the group which was introduced into the study at an age of 120 days and the average latent period was about 11 months, the authors suggested that some oncogenic effect was apparent (Mitrou et al., 1979a). The detailed histology of the types of tumours observed was reported later: tumours were observed in 43 treated animals in all groups [however, they were not tabulated according to individual groups] and consisted of 33 lymphomas, 3 undifferentiated sarcomas, 4 squamous-cell carcinomas of the anal region and 2 adenocarcinomas of the lung (Mitrou et al., 1979b). [The Working Group noted that in the absence of age-adjusted comparisons, early death of NZB hybrid mice from autoimmune disease precluded direct comparison with treated mice.]

A similar study was carried out with younger female mice of the same strain. Four groups of 9 - 10 mice, 6, 7, 8 or 12 weeks of age, were given s.c. injections of 0.2 mg azathioprine 5 times per week. The study was terminated after 7 or 8 months. The same control group as that described in the previous study (Mitrou et al., 1979a) was used. Ten treated animals developed 11 tumours, which were, histologically, 9 lymphomas, 1 mammary adenocarcinoma and 1 adenocarcinoma of the lung. The incidence of neoplasms in treated animals (10/39, 26%) was significantly higher than that in controls. Tumours occurred in each of the four groups of treated mice [however, these were not tabulated according to individual groups] (Mitrou et al., 1979b). [The Working Group noted that in the absence of age-adjusted comparisons, early death of NZB hybrid mice from auto-immune disease precluded direct comparison with treated mice.]

Azathioprine was administered intramuscularly into the thigh muscles of male inbred NZB mice before onset of autoimmune haemolytic anaemia, which develops spontaneously in mice of this strain. Azathioprine was dissolved in 0.1N NaOH and then diluted with physiological saline to a final concentration of 10 mg/ml azathioprine; single doses corresponded to 100 mg/kg bw. The 16 mice, aged 2 months, were matched into two similar groups on the basis of body weight and haematocrit readings; 8 mice were injected 3 times a week for 4 weeks, followed by 2 injections during the 5th week and then one injection a week, for a total treatment period of 6 months; 8 controls were given the solvent only. Of the treated mice, 6/8 (75%) had malignant thymic lymphomas; 4 of these died during treatment, and in the other 2 animals the tumours were diagnosed after termination of the experiment. No lymphoma was seen in the 6 control mice examined histologically at the end of the study (Casey, 1968a,b). [The Working Group noted that in the absence of age-adjusted comparisons, early death of NZB mice from autoimmune disease precluded direct comparison with treated mice.]

A similar study was carried out with 12 female NZB/NZW hybrid mice. Azathioprine solutions were prepared as described above (Casey, 1968a);   single doses again corresponded to 100 mg/kg bw. Twelve mice, aged 3 months, were given 3 doses per week for 3 weeks, 2 doses a week for one week and then 1 dose a week, for a total treatment period of 10 months. Three surviving mice were killed at the end of the treatment period. Twelve mice served as controls [no further details reported]. Of the treated mice, 7/12 (58%) developed malignant thymic lymphomas, the first after 4 months. No tumour was seen in controls (Casey, 1968b). [Mean survival times and latent periods were not specified. The Working Group noted that in the absence of age-adjusted comparisons, early death of NZB hybrid mice from autoimmune disease precluded direct comparison with treated mice.]

(c)   Intraperitoneal administration

Mouse: Two groups, each of 25 male and 25 female outbred Swiss-Webster-derived mice, 6 weeks old, were given i.p. injections of either 7.5 or 15 (females, 30) mg/kg bw azathioprine as an NaOH-stabilized solution in physiological saline 3 times a week for 6 months. Animals that survived over 100 days were observed for up to 12 further months, at which time they were killed. Controls consisted of 254 untreated mice. The survival times of the treated animals were reported as percentages of that of the controls [no precise definition of the mode of calculation was given] : the survival times of treated male mice were reported to be 51 - 77% that of untreated controls, and the corresponding figures for females were 23 - 75%. Animals that died before day 100 on test were excluded from evaluation. The incidence of 9/21 (43%) tumour-bearing males and of 25/40 (63%) tumour-bearing females was 1.5 - 2 times higher than that in controls (26%), in which there was only a small difference between males (28/101) and females (38/153). Histologically, 4 lymphosarcomas and 5 lung tumours were reported in treated males, and 11 lympho-sarcomas and 6 lung and 2 uterine tumours in females (Weisburger, 1977). [The Working Group considered that the inadequate reporting of certain items, such as survival times, the amalgamation of various experimental groups and tumour types, as well as the lack of age-adjustment in the analyses precluded a complete evaluation of this study.]

Rat: Two groups, each of 25 male and 25 female Sprague-Dawley-derived Charles River (CD) rats, about 6 weeks old, were given i.p. injections of 18 or 37 mg/kg bw azathioprine, stabilized with NaOH and dissolved in physiological saline, 3 times a week for 6 months. Animals that survived over 100 days were observed for up to 12 further months, at which time they were killed. Spontaneous tumours were seen in 60/179 untreated males and 105/181 untreated females. The survival times of the treated animals were reported as percentages of that of the controls [no precise definition of the mode of calculation was given] :   the survival times of treated males were reported to be 83 - 100% that of controls; in females the survival time corresponded to 100%. Animals that died before day 100 on test were excluded from evaluation. Tumours developed in 15/34 males and 22/44 females that received azathioprine. Histological examination of the males showed 4 skin tumours (unspecified), 4 pituitary tumours, 2 lymphosarcomas and 2 sarcomas; females had 10 pituitary tumours, 5 breast tumours (unspecified), 2 skin tumours (unspecified), 1 leukaemia and 2 sarcomas. The author stated that azathioprine caused either only a slight increase in tumour incidence or the same tumour incidences as observed in controls (Weisburger, 1977). [The Working Group considered that the inadequate reporting of certain items, such as survival times, the amalgamation of various experimental groups and tumour types, as well as the lack of age-adjustment in the analyses precluded a complete evaluation of this study.]

Newborn mouse: Of 60 newborn, random-bred Swiss mice of both sexes, 22 survived day 30 after i.p. administration of 40 mg/kg bw azathioprine (dissolved in 0.1N NaOH and diluted in physiological saline) once a day on days 1 - 4 after birth. The experiment was terminated after 180 - 200 days. Of 135 controls treated with identical amounts of physiological saline, 124 survived day 30. Leukaemia developed in 4/20 treated mice (20%), and in only 1 of 119 controls. This difference was reported to be statistically significant (P < 0.001). Azathioprine was administered under identical conditions to an additional group of 17 newborn mice as 4 single doses of 10 mg/kg on days 1 - 4 after birth. In the 14 animals that survived day 30, no leukaemia occurred; 2 (14%) animals developed lung adenomas, and this type of tumour was reported in 10/119 (8%) controls. The authors concluded that azathioprine is tumorigenic only at high doses (40 mg/kg bw) under the conditions of the test system used (Brambilla *et al.*, 1971).

(d) Effects of combinations

A variety of studies have been conducted in which azathioprine has been administered in conjunction with other chemical or biological agents.

To model the effect of azathioprine in the presence of antigenic stimulation, as would occur during transplantation, Krueger *et al.* (1971) gave daily doses of 15 mg/kg bw azathioprine in drinking-water, alone or in combination with antigenic stimulation in the form of a single i.p. injection of lactic dehydrogenase elevating virus, 2 s.c. injections per week of complete Freund's adjuvant, 2 i.m. injections of HeLa cells, or twice weekly footpad vaccination with smallpox vaccine. Neither the antigenic stimuli alone nor azathioprine alone led to tumours, and untreated mice were reported to be tumour-free. Combined treatment with antigenic stimuli and azathioprine resulted in malignant lymphomas of the lymphoblastic type in 23% (11/47) of mice.

In studies to examine the effect of azathioprine on the chemical induction of tumours, a group of 30 male and 30 female Fischer 344 rats were fed 150 mg/kg of diet azathioprine plus 160 mg/kg of diet N-hydroxy-N-2-fluorenyl-acetamide for 16 weeks, followed by a diet containing the same dose of azathioprine alone for a further 36 weeks. A group of 10 males and 10 females were fed a diet containing N-hydroxy-N-2-fluor-enyl-acetamide alone for 16 weeks, followed by a control diet for the next 36 weeks. Azathioprine did not enhance the hepatocarcinogenesis of N-hydroxy-N-2-fluorenyl-acetamide (Frankel et al., 1970).

In another study (Dargent et al., 1972), female Sprague-Dawley rats, 8 weeks old, were given 0.05 mg/rat azathioprine intragastrically twice weekly either together with 7,12-dimethylbenz(a)anthracene (DMBA), or 10 days before and during DMBA exposure, or following the appearance of the first DMBA-induced tumour. Additional groups received DMBA alone, azathioprine alone, or no treatment. The animals were maintained for 300 days. Although prior or concurrent administration of azathioprine appeared to modify carcinogenesis, under none of the conditions did it enhance overall tumour yield.

Koranda et al. (1975) exposed 5 - 8-week-old hr/hr hairless female albino mice to ultra-violet radiation or to ultra-violet radiation followed by azathioprine for 4 months at a level of 75 mg/kg of diet and then at a level of 50 mg/kg for the remainder of the 220-day experiment. Azathioprine increased the incidence of squamous-cell carcinomas of the skin from 18% to 57%.

The combined effects of azathioprine and other chemotherapeutic agents have also been investigated. In a large study of the carcinogenic hazards of anticancer drugs, a series of combinations were tested (Weisburger, 1977). Weanling Swiss mice were given either 5 mg/kg bw or 2.5 mg/kg bw of both azathioprine and prednisone intraperitoneally 3 times weekly for 6 months. After one additional year, the tumour incidences in mice receiving either dosage regimen were no greater than those produced by individual drugs in the study.

In similar studies in weanling Sprague-Dawley rats (Weisburger, 1977), animals were given either 10 or 20 mg/kg bw azathioprine intraperitoneally together with equal doses of prednisone. The overall incidence of tumours in the small number of animals studied was not increased compared with those produced by individual drugs in the study.

3.2 Other relevant biological data

(a) Experimental systems

Toxic effects

The single-dose oral LD_{50} for azathioprine was 2500 mg/kg bw in mice and 400 mg/kg bw in rats; and the i.p. LD_{50} was 650 mg/kg bw in mice and 310 mg/kg bw in rats (Elion *et al*., 1961).

Maximum tolerated doses after chronic daily treatment were 20 mg/kg bw in mice (Elion & Hitchings, 1975); 2 mg/kg bw in dogs (Elion *et al*., 1961); 1 mg/kg bw in Patas monkeys (Elion & Hitchings, 1975); and about 20 mg/kg bw in male rats (Frankel *et al*., 1970). Guinea-pigs are much less sensitive to the toxic effects of azathioprine than other animals and can tolerate 5 i.p. injections of 175 mg/kg bw (Elion & Hitchings, 1975).

The main toxic effect of azathioprine (after, e.g., 45 mg/kg bw per day in rats or 4 mg/kg bw per day in dogs) is bone-marrow depression (Elion *et al*., 1961; Starzl *et al*., 1965; Hunstein *et al*., 1967). Lymphocyte depletion in lymphoid tissues has also been observed in mice following chronic administration (Gabor & Scott, 1968). Infections have been a frequent complication, especially in animals receiving large doses for a prolonged period, and germ-free mice tolerated larger doses than mice in a conventional environment (Silas & Nance, 1968). Such infections can develop with a large variety of organisms, including those with a facultative intracellular parasitism (Touraine *et al*., 1972).

Whether or not azathioprine is hepatotoxic is controversial. In dogs, histological and biochemical liver damage has been observed after 40 days of azathioprine therapy (Starzl *et al*., 1965). Liver function changes in treated dogs have also been reported by other investigators (Haxhe *et al*., 1967; Aronsen *et al*., 1969; Filipowicz, 1972). However, when administration of azathioprine has been continued, recovery of normal hepatic function has been recorded (Worth, 1968; Aronsen *et al*., 1969). At moderate doses, azathioprine induced little hepatic damage in rats; but at relatively high doses for 3 - 4 weeks, and in association with phenobarbital, it induced hepatic lesions documented by light and electron microscopy and by biochemical modifications (Watanabe *et al*., 1979). In rats that received a liver transplant, 10 mg/kg per day of azathioprine for 20 days given intravenously produced no significant lesions of hepatocytes except when biliary stasis was induced experimentally (Hess *et al*., 1976).

Azathioprine did not directly induce lesions of the oesophagus, stomach, large bowel or pancreas (the only organs examined) in rats (Mansi *et al*., 1979).

Effects on reproduction and prenatal toxicity

Azathioprine was shown to induce embryolethality in Wistar rats and Swiss albino mice when given at doses of 1 - 20 mg/kg bw on days 3-12 of pregnancy. No gross malformations were noted in the surviving fetuses. Intragastric doses of 5 - 15 mg/kg bw azathioprine to rabbits on days 6 - 14 of gestation induced a large variety of skeletal malformations. Under these experimental conditions in rabbits, the rate of resorptions was not increased when compared with controls (Tuchmann-Duplessis & Mercier-Parot, 1964, 1966, 1968).

In Swiss-Webster mice, i.p. injections of 10 - 30 mg/kg bw azathioprine (dissolved in dilute NaOH) given over 2-3 consecutive days during days 6-11 of pregnancy induced a large variety of structural abnormalities (encephalocele, cleft palate, vertebral anomalies, oligodactyly, micrognathia) in up to 100% of the fetuses. Embryomortality occurred particularly with the higher doses. Hydrops and reduced haematocrit were found in fetuses that were exposed *in utero* on days 12 - 14 of gestation (Rosenkrantz *et al.*, 1967).

I.p. or s.c. treatment with 30 mg/kg bw azathioprine on days 6 - 11 of pregnancy was shown to induce malformations in 30 - 80% of fetuses of Swiss mice; no teratogenic effects were seen with doses of 20 mg/kg bw or lower given on days 6-10 of pregnancy, although embryomortality was striking with 20 mg/kg bw. When the drug was given orally on days 8 - 12 of pregnancy, 100% embryomortality was seen with 50 mg/kg bw and 36% with 20 mg/kg bw. Among the fetuses which survived after the smaller dose, two were found to be malformed. When Wistar rats received i.p. injections of 20 or 30 mg/kg bw azathioprine on days 10 and 11 of pregnancy, 12 - 14% of fetuses were malformed. When these doses were given over 5 days (days 8 - 12 of pregnancy), embryomortality was 100%, but no teratogenic effect was seen. The teratogenic effect of azathioprine was also confirmed in hybrid rabbits given 5 - 10 mg/kg bw intraperitoneally on days 12-16 of pregnancy and in *Ochotona rufescens,* a small hare, given 10 - 20 mg/kg bw intraperitoneally on days 10, 11 or 12 of pregnancy (Puget *et al.*, 1975).

A single s.c. dose of 50 mg/kg bw azathioprine given on day 10 of gestation was teratogenic in NMRI mice, inducing cleft palates in 90%, malformations of the vertebrae in 70%, malformations of the upper extremities in about 75% and malformations of the lower extremities in 50% of the fetuses. When the same dose was administered orally at the same gestational stage, 80% of fetuses showed cleft palates and about 20% showed abnormalities of the lower extremities; embryomortality was approximately 20% in both treated groups, in comparison to 6% in the control series (Neubert *et al.*, 1977).

When the 'teratogenic' effect of azathioprine was studied in an organ culture system that allowed differentiation of embryonic mouse limb buds, azathioprine was able to induce abnormal development *in vitro* at an identical concentration ($\sim$ 50% at 5 μg/ml) as 6-mercaptopurine (see p. 257   ), indicating that differences in the teratogenic potential of azathioprine and 6-mercaptopurine may be due to pharmacokinetic rather than to pharmacodynamic parameters (Lessmöllmann *et al.*, 1975; Neubert *et al.*, 1977).

Absorption, distribution, excretion and metabolism

Following i.p. injection of ^{35}S-azathioprine to mice, the level of radioactivity in liver exceeded that in plasma during the first 2 hours, while levels in the kidney, spleen, lung, muscle and brain were lower (Elion & Hitchings, 1975).

The metabolism of azathioprine has been studied by administering compounds labelled with either ^{35}S or ^{14}C to rats and dogs (de Miranda & Chu, 1970; Bach & Dardenne, 1972; de Miranda *et al.*, 1973, 1975). Most of the biological and biochemical effects of azathioprine depend on its conversion *in vivo* to 6-mercaptopurine, primarily by chemical conversion (Elion & Hitchings, 1975) but possibly also by enzymatic conversion (Watanabe *et al.*, 1978), and subsequent anabolism of the free purine to its ribonucleotide, thioinosinic acid, and other thioanalogues of purine derivatives. 6-Mercaptopurine is a competitive inhibitor of, and a substrate for hypoxanthine-guanine phosphoribosyltransferase. 6-Thioinosinic acid is an inhibitor of succinoadenylate synthetase and lyase, and of inosinate dehydrogenase.

In rats, the biotransformation of the methylnitroimidazole moiety of azathioprine in the presence of glutathione appears to give rise to 1-methyl-4-nitro-5-(*S*-glutathionyl)-imidazole (MNGI), then to 1-methyl-4-nitro-5-(*N*-acetyl-*S*-cysteinyl)imidazole (MNACI) and 1-methyl-4-nitro-5-thioimidazole (MNTI) (de Miranda *et al.*, 1973). The metabolic pathway proposed by de Miranda *et al.* (1975) for the conversion of azathioprine into its principal methylnitroimidazole metabolites in dogs is represented schematically in Figure 1. Azathioprine is cleaved by a nucleophilic attack on carbon 5 of the imidazole ring, primarily by glutathione *via* its sulphydryl group, giving rise to 6-mercaptopurine and MNGI. To a lesser extent, proteins, peptides and amino acids can also split azathioprine. MNGI is not excreted as such but is the precursor of the urinary metabolites MNACI, *N,N'*-[5-(1-methyl-4-nitro)imidazolyl] cystine and MNTI.

Fig. 1. Conversion of azathioprine into its principal methylnitroimidazole metabolites in dogs[a]

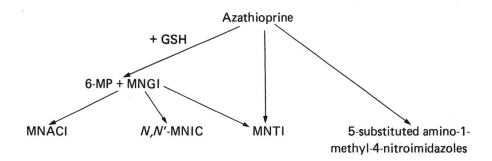

Azathioprine	=	6-(1-methyl-4-nitro-5-imidazoyl)thiopurine
GSH	=	glutathione
6-MP	=	6-mercaptopurine
MNGI	=	1-methyl-4-nitro-5-(S-glutathionyl)imidazole
MNACI	=	1-methyl-4-nitro-5-(N-acetyl-S-cysteinyl)imidazole
N,N'-MNIC	=	N,N'-[5-(1-methyl-4-nitro)imidazoyl] cystine
MNTI	=	1-methyl-4-nitro-5-thioimidazole

[a]From de Miranda et al. (1975)

These metabolic data are very likely to account for: (i) an immunosuppressive efficacy/toxicity ratio higher than that of 6-mercaptopurine (Chalmers et al., 1967); and (ii) increased toxicity and efficacy when allopurinol is given simultaneously with azathioprine, although the efficacy is decreased by prior administration of cysteine or glutathione (Watanabe et al., 1979).

Mutagenicity and other short-term tests

Azathioprine was mutagenic in Salmonella typhimurium strains his G46 and TA1535 only, with metabolic activation by mouse liver microsomes (Herbold & Buselmaier, 1976). Under anaerobic conditions, it was mutagenic to strain TA100 without such activation (Speck & Rosenkranz, 1976). The drug induced recessive lethal mutations in Neurospora crassa and dominant lethal mutations and nondisjunctions in Drosophila melanogaster (Clark, 1975).

Azathioprine induced dominant lethal mutations in Swiss albino mice (Clark, 1975) and in ICR/Ha Swiss mice (Epstein et al., 1972), although the authors of the latter study considered the data to be equivocal due to experimental inconsistencies.

Azathioprine induced morphological abnormalities in spermatids in mice (Wyrobeck & Bruce, 1975) and a dose-dependent increase in the number of micronuclei in mice and rats (van Went, 1979).

At high concentrations (10 - 90 µg/ml), azathioprine was clastogenic to human lymphocytes in vitro (Hampel et al., 1971; Obe, 1971; van Zyl & Wissmüller, 1974; Kučerová et al., 1979).

(b) Humans

Toxic effects

Complications are more likely to occur with large daily doses (3 - 5 mg/kg bw), particularly if excretion of metabolites is impaired by renal insufficiency (Burroughs Wellcome & Co. (USA) Inc., 1969; Penn, 1971). Most side effects are reversible on stopping the drug (Harris et al., 1971).

The major toxic effect of azathioprine is bone-marrow depression (Starzl, 1964). Three phases of marrow toxicity have been described: (i) megaloblastic erythropoiesis, (ii) defective granulopoiesis, and (iii) toxic panmyelopathy leading to leucopenia, anaemia, thrombocytopenia and bleeding (Gjone et al., 1973). In one study, two-thirds of 70 renal transplant recipients had erythrocyte macrocytosis. Its severity correlated with the dose of azathioprine and was associated with normoblastic or megaloblastic changes in the bone marrow. In two cases, macrocytosis was followed later by red-cell hypoplasia (McGrath et al., 1975). Fatal pancytopenia and agranulocytosis may also occur (Gjone et al., 1973).

Bone-marrow depression and lymphocyte depletion predispose to infection. There have been reports of fungal, protozoal, viral and uncommon bacterial infections, some of which have been fatal; and the major cause of death after renal transplantation, associated with therapy using azathioprine and prednisone, is infection (Starzl, 1964; Penn, 1971; Simmons et al., 1972).

Whether azathioprine and 6-mercaptopurine cause hepatotoxicity in humans is controversial (Krawitt et al., 1967; Ireland et al., 1973; Starzl & Putnam, 1969). Changes described include intrahepatic cholestasis, a zonal carbon tetrachloride-like injury with centrilobular fatty metamorphosis, nuclear pyknosis and cytoplasmic basophilia of hepatocytes or frank necrosis, occasional pigment macrophages containing periodic-acid-Schiff-positive material, and sparse or absent inflammatory infiltrates. Patients may have extremely high alkaline phosphatase levels with slightly elevated bilirubin levels. Some authors believe that these changes are due to hepatitis (Hamburger *et al.*, 1972).

Occasional complications attributed to azathioprine therapy include anorexia and gastric haemorrhage (Harris *et al.*, 1971; Gjone *et al.*, 1973); formication (Brandt, 1977); meningitic reactions (Lockshin & Kagen, 1972; Sergent & Lockshin, 1978); oral lesions, skin rashes, drug fever, alopecia, arthralgia and steatorrhoea (Burroughs Wellcome & Co. (USA) Inc., 1969). A unique case has been reported of a renal transplant recipient who received a single massive overdose of 7500 mg azathioprine during immunosuppressive therapy: the immediate toxic reactions were nausea, vomiting and diarrhoea, followed by mild leucopenia, mild abnormalities in liver function and improved homograft function (Carney *et al.*, 1974).

Dysplasia of the uterine cervical epithelium has been described in several reports (Gupta *et al.*, 1969; Kay *et al.*, 1970; Schramm, 1970).

Effects on reproduction and prenatal toxicity

Azathioprine is known to cross the human placenta (Saarikoski & Seppälä, 1973).

Many cases of prenatal exposure to azathioprine have been reported; in about half of these it was administered in conjuction with prednisone. In a series of 56 pregnancies in women who had received a renal homograft and were taking azathioprine (37.5 - 150 mg/day) and prednisone (0 - 35 mg/day) during the entire pregnancy, 4 of 44 live newborns had major congenital anomalies. Two had pulmonary arterial stenosis, one a deformed hand and one bilaterial inguinal hernias. Another infant had seizures of unknown etiology. Ten of the 44 live born infants (23%) were premature (gestational age, < 36 weeks); and 8 of 34 (24%) full-term infants (gestational age, 36 weeks) had a birth weight of < 2500 g; the mean birth weight of full-term infants was 3030 g (Penn *et al.*, 1980). Of 5 women treated with azathioprine during pregnancy (2.5 mg/kg bw per day), 3 had normal infants but with birth weights of less than 2500 g; the other 2 aborted (Sharon *et al.*, 1974).

Transient lymphopenia was reported in an infant whose mother was treated with 150 mg azathioprine and 30 mg prednisone throughout pregnancy (Coté *et al.*, 1974). Two cases of hypoplasia of the lymphatic system were reported in twins born to a mother who was treated with 100 mg/day azathioprine and 12.5 mg/day prednisone throughout pregnancy (Lower *et al.*, 1971).

Chromosome breaks, bridgings and translocations were observed in a newborn infant whose mother had been treated with high doses of azathioprine and prednisone, 400 mg actinomycin C and 450 roëntgens to the area of a renal homograft. These abnormalities were not evident after one week of age (Leb et al., 1971). Chromosome abnormalities were reported in 3 children whose parents had been treated with azathioprine: 1 mother during her pregnancy, and 2 fathers before and around the time of conception (Zeuthen & Friedrich, 1971).

Penn et al. (1980) have reported on 60 infants whose fathers were kidney transplant recipients being maintained on azathioprine and prednisone. Two of the infants had birth defects. One had a myelomeningocele, with its associated talipes equinovarus, and bilateral dislocated hips; there was a positive family history of spina bifida. The other infant had microcephaly, polycystic kidneys and other multiple congenital anomalies and died at birth.

Absorption, distribution, excretion and metabolism

Azathioprine is readily absorbed from the gut. In studies with ^{35}S-azathioprine, a 48-hour fecal specimen contained 12% of presumably unabsorbed material; 50% of the administered dose was found in the urine over 24 hours. Following oral administration of 100 mg, blood levels of azathioprine seldom exceeded 1-2 μg/ml; however, as purine antagonists rapidly enter into anabolic and catabolic pathways of purines, the level of radioactivity in the blood may represent several compounds. The significance of blood levels is therefore questionable. About 30% of azathioprine is bound to serum proteins, but it appears to be dialysable (Elion, 1972).

In vivo, azathioprine is split in two ways. In one, the S-linkage is split by thio-glucosidases, with the release of 6-mercaptopurine (Jensen, 1970), which competes with hypoxanthine for hypoxanthine-guanine phosphoribosyltransferase (Elion & Hitchings, 1975). It therefore inhibits both RNA and DNA synthesis and leads to formation of altered nucleotides (Zimmerman et al., 1974). In addition, some splitting occurs such that the sulphur is left with the methyl-nitro-imidazole ring (Elion, 1972). Azathioprine is catabolized to a variety of oxidized and methylated derivatives, which are excreted by the kidneys; very little azathioprine and 6-mercaptopurine are excreted intact. At least 11 different metabolites have been obtained, of which 6-thiouric acid is the major one found in the urine. Other metabolites include 5-mercapto-1-methyl-4-nitroimidazole, 1-methyl-4-nitro-5-thioimidazole, 8-hydroxyazathioprine and inorganic sulphate (Chalmers et al., 1967; Elion, 1972; Elion & Hitchings, 1975).

Mutagenicity and chromosomal effects

In various reports, clastogenic activity has been shown in peripheral lymphocytes of non-cancer patients treated with azathioprine alone or with prednisone (Jensen & Søborg, 1966: cumulative doses ranging from 1.8 - 5.9 g; Jensen, 1967: cumulative doses ranging from 1 - 18 g; Jensen, 1970: 50 - 150 mg/day for 7 to 462 days; Ganner *et al.*, 1973: 100 - 150 mg/day for weeks to years; Rossi *et al.*, 1973: cumulative doses of 4.4 - 7.2 g; van Went, 1979: cumulative doses of 4.4 - 38.2 g). Significant increases in sister chromatid exchanges have been reported in the peripheral lymphocytes of children with nephrotic syndrome treated with azathioprine (cumulative dose, 1.7 - 19.7 g) and prednisone (Torigoe, 1980).

3.3 Case reports and epidemiological studies of carcinogenicity in humans

Most of the literature on cancers in relation to azathioprine treatment concerns case reports of cancer in transplant patients; this has been regularly summarized by Penn, who collects details of such cases for an informal registry (e.g., Penn, 1970, 1979). Thus, by August 1978 the following numbers of malignancies had been recorded in organ transplant recipients: 277 cancers of skin and lips, 150 lymphomas (of which 3 were Hodgkin's disease and 20 Kaposi's sarcomas), 49 carcinomas of the cervix (including *in situ* cases), 36 lung cancers, 24 cancers of the head and neck, 21 colorectal cancers, 18 breast cancers, 17 leukaemias, 16 kidney cancers, 14 bladder cancers, 12 hepatobiliary cancers and 78 malignancies at other or unknown primary sites (Penn, 1979).

At least 81 cases of malignancy have been reported in non-transplant patients treated with azathioprine for nonmalignant disorders; of these 15 were *non-Hodgkin's lymphomas*. The underlying disorder was *systemic lupus erythematosus* in 4 cases (Goldenberg *et al.*, 1971; Lipsmeyer, 1972; Walden *et al.*, 1977; Hehir *et al.*, 1979) and *idiopathic thrombocytopenic purpura* in 2 (Nord *et al.*, 1976; Varadachari *et al.*, 1978); and there was 1 *lupus nephritis* (Lindeman *et al.*, 1976), 1 *proliferative glomerulonephritis* (Sharpstone *et al.*, 1969), 1 *nephrotic syndrome* (Rabkin *et al.*, 1973), 1 *dermatomyositis* (Sneddon & Wishart, 1972); 1 *Sjögren's syndrome* (Slater *et al.*, 1976), 1 *rheumatoid arthritis* (Neuhaus *et al.*, 1976), 1 *chronic active hepatitis* (Chaput *et al.*, 1978), 1 *multiple sclerosis* (Ulrich & Wüthrich, 1974) and 1 unspecified disorder (Aptekar *et al.*, 1973). In addition, 6 cases of *Hodgkin's disease* following azathioprine treatment have been reported (Michlmayr *et al.*, 1973; Scholz *et al.*, 1973; Pirotte, 1974; Green *et al.*, 1978; Hecker *et al.*, 1978; Orbuch & Findor, 1979); the case reported by Green *et al.* was in a patient with systemic lupus erythematosus. An association between systemic lupus erythematosus and lymphomas has been reported in the absence of immunosuppressive therapy (Green *et al.*, 1978).

There have been 12 reports of *myeloid leukaemia*, also in non-transplant patients, following azathioprine treatment for nonmalignant disease (Cobau *et al.*, 1973; Hicks, 1973; Silvergleid & Schrier, 1974; Rosner & Grünwald, 1975; Battin *et al.*, 1976; Roberts & Bell, 1976; Seidenfeld *et al.*, 1976; Alexon & Brandt, 1977; Gilmore *et al.*, 1977; Uszyński *et al.*, 1978; Vismans *et al.*, 1980): 2 *Kaposi's sarcomas* (Turnbull & Almeyda, 1970; Klein *et al.*, 1974), 3 *bladder cancers* (Scharf *et al.*, 1977; Summerskill *et al.*, 1975), 4 *cervical carcinomas* (Canoso & Cohen, 1974: *in situ*; Cade *et al.*, 1976; Abel *et al.*, 1978: *in situ*; Norfleet & Sampson, 1978: *in situ*), 4 cases of *endometrial cancer* (Hodgkinson & Williams, 1977; Abel *et al.*, 1978), 4 cases of *breast cancer* (Pinals, 1976; Viteri *et al.*, 1976; Krutchik *et al.*, 1978), 11 *squamous-cell cancers of skin or lip* (Marshall, 1974; Lindeman *et al.*, 1976; Neuhaus *et al.*, 1976; Seidenfeld *et al.*, 1976; Symington *et al.*, 1977), 2 cases of *basal-cell skin cancer* (Summerskill *et al.*, 1975; Symington *et al.*, 1977), 3 cases of *lung cancer* (McAdam *et al.*, 1974; Neuhaus *et al.*, 1976; Pinals, 1976), 3 cases of *renal-cell carcinoma* (Metz *et al.*, 1974; Gärtner *et al.*, 1975) and 1 *colonic cancer* (Patterson *et al.*, 1971), 1 *rectal cancer* (Gärtner *et al.*, 1975), 1 *small-bowel cancer* (Westaby *et al.*, 1977), 1 *pancreatic cancer* (Fusco *et al.*, 1971), 1 *Bowen's disease of the skin* (Canoso & Cohen, 1974), 1 *uterine cervical plasmacytoma* (Neuberg, 1974), 1 *gall-bladder cancer* (De Groote *et al.*, 1978), 1 *malignant melanoma* (Manny *et al.*, 1972), 1 *giant-cell tumour of the tendon sheath* (Aptekar *et al.*, 1973), 1 *tongue cancer* (Chaput *et al.*, 1978), 1 *adrenocortical carcinoma* (Wallace *et al.*, 1979) and 1 *latent prostatic carcinoma* (Elliott *et al.*, 1977).

Most of the patients also received corticosteroids, and the following 9 cases involved exposure to other cytotoxic agents in addition to azathioprine: 5 *myeloid leukaemias* (Cobau *et al.*, 1973; Hicks, 1973; Roberts & Bell, 1976; Seidenfeld *et al.*, 1976; Uszyński *et al.*, 1978), 1 *squamous-cell cancer of the skin* (Marshall, 1974), 1 *melanoma* (Manny *et al.*, 1972), 1 *renal-cell carcinoma* (Gärtner *et al.*, 1975) and 1 *latent prostatic cancer* (Elliott *et al.*, 1977).

Two prospective studies have investigated the incidence of cancer in transplant patients.

Hoover (1977) reported an updated analysis of a study by Hoover & Fraumeni (1973) of 16,290 patients who survived for at least 1 month after transplantation in the period 1951 - 1975 and who were notified on a voluntary basis to the Human Renal Transplant Registry of the American College of Surgeons. Most of the patients were followed up to the end of 1975. The incidence of different types of cancer was compared with the numbers that would have been expected if the incidence rates recorded by the Connecticut Cancer Registry had obtained. Fifty-two cases of non-Hodgkin's lymphoma (mainly reticulum-cell sarcomas) were observed, compared with 1.62 expected, a relative risk of 32; 50% of these occurred in the brain. There were also significantly increased incidences of hepato-biliary carcinomas (7 observed, 0.23 expected); lung cancer, mainly adeno-carcinoma (12 observed, 4.96 expected); bladder cancer (9 observed, 1.65 expected); melanoma (6 observed, 1.55 expected); and thyroid cancer (4 observed, 1.01 expected). The observed excess of leukaemia was not statistically significant (4 observed, 1.5 expected). Three soft-tissue sarcomas were observed, indicating an excess, although expected numbers could not be calculated. The authors noted that 2 of the patients with leukaemia had also received appreciable radiation therapy. The excess lymphoma risk appeared within a year of transplantation and remained at the same high level for the period of follow-up. In the earlier study (Hoover & Fraumeni, 1973), 21 cases of skin cancer were observed, compared with 5.0 cases expected on the basis of rates in a low-incidence area of the USA and compared with 16.2 cases expected on the basis of rates in a high-incidence area of the USA.

Kinlen et al. (1979) investigated the cancer incidence and mortality in 3823 renal transplant patients in Australia, New Zealand and the UK. Ascertainment and follow-up were complete. The numbers of cases of cancer and deaths from cancer of different types were compared with expected numbers based on incidence and mortality rates for the relevant country. A 58-fold increase in non-Hodgkin's lymphoma was recorded (34 observed, 0.58 expected). No clear relationship between azathioprine dosage and the risk of lymphoma could be detected. Squamous-cell carcinoma of the skin was increased in incidence; an estimate of risk was computed only for the UK series, since incidence data were not available for the Australasian population; thus, in the UK, 3 cases of squamous-cell skin cancer were observed compared with 0.13 expected. An excess of mesenchymal tumours was also noted (3 cases, a rhabdomyosarcoma, a mesothelioma and a Kaposi's sarcoma, compared with < 0.1 expected). There were no excesses of such common tumour types as those of colon, lung and breast.

The lymphomas that occur in transplant recipients are often of the immunoblastic sarcoma type (Lukes & Collins, 1975). They also show an unusual tendency to involve the brain. The origin of 7 lymphomas was determined: 6 were of host origin, and 1 (involving a marrow transplant) was of donor origin (Gossett et al., 1979; Penn, 1979).

A study of 1254 transplant recipients covered by the Scandia Transplant Programme in Denmark reported excesses of non-Hodgkin's lymphoma (based on 5 cases) and of melanoma (based on 2 cases) (Birkeland et al., 1975).

In the only epidemiological study that has been reported in which the incidence of cancer has been investigated in a group of non-transplant patients treated with azathioprine (Kinlen *et al.*, 1979, 1981), 1349 patients without transplants were followed who had received at least 3 months' treatment with azathioprine, cyclophosphamide or chlorambucil for such disorders as chronic glomerulonephritis, rheumatoid arthritis and collagen diseases. Of these patients, 64% (870) had received azathioprine. In the group that received azathioprine, excesses were noted for the same tumours that showed an excess in transplant patients, namely, non-Hodgkin's lymphoma (3 observed, compared with 0.23 expected) and squamous-cell carcinoma of the skin (1 observed compared with 0.27 expected); 1 bladder tumour (0.70 expected) was seen. The increase in these tumours was, however, of a lesser degree than in the transplant group.

[The fact that an excess of non-Hodgkin's lymphoma occurs In transplant patients with several different underlying renal diseases as well as in non-transplant patients treated with azathioprine suggests that the association is not due to the basic renal disorders or entirely to the presence of foreign antigens. It may be noted that an excess of non-Hodgkin's lymphomas has been reported in dialysis patients, who had received neither a transplant nor immunosuppressive drugs, but who show an appreciable impairment of immune function (Kinlen *et al.*, 1980).]

4. SUMMARY OF DATA REPORTED AND EVALUATION

4.1   Experimental data

Azathioprine was tested by intraperitoneal, subcutaneous and/or intramuscular administration in mice and by oral and intraperitoneal administration in rats. Suggestive evidence was obtained for the induction of lymphomas after intraperitoneal, subcutaneous or intramuscular injection in mice and for ear-duct carcinomas in rats after oral administration. Because of limitations in design and reporting, however, the results were considered to be inconclusive.

Studies in which azathioprine was tested in combination with other agents were inadequate for evaluation.

Azathioprine is embryolethal at doses nontoxic to the mother and can induce a variety of severe teratogenic effects in several animal species. It is mutagenic in bacteria and yeast *in vitro* and in *Drosophila melanogaster* and mice *in vivo*. At high concentrations, the drug is clastogenic to human lymphocytes *in vitro*.

4.2 Human data

Azathioprine has been widely used since the 1970s to prevent rejection following organ transplantation. It is also used to treat a variety of autoimmune diseases.

Use of azathioprine during pregnancy may reduce birth weight significantly. The data were insufficient to evaluate the teratogenic potential of this drug to humans. Azathioprine produces chromosomal abnormalities and increases in sister chromatid exchanges in the peripheral lymphocytes of non-cancer patients. No data were available to evaluate the mutagenic potential of this drug to humans.

There is evidence that azathioprine, often combined with prednisone, is associated with an increased incidence of non-Hodgkin's lymphoma, squamous-cell cancers of the skin, hepato-biliary carcinomas, mesenchymal tumours, and perhaps certain other rare neoplasms. The risk of non-Hodgkin's lymphoma is higher in organ transplant recipients; the presence of the graft may make some contribution to this increased incidence.

4.3 Evaluation

There is *limited evidence*[1] for the carcinogenicity of azathioprine in mice and rats. There is *sufficient evidence*[2] that azathioprine is carcinogenic in humans.

---

[1] See preamble, p. 19.

[2] See preamble, p. 17.   This evaluation is not the result of the consensus of the group but of a majority vote. A minority of three voted for 'limited evidence'.

5. REFERENCES

Abel, T., Urowitz, M.B., Smythe, H.A., Keystone, E.C. & Norman, C.S. (1978) Long-term effects of azathioprine in rheumatoid arthritis (Abstract). *Arthritis Rheum., 21,* 539

Alexon, E. & Brandt, K.D. (1977) Acute leukemia after azathioprine treatment of connective tissue disease. *Am. J. med. Sci., 273,* 335-340

Aptekar, R.G., Steinberg, A.D. & Decker, J.L. (1973) Complications of cytotoxic agents in systemic lupus erythematosus and rheumatoid arthritis (Abstract). *Arthritis Rheum., 16,* 533

Aronsen, K.F., Husberg, B. & Pihl, B. (1969) Immunosuppressive treatment in non-transplanted dogs. Azathioprine *versus* azathioprine-antilymphocyteimmuno-globulin-G. *Acta chir. scand., 135,* 475-481

Bach, J.F. & Dardenne, M. (1972) Serum immunosuppressive activity of azathioprine in normal subjects and patients with liver diseases. *Proc. R. Soc. Med., 65,* 260-263

Baker, C.E., Jr, ed. (1980) *Physicians' Desk Reference,* 34th ed., Oradell, NJ, Medical Economics Co., pp. 751-753

Battin, J., Hehunstre, J.-P., Bui, N.-B., Auzerie, J. & Colle, M. (1976) Chronic myeloid leukaemia after immunosuppressive treatment for chronic nephropathy (Fr.). *Nouv. Presse méd., 5,* 2632

Birkeland, S.A., Kemp, E. & Hauge, M. (1975) Renal transplantation and cancer. The Scandia Transplant material. *Tissue Antigens, 6,* 28-36

Brambilla, G., Careceni, C.E., Cavanna, M. & Parodi, S. (1971) Evaluation, in Swiss neonatal mice, of the carcinogenic activity of some antineoplastic and immunosuppressive compounds (Ital.). *Boll. Soc. Ital. Biol. sper., 47,* 418-422

Brandt, L.J. (1977) Formication and azathioprine therapy (Letter to the Editor). *Ann. intern. Med., 87,* 458

Burroughs Wellcome & Co. (USA), Inc. (1969) Azathioprine (Imuran) 50 mg scored tablets: an adjunct for the prevention of rejection in renal homotransplantation. *Clin. Pharmacol. Ther., 10,* 136-141

Cade, R., Stein, G., Pickering, M., Schlein, E. & Spooner, G. (1976) Low dose, long-term treatment of rheumatoid arthritis with azathioprine. *South. med. J., 69,* 388-392

Canoso, J.J. & Cohen, A.S. (1974) Malignancy in a series of 70 patients with systemic lupus erythematosus. *Arthritis Rheum., 17,* 383-390

Carney, D.M., Zukiski, C.F. & Ogden, D.A. (1974) Massive azathioprine overdose. Case report and review of the literature. *Am. J. Med., 56,* 133-136

Casey, T.P. (1968a) Azathioprine (Imuran) administration and the development of malignant lymphomas in NZB mice. *Clin. exp. Immunol., 3,* 305-312

Casey, T.P. (1968b) The development of lymphomas in mice with autoimmune disorders treated with azathioprine. *Blood, 31,* 396-399

Chalmers, A.H. (1975) A spectrophotometric method for the estimation of urinary azathioprine, 6-mercaptopurine, and 6-thiouric acid. *Biochem. Med., 12,* 234-241

Chalmers, A.H., Knight, P.R. & Atkinson, M.R. (1967) Conversion of azathioprine into mercaptopurine and mercaptoimidazole derivatives *in vitro* and during immunosuppressive therapy. *Aust. J. exp. Biol. med. Sci., 45,* 681-691

Chaput, J.C., Buffet, C., Papoz, L. & Etienne, J.P. (1978) Chronic active hepatitis and extrahepatic malignancy. *Lancet, i,* 1367

Clark, J.M. (1975) The mutagenicity of azathioprine in mice, *Drosophila melanogaster* and *Neurospora crassa. Mutat. Res., 28,* 87-99

Cobau, C.D., Sheon, R.P. & Kirsner, A.B. (1973) Immunosuppressive drugs and acute leukemia. *Ann. intern. Med., 79,* 131-132

Coté, C.J., Meuwissen, H.J. & Pickering, R.J. (1974) Effects on the neonate of prednisone and azathioprine administered to the mother during pregnancy. *J. Pediatr., 85,* 324-328

Dargent, M., Bourgoin, J.-J., Noel, P. & Weissbrod, R. (1972) The influence of azathioprine on tumorigenesis by 7-12 dimethylbenz(a)anthracene in rats. *Eur. J. Cancer, 8,* 605-609

De Groote, J., Fevery, J. & Lepoutre, L. (1978) Long-term follow-up of chronic active hepatitis of moderate severity. *Gut, 19,* 510-513

Ding, T.L. & Benet, L.Z. (1979) Determination of 6-mercaptopurine and azathioprine in plasma by high-performance liquid chromatography. *J. Chromatogr., 163,* 281-288

Elion, G.B. (1972) Significance of azathioprine metabolites. *Proc. R. Soc. Med., 65,* 257-260

Elion, G.B. & Hitchings, G.H. (1975) *Azathioprine.* In: Eichler, O., Farah, A., Heiken, H. & Welch, A.D., eds, *Handbook of Experimental Pharmacology,* Vol. 38, No. 2, Berlin, Springer, pp. 404-425

Elion, G.B., Callahan, S., Bieber, S., Hitchings, G.H. & Rundles, R.W. (1961) A summary of investigations with 6-[(1-methyl-4-nitro-5-imidazolyl)thio]purine (B.W. 57-322). *Cancer Chemother. Rep., 14,* 93-98

Elliott, G.B., Silverberg, D.S., Dossetor, J.B. & Muir, C.S. (1977) Latent carcinoma of the prostate in a 24-year-old man receiving cyclophosphamide and azathioprine. *Can. med. Assoc. J., 116,* 651-652

Epstein, S.S., Arnold, E., Andrea, J., Bass, W. & Bishop, Y. (1972) Detection of chemical mutagens by the dominant lethal assay in the mouse. *Toxicol. appl. Pharmacol., 23,* 288-325

Filipowicz, Z. (1972) The effect of long-term administration of azathioprine to healthy dogs (Pol.). *Pol. Arch. Med. Wewn., 49,* 239-248

Frankel, H.H., Yamamoto, R.S., Weisburger, E.K. & Weisburger, J.H. (1970) Chronic toxicity of aza-thioprine and the effect of this immunosuppressant on liver tumor induction by the carcinogen *N*-hydroxy-*N*-2-fluorenyl-acetamide. *Toxicol. appl. Pharmacol., 17,* 462-480

Fusco, F.A., Mattioli, F. & Bertocchi, J. (1971) *Development of malignancy after immunosuppressive treatment (azathioprine) (Abstract no. 343).* In: *First Meeting of European Division of International Society of Haematology, Milan*

Gabor, E.P. & Scott, J.L. (1968) Effect of thiopurines on rat lymphoid tissues (Abstract). *Clin. Res., 16,* 154

Ganner, E., Osment, J., Dittrich, P. & Huber, H. (1973) Chromosomes in patients treated with azathio-prine. *Humangenetik, 18,* 231-236

Gärtner, U., Schief, A. & Stocker, W.G. (1975) The problem of malignant deuteropathy following cyto-static therapy (Ger.). *Münch. med. Wochenschr., 117,* 671-676

Gilmore, I.T., Holden, G. & Rodan, K.S. (1977) Acute leukaemia during azathioprine therapy. *Postgrad. med. J., 53,* 173-174

Gjone, E., Boye, N.P. & Blomhoff, J.P. (1973) Azathioprine treatment in chronic active hepatitis. Evalu-ation of dose levels. *Acta med. scand., 193,* 109-112

Goldenberg, G.J., Paraskevas, F. & Israels, L.G. (1971) Lymphocyte and plasma cell neoplasms associated with autoimmune diseases. *Semin. Arthritis Rheum., 1,* 174-193

Goodman, L.S. & Gilman, A., eds (1970) *The Pharmacological Basis of Therapeutics*, 4th ed., New York, Macmillan, p. 1375

Goodman, L.S. & Gilman, A., eds (1975) *The Pharmacological Basis of Therapeutics,* 5th ed., New York, Macmillan, pp. 1281-1283

Gossett, T.C., Gale, R.P., Fleischman, H., Austin, G.E., Sparkes, R.S. & Taylor, C.R. (1979) Immuno-blastic sarcoma in donor cells after bone-marrow transplantation. *New Engl. J. Med., 300,* 904-907

Green, J.A., Dawson, A.A. & Walker, W. (1978) Systemic lupus erythematosus and lymphoma. *Lancet, ii,* 753-756

Gupta, P.K., Pinn, V.M. & Taft, P.D. (1969) Cervical dysplasia associated with azathioprine (Imuran) therapy. *Acta cytol., 13,* 373-376

Hamburger, J., Crosnier, J., Dormont, J. & Bach, J.F. (1972) *Renal Transplantation. Theory and Prac-tice*, Baltimore, Williams & Wilkins

Hampel, K.E., Lackner, A., Schulz, G. & Busse, V. (1971) Chromosomal mutations by azathioprine in human leukocytes *in vitro* (Ger.). *Z. Gastroenterol., 9,* 47-51

Harber, M.J. & Maddocks, J.L. (1973) Microbiological assay for purine analogues with *Lactobacillus casei. J. gen. Microbiol., 79,* 351-353

Harris, J., Jessop, J.D. & Chaput de Saintonge, D.M. (1971) Further experience with azathioprine in rheumatoid arthritis. *Br. med. J., iv,* 463-464

Harvey, S.C. (1975) *Antineoplastic and immunosuppressive drugs.* In: Osol, A., ed., *Remington's Pharmaceutical Sciences,* 15th ed., Easton, PA, Mack Publishing Co., pp. 1075-1076

Haxhe, J.J., Alexandre, G.P.J. & Kestens, P.J. (1967) The effect of Imuran and azaserine on liver function tests in the dog. Its relation to the detection of graft rejection following liver transplantation. *Arch. int. Pharmacodyn., 168,* 366-372

Hecker, R., Sheers, R. & Thomas, D. (1978) Hodgkin's disease as a complication of Crohn's disease. *Med. J. Aust., 2,* 603

Hehir, M.E., Sewell, J.R. & Hughes, G.R.V. (1979) Reticulum cell sarcoma in azathioprine-treated systemic lupus erythematosus. *Ann. rheum. Dis., 38,* 94-95

Herbold, B. & Buselmaier, W. (1976) Induction of point mutations by different chemical mechanisms in the liver microsomal assay. *Mutat. Res., 40,* 73-84

Hess, F., Jerusalem, C. & Polak, M. (1976) Azathioprine hepatotoxicity, direct complication or secondary effect in rat liver transplantation. *Eur. surg. Res., 8,* 156-165

Hicks, N.D. (1973) An unusual form of leukaemia associated with immunosuppressive therapy. *Pathology, 5,* 77

Hitchings, G.H. & Elion, G.B. (1962) *Purines.* US Patent 3,056,785, Burroughs Wellcome Co., Inc. [*Chem. Abstr., 48,* 5701e]

Hodgkinson, D.J. & Williams, T.J. (1977) Endometrial carcinoma associated with azathioprine and cortisone therapy. A case report. *Gynecol. Oncol., 5,* 308-312

Hoover, R. (1977) *Effects of drugs - immunosuppression.* In: Hiatt, H.H., Watson, J.D. & Winsten, J.A., eds, *Origins of Human Cancer,* Cold Spring Harbor, NY, Cold Spring Harbor Laboratory, pp. 369-379

Hoover, R. & Fraumeni, J.F., Jr (1973) Risk of cancer in renal transplant recipients. *Lancet, ii,* 55-57

Hunstein, W., Perings, E. & Klose, U. (1967) Long-term animal experiments with azathioprine (Imuran) to test its myelotoxic effect (Ger.). *Vehr. dtsch. Ges. inn. Med., 73,* 450-453

Imamura, N., Nakano, M., Kawase, A., Kawamura, Y. & Yokoro, K. (1973) Synergistic action of *N*-nitrosobutylurea and azathioprine in induction of leukemia in C57BL mice. *Gann, 64,* 493-498

Ireland, P., Rashid, A., von Lichtenberg, F., Cavallo, T. & Merrill, J.P. (1973) Liver disease in kidney transplant patients receiving azathioprine. *Arch. intern. Med., 132,* 29-37

Jensen, M.K. (1967) Chromosome studies in patients treated with azathioprine and amethopterin. *Acta med. scand., 182,* 445-455

Jensen, M.K. (1970) Effect of azathioprine on the chromosome complement of human bone marrow cells. *Int. J. Cancer, 5,* 147-151

Jensen, M.K. & Søborg, M. (1966) Chromosome aberrations in human cells following treatment with Imuran. Preliminary report. *Acta med. scand., 179,* 249-250

Kay, S., Frable, W.J. & Hume, D.M. (1970) Cervical dysplasia and cancer developing in women on immunosuppression therapy for renal homotransplantation. *Cancer, 26,* 1048-1052

Kinlen, L.J., Sheil, A.G.R., Peto, J. & Doll, R. (1979) Collaborative United Kingdom-Australasian study of cancer in patients treated with immunosuppressive drugs. *Br. med. J., iv,* 1461-1466

Kinlen, L.J., Eastwood, J.B., Kerr, D.N.S., Moorhead, J.F., Oliver, D.O., Robinson, B.H.B., de Wardener, H.E. & Wing, A.J. (1980) Cancer in patients receiving dialysis. *Br. med. J., ii,* 1401-1403

Kinlen, L.J., Peto, J., Doll, R. & Sheil, A.G.R. (1981) Cancer in patients treated with immunosuppressive drugs. *Br. med. J., i,* 474

Klein, M.B., Pereira, F.A. & Kantor, I. (1974) Kaposi sarcoma complicating systemic lupus erythematosus treated with immunosuppression. *Arch. Dermatol., 110,* 602-604

Koranda, F.C., Loeffler, R.T., Koranda, D.M. & Penn, I. (1975) Accelerated induction of skin cancers by ultraviolet radiation in hairless mice treated with immunosuppressive agents. *Surg. Forum, 26,* 145-146

Krawitt, E.L., Stein, J.H., Kirkendall, W.M. & Clifton, J.A. (1967) Mercaptopurine hepatotoxicity in a patient with chronic active hepatitis. *Arch. intern. Med., 120,* 729-734

Krueger, G.R.F., Malmgren, R.A. & Berard, C.W. (1971) Malignant lymphomas and plasmacytosis in mice under prolonged immunosuppression and persistent antigenic stimulation. *Transplantation, 11,* 138-144

Krutchik, A.N., Buzdar, A.U. & Tashima, C.K. (1978) Azathioprine and breast carcinoma. *J. Am. med. Assoc., 239,* 107-108

Kučerová, M., Polivková, Z. & Budínská, B. (1979) *Mutagenic effect of Imuran.* In: Benešová, O., Rychter, Z. & Jelínek, R., eds, *Evaluation of Embryotoxicity, Mutagenicity and Carcinogenicity Risks in New Drugs,* Prague, Universita Karlova, pp. 257-261

Leb, D.E., Weisskopf, B. & Kanovitz, B.S. (1971) Chromosome aberrations in the child of a kidney transplant recipient. *Arch. intern. Med., 128,* 441-444

Lessmöllmann, U., Neubert, D. & Merker, H.-J. (1975) *Mammalian limb buds differentiating* in vitro *as a test system for the evaluation of embryotoxic effects.* In: Neubert, D. & Merker, H.J., eds, *New Approaches to the Evaluation of Abnormal Embryonic Development,* Stuttgart, Georg Thieme, pp. 99-113

Lindeman, R.D., Pederson, J.A., Matter, B.J., Laughlin, L.O. & Mandal, A.K. (1976) Long-term azathio-prine-corticosteroid therapy in lupus nephritis and idiopathic nephrotic syndrome. *J. chronic Dis., 29,* 189-204

Lipsmeyer, E.A. (1972) Development of malignant cerebral lymphoma in a patient with systemic lupus erythematosus treated with immunosuppression. *Arthritis Rheum., 15,* 183-186

Lockshin, M.D. & Kagen, L.J. (1972) Meningitic reactions after azathioprine (Letter to the Editor). *New Engl. J. Med., 286,* 1321-1322

Lower, G.D., Stevens, L.E., Najarian, J.S. & Reemtsma, K. (1971) Problems from immunosuppressives during pregnancy. *Am. J. Obstet. Gynecol., 111,* 1120-1121

Lukes, R.J. & Collins, R.D. (1975) *A functional classification of malignant lymphomas.* In: Rebuck, J.W., Berard, C.W. & Abell, M.R., eds, *The Reticuloendothelial System,* Baltimore, Williams & Wilkins, p. 224

Manny, N., Rosenman, E. & Benbassat, J. (1972) Hazard of immunosuppressive therapy. *Br. med. J., ii,* 291

Mansi, C., Dodero, M., Savarino, V., Picciotto, A., Ciravegna, G., Testa, R. & Celle, G. (1979) Toxic effects on mucosa of the oesophagus, stomach and colon and on the pancreas after chronic adminis-tration of azathioprine and cyclophosphamide to rats (Ital.). *Pathologica, 71,* 235-241

Marshall, V. (1974) Premalignant and malignant skin tumours in immunosuppressed patients. *Transplantation, 17,* 272-275

McAdam, L., Paulus, H.E. & Peter, J.B. (1974) Adenocarcinoma of the lung during azathioprine therapy. *Arthritis Rheum., 17,* 92-94

McGrath, B.P., Ibels, L.S., Raik, E., Hargrave, M., Mahony, J.F. & Stewart, J.H. (1975) Erythroid toxicity of azathioprine. Macrocytosis and selective marrow hypoplasia. *Q. J. Med. (New Series), 44,* 57-63

Metz, G., Lurz, C. & Metz, J. (1974) Effects and side-effects of immunosuppressive therapy in various dermatoses (Ger.). *Münch. med. Wochenschr., 116,* 1329-1338

Michlmayr, G., Günther, R., Lederer, B. & Huber, H. (1973) Malignant lymphoma after two years' immunosuppressive therapy of periarteritis nodosa (Ger.). *Med. Klin., 68,* 180-182

de Miranda, P. & Chu, L.-C. (1970) Reaction of azathioprine (Imuran) with ^{14}C-glycine in the rat (Abstract no. 2028). *Fed. Proc., 29,* 608

de Miranda, P., Beacham, L.M., III, Creagh, T.H. & Elion, G.B. (1973) The metabolic fate of the methyl-nitroimidazole moiety of azathioprine in the rat. *J. Pharmacol. exp. Ther., 187,* 588-601

de Miranda, P., Beacham, L.M., III, Creagh, T.H. & Elion, G.B. (1975) The metabolic disposition of ^{14}C-azathioprine in the dog. *J. Pharmacol. exp. Ther., 195,* 50-57

Mitrou, P.S., Fischer, M., Mitrou, G., Röttger, P. & Holtz, G. (1979a) The oncogenic effect of immuno-suppressive (cytotoxic) agents in (NZB x NZW) mice. I. Long-term treatment with azathioprine and ifosfamide. *Arzneimittel-Forsch./Drug Res., 29,* 483-488

Mitrou, P.S., Fischer, M., Mitrou, G. & Röttger, P. (1979b) The oncogenic effect of immunosuppressive (cytotoxic) agents in (NZB x NZW) mice. II. Emergence of tumors in young animals treated with azathioprine and ifosfamide, including a histologic assessment of the neoplasms. *Arzneimittel-Forsch./Drug Res., 29,* 662-667

Neuberg, R. (1974) Immunosuppression and plasmocytoma of the cervix. *J. Obstet. Gynaecol. Br. Commonw., 81,* 165-167

Neubert, D., Lessmöllmann, U., Hinz, N., Dillmann, I. & Fuchs, G. (1977) Interference of 6-mercapto-purine riboside, 6-methylmercaptopurine riboside and azathioprine with the morphogenetic differ-entiation of mouse extremities *in vivo* and in organ culture. *Naunyn-Schmiedeberg's Arch. Pharmacol., 298,* 93-105

Neuhaus, K., Thorhorst, J., Bertel, O. & Speck, B. (1976) Multiple neoplasms in a case of rheumatoid arthritis treated with azathioprine (Ger.). *Schweiz. Rundsch. Med. (Praxis), 65,* 213-221

Nord, E., Douer, D., Kessler, E., Pinkhas, J. & de Vries, A. (1976) Sclerosing reticulum cell sarcoma following prolonged treatment with azathioprine for idiopathic thrombocytopenic purpura. *Scand. J. Haematol., 17,* 321-325

Norfleet, R.G. & Sampson, C.E. (1978) Carcinoma of the cervix after treatment with prednisone and azathioprine for chronic active hepatitis. *Am. J. Gastroenterol., 70,* 383-384

Obe, G. (1971) The effect of 6-mercaptopurine and azathioprine on human chromosomes *in vitro* (Ger.). *Arzneimittel-Forsch., 21,* 504-505

Orbuch, D. S.J. & Findor, J.A. (1979) Hodgkin's disease in a patient with ulcerative colitis and chronic hepatitis treated with the immunosuppressive azathioprine (Sp.). *Acta gastroenterol. lat. am., 9,* 73-80

Patterson, J.F., Norton, R.A. & Schwartz, R.S. (1971) Azathioprine treatment of ulcerative colitis, granulomatous colitis and regional enteritis. *Dig. Dis., 16,* 327-332

Penn, I. (1970) Malignant tumors in organ transplant recipients. *Recent Results Cancer Res., 35,* 1-47

Penn, I. (1971) Complications of immunosuppression. *Minerva Chir., 26,* 718-720

Penn, I. (1979) Tumor incidence in human allograft recipients. *Transplant. Proc., 11,* 1047-1051

Penn, I., Makowski, E.L. & Harris, P. (1980) Parenthood following renal transplantation. *Kidney Int., 18,* 221-233

Pinals, R.S. (1976) Azathioprine in the treatment of chronic polyarthritis: longterm results and adverse effects in 25 patients. *J. Rheumatol., 3,* 140-144

Pirotte, J.H. (1974) Development of Hodgkins disease in the course of active chronic hepatitis treated by immunosuppressive drugs. *Am. J. Gastroenterol., 62,* 230-239

Puget, A., Cros, S., Oreglia, J. & Tollon, Y. (1975) Study of the embryonal sensitivity of the Afghan pika (*Ochotona rufescens rufescens*) to two teratogenic agents, azathioprine and 6-mercaptopurine (Fr.). *Zbl. vet. Med. A, 22,* 38-56

Rabkin, R., Thatcher, G.N., Diamond, L.H. & Eales, L. (1973) The nephrotic syndrome, malignancy and immunosuppression. *S. Afr. med. J., 47,* 605-606

Roberts, M.M. & Bell, R. (1976) Acute leukaemia after immunosuppressive therapy. *Lancet, ii,* 768-770

Rosenkrantz, J.G., Githens, J.H., Cox, S.M. & Kellum, D.L. (1967) Azathioprine (Imuran) and pregnancy. *Am. J. Obstet. Gynecol., 97,* 387-394

Rosner, F. & Grünwald, H. (1975) Hodgkin's disease and acute leukemia. Report of eight cases and review of the literature. *Am. J. Med., 58,* 339-353

Rossi, A., Sebastio, L. & Ventruto, V. (1973) Chromosomal study in 14 psoriatic subjects treated with hydroxyurea or azathioprine (Ital.). *Minerva Med., 64,* 1728-1732

Saarikoski, S. & Seppälä, M. (1973) Immunosuppression during pregnancy: transmission of azathioprine and its metabolites from the mother to the fetus. *Am. J. Obstet. Gynecol.,115,* 1100-1106

Scharf, J., Nahir, M., Eidelman, S., Jacobs, R. & Levin, D. (1977) Carcinoma of the bladder with azathioprine therapy. *J. Am. med. Assoc., 237,* 152

Scholz, G., Rehn, K. & Hunstein, W. (1973) Hodgkin's sarcoma after immunosuppressive treatment of erythema visceralis (Ger.). *Verh. Dtsch. Ges. Inn. Med., 79,* 1376-1378

Schramm, G. (1970) Development of severe cervical dysplasia under treatment with azathioprine (Imuran). *Acta cytol., 14,* 507-509

Seidenfeld, A.M., Smythe, H.A., Ogryzlo, M.A., Urowitz, M.B. & Dotten, D.A. (1976) Acute leukemia in rheumatoid arthritis treated with cytotoxic agents. *J. Rheumatol., 3,* 295-304

Sergent, J.S. & Lockshin, M. (1978) Azathioprine-induced meningitis in systemic lupus erythematosus (Letter to the Editor). *J. Am. med. Assoc., 240,* 529

Sharon, E., Jones, J., Diamond, H. & Kaplan, D. (1974) Pregnancy and azathioprine in systemic lupus erythematosus. *Am. J. Obstet. Gynecol., 118,* 25-28

Sharpstone, P., Ogg, C.S. & Cameron, J.S. (1969) Nephrotic syndrome due to primary renal disease in adults. II. A controlled trial of prednisolone and azathioprine. *Br. med. J., ii,* 535-539

Silas, D.E. & Nance, F.C. (1968) Increased tolerance to high doses of azathioprine by germfree animals (Abstract). *Clin. Res., 16,* 84

Silvergleid, A.J. & Schrier, S.L. (1974) Acute myelogenous leukemia in two patients treated with azathioprine for nonmalignant diseases. *Am. J. Med., 57,* 885-888

Simmons, R.L., Kjellstrand, C.-M. & Najarian, J.S. (1972) *Technique, complications, and results.* In: Najarian, J.S. & Simmons, R.L., eds, *Transplantation,* Philadelphia, PA, Lea & Febiger, pp. 445-495

Slater, A., Whittaker, J.A. & Fisher, D.J.H. (1976) Reticulum-cell sarcoma and Sjögren's syndrome in a patient treated with azathioprine. *New Engl. J. Med., 294,* 51

Sneddon, I. & Wishart, J.M. (1972) Immunosuppression and malignancy. *Br. med. J., iv,* 235

Speck, W.T. & Rosenkranz, H.S. (1976) Mutagenicity of azathioprine. *Cancer Res., 36,* 108-109

Starzl, T.E. (1964) *Experience in Renal Transplantation,* Philadelphia, W.B. Saunders, p. 181

Starzl, T.E. & Putnam, C.W. (1969) *Experience in Hepatic Transplantation,* Philadelphia, W.B. Saunders, pp. 194-201

Starzl, T.E., Marchioro, T.L., Porter, K.A., Taylor, P.D., Faris, T.D., Hermann, T.J., Hlad, C.L. & Waddell, W.R. (1965) Factors determining short- and long-term survival after orthotopic liver homotransplantation in the dog. *Surgery, 58,* 131-155

Summerskill, W.H.J., Korman, M.G., Ammon, H.V. & Baggenstoss, A.H. (1975) Prednisone for chronic active liver disease: dose titration, standard dose, and combination with azathioprine compared. *Gut, 16,* 876-883

Symington, G.R., Mackay, I.R. & Lambert, R.P. (1977) Cancer and teratogenesis: infrequent occurrence after medical use of immunosuppressive drugs. *Aust. N.Z. J. Med., 7,* 368-372

Torigoe, K. (1980) Sister chromatid exchanges in children treated with azathioprine and cyclophosphamide, and effect of protein-bound polysaccharide (PS-K). *Jpn. J. Hum. Genet., 25,* 15-21

Touraine, J.L., Revillard, J.P. & Traeger, J. (1972) Biology of Listerian infection. Influence of immunosuppression (Fr.). *Nouv. Presse méd., 1,* 2827-2832

Tuchmann-Duplessis, H. & Mercier-Parot, L. (1964) Production of limb malformations in rabbits by administration of an antimetabolite: azathioprine (Fr.). *C.R. Acad. Sci. (Paris), 259,* 3648-3651

Tuchmann-Duplessis, H. & Mercier-Parot, L. (1966) Production of limb malformations in rabbits by administration of azathioprine and 6-mercaptopurine (Fr.). *C.R. Soc. Biol., 160,* 501-506

Tuchmann-Duplessis, H. & Mercier-Parot, L. (1968) Experimental production of limb malformations (Fr.). *Union méd. Can., 97,* 283-288

Turnbull, A. & Almeyda, J. (1970) Idiopathic thrombocytopenic purpura and Kaposi's sarcoma. *Proc. R. Soc. Med., 63,* 603-605

Ulrich, J. & Wüthrich, R. (1974) Multiple sclerosis: reticulum cell sarcoma of the nervous sytem in a patient treated with immunosuppressive drugs. *Eur. Neurol., 12,* 65-78

US International Trade Commission (1979) *Synthetic Organic Chemicals, US Production and Sales, 1978,* TC Publication 1001, Washington DC, US Government Printing Office, p. 173

US Pharmacopeial Convention, Inc. (1980) *The US Pharmacopeia,* 20th rev., Rockville, MD, pp. 61-62

US Tariff Commission (1972) *Synthetic Organic Chemicals, US Production and Sales, 1970,* TC Publication 479, Washington DC, US Government Printing Office, p. 120

Uszyński, L., Szczecińska, M., Dudkiewicz, H. & Śliwowski, A. (1978) Acute leukaemia during immunosuppressive therapy of glomerulonephritis. *Mater Med. Pol., 10,* 226-227

Varadachari, C., Palutke, M., Climie, A.R.W., Weise, R.W. & Chason, J.L. (1978) Immunoblastic sarcoma (histiocytic lymphoma) of the brain with B cell markers. *J. Neurosurg., 49,* 887-892

Vismans, J.J., Briët, E., Meijer, K. & den Ottolander, G.J. (1980) Azathioprine and subacute myelomonocytic leukemia. *Acta med. scand., 207,* 315-319

Viteri, A., Vernace, S.J. & Schaffner, F. (1976) Extrahepatic malignancy in chronic liver disease: report of six cases. *Gastroenterology, 71,* 1075-1078

Wade, A., ed. (1977) *Martindale, The Extra Pharmacopoeia,* 27th ed., London, The Pharmaceutical Press, pp. 123-127

Walden, P.A.M., Philalithis, P.E., Joekes, A.M. & Bagshawe, K.D. (1977) Development of a lymphocytic lymphoma during immunosuppressive therapy with azathioprine for systemic lupus erythematosus with renal involvement induced by phenylbutazone. *Clin. Nephrol., 8,* 317-320

Wallace, E.Z., Rosman, P.M., Balthazar, A. & Sacerdote, A. (1979) Adrenocortical carcinoma in a patient with systemic lupus erythematosus treated with azathioprine. *Arthritis Rheum., 22,* 937-938

Watanabe, A., Hobara, N. & Nagashima, H. (1978) Demonstration of enzymatic activity converting azathioprine to 6-mercaptopurine. *Acta med. Okayama, 32,* 173-179

Watanabe, A., Hobara, N., Tobe, K., Endo, H. & Nagashima, H. (1979) Biochemical and morphological study on hepatotoxicity of azathioprine in rat. *Acta med. Okayama, 33,* 5-14

Weisburger, E.K. (1977) Bioassay program for carcinogenic hazards of cancer chemotherapeutic agents. *Cancer, 40,* 1935-1951

van Went, G.F. (1979) Investigation into the mutagenic activity of azathioprine (Imuran®) in different test systems. *Mutat. Res., 68,* 153-162

Westaby, S., Everett, W.G. & Dick, A.P. (1977) Adenocarcinoma of the small bowel complicating Crohn's disease in a patient treated with azathioprine. *Clin. Oncol., 3,* 377-381

Windholz, M., ed. (1976) *The Merck Index,* 9th ed., Rahway, NJ, Merck & Co., p. 120

Worth, W.S. (1968) Azathioprine effect on normal canine liver and kidney function. *Toxicol. appl. Pharmacol., 12,* 1-6

Wyrobek, A.J. & Bruce, W.R. (1975) Chemical induction of sperm abnormalities in mice. *Proc. natl Acad. Sci. USA, 72,* 4425-4429

Zeuthen, E. & Friedrich, U. (1971) Chromosome examination in children of parents treated with Imuran® (Ger.). *Humangenetik, 12,* 74-76

Zimmerman, T.P., Chu, L.-C., Buggé, C.J.C., Nelson, D.J., Miller, R.L. & Elion, G.B. (1974) Formation of 5'-nucleotides of 6-methylmercaptopurine ribonucleoside in human tissues *in vitro. Biochem. Pharmacol., 23,* 2737-2749

van Zyl, J. & Wissmüller, H.F. (1974) The clastogenic effect of azathioprine on human chromosomes *in vitro. Humangenetik, 21,* 153-165

1. CHEMICAL AND PHYSICAL DATA

1.1 Synonyms and trade names

Chem. Abstr. Services Reg. No.: 154-93-8

Chem. Abstr. Name: Urea, *N,N'*-bis(2-chloroethyl)-*N*-nitroso-

IUPAC Systematic Name: 1,3-Bis(2-chloroethyl)-1-nitrosourea

Synonyms: BCNU; bis(2-chloroethyl)nitrosourea; 1,3-bis(2-chloroethyl)nitrosourea; 1,3-bis(β-chloroethyl)-1-nitrosourea; carmustin; carmustine; 1,3-di(2-chloroethyl)-1-nitrosourea

Trade names: BiCNU; Nitrumon; NSC 409962

1.2 Structural and molecular formulae and molecular weight

$$\begin{array}{c} NO\;\;O \\ |\quad \| \\ ClCH_2CH_2N-C-NHCH_2CH_2Cl \end{array}$$

$C_5H_9Cl_2N_3O_2$ Mol. wt: 214.0

1.3 Chemical and physical properties of the pure substance

From Wade (1977) or Windholz (1976), unless otherwise specified

(a) *Description*: Light-yellow powder
(b) *Melting-point*: 30-32°C
(c) *Solubility*: Slightly soluble in water (4 mg in 1 ml) and 50% ethanol (150 mg in 1 ml); soluble in ethanol (1 in 2); highly soluble in lipids
(d) *Stability*: Sensitive to oxidation and hydrolysis, forming alkylating and carbamoylating intermediates. Its half-life at neutral pH is 98 minutes (Schein *et al.*, 1978).

1.4 Technical products and impurities

BCNU is available in the US in vials containing 100 mg (Baker, 1980).

2. PRODUCTION, USE, OCCURRENCE AND ANALYSIS

2.1 Production and use

(a) Production

Synthesis of BCNU was reported (Johnston *et al.*, 1963) to have been carried out by the reaction of sodium nitrite with a solution of 1,3-bis(2-chloroethyl)urea in formic acid. It is believed to be produced commercially by the same process.

The information available to the Working Group indicated that BCNU is currently produced only by one company in the US, in an undisclosed amount (see preamble, pp. 20-21).

(b) Use

BCNU has been used in human medicine since 1971 as an antineoplastic agent (alone or in combination with other agents) in the treatment of Hodgkin's lymphoma, multiple myeloma and primary or metastatic brain tumours. It is given in doses of 100-250 mg/m^2 body surface by i.v. injection daily, for courses of 2 or 3 days (Wade, 1977).

BCNU has also been reported to have antiviral (Sidwell *et al.*, 1965), antibacterial (Pittillo *et al.*, 1964) and antifungal activity (Hunt & Pittillo, 1966), but no evidence was found that it is used in these ways.

2.2 Occurrence

BCNU is not known to be produced in Nature.

2.3 Analysis

Typical methods for the analysis of BCNU in blood plasma are summarized in Table 1.

Table 1. Methods for the analysis of BCNU

Sample matrix	Sample preparation	Assay procedure[a]	Limit of detection	Reference
Blood plasma	Mix with citric acid; extract with pentane	DPP	1 μg/ml	Bartošek et al. (1978)
	Extract with diethyl ether; evaporate; dissolve in dichloromethane	CIMS	0.85 ng/ml	Weinkam et al. (1978)

[a]Abbreviations: DPP, differential pulse polarography; CIMS, chemical ionization-mass spectrometry

3. BIOLOGICAL DATA RELEVANT TO THE EVALUATION OF CARCINOGENIC RISK TO HUMANS

3.1 Carcinogenicity studies in animals

(a)   Oral administration

Rat: Two groups, each of 20 female Sprague-Dawley rats, 50 - 55 days old, were administered a single oral dose by gavage of 4 mg/rat or 2 mg/rat BCNU suspended in 1 ml sesame oil.   The higher dose corresponded to the maximum tolerated dose determined in 45-day-old female Sprague-Dawley rats in the same laboratory.   Twenty rats that received 18 mg/rat 7,12-dimethylbenz[a]anthracene (DMBA) served as positive controls; 89 rats that received sesame oil alone were used as solvent controls.   The cumulative 6-month mortality was 4/20 (20%) in DMBA-treated animals, 5/89 (4%) in solvent controls, 20/20 (100%) in the group that received the high dose of BCNU, and 2/20 (10%) in the low-dose group.   All of the tumours seen in 18 (90%) positive control rats were multiple breast tumours, of which 13 (65%) were mammary carcinomas.   Of the solvent controls, 1 rat had a fibroadenomatous hyperplasia of the mammary gland; in addition, 1 kidney carcinoma, 1 lung carcinoma and 1 precancerous change in the bronchus were reported.   No tumour was seen in the 18 BCNU-treated rats that survived the 6-month experimental period (Griswold et al., 1966).   [Because of limitations in experimental design, the Working Group considered the absence of carcinogenic effect to be inconclusive.]

(b)   Skin application

Mouse: In a study on the synergistic effects of ultra-violet light and BCNU [see below, section (*e*)] , a group of 29 female Uscd:(HR) hairless mice, 3 - 4 months old, received a single weekly application of 0.5 mg BCNU in 0.1 ml acetone solution to the posterior parts of their backs.   Another group of 40 mice received applications of acetone solution.   No skin tumour occurred in either of these groups (Epstein, 1979).   [The duration of observation was not stated.]

(c)   Intraperitoneal administration

Mouse: Two groups, each of 25 male and 25 female outbred Swiss-Webster-derived mice, 6 weeks old, were given i.p. injections of 1.25 or 2.5 mg/kg bw BCNU in 10 ml/kg bw physiological saline 3 times weekly for 6 months.   Animals that survived over 100 days were observed for up to 12 further months.   Controls consisted of 254 untreated mice. The survival times of the treated animals were reported as percentages of that of the controls [no precise definition of the mode of calculation was given] : the survival times of male mice were reported to be 41% and 45%, respectively, that of untreated controls; and the corresponding figures for females were 32% and 53%.   Animals that died before day 100 on test were excluded from evaluation. The incidence of 9/21 (43%) female tumour-bearing mice was 1.5 - 2 times higher than that in controls (38/153, 25%); 4 lung tumours and 4 lymphosarcomas were described.   Of treated males, 4/34 (12%) had 2 lymphosarcomas, 1 lung tumour and 1 reticuloendothelioma;   this incidence was comparable to that in controls (28/101, 28%) (Weisburger, 1977).   [The Working Group considered that the inadequate reporting of certain items, such as survival times, the amalgamation of various experimental groups and tumour types, as well as the lack of age-adjustment in the analyses precluded a complete evaluation of this study.]

Rat: Two groups, each of 25 male and 25-28 female Sprague-Dawley-derived Charles River (CD) rats, about 30 days old, were given i.p. injections of 0.75 or 1.5 mg/kg bw BCNU as a 2.5 ml/kg bw dilution in physiological saline 3 times a week for 6 months. Animals that survived over 100 days were observed for up to 12 further months, at which time they were killed.   Tumours were seen in 60/179 (34%) untreated males and in 105/181 (58%) untreated females.   The survival times of the treated animals were reported as percentages of that of the controls [no precise definition of the mode of calculation was given] : the survival times of treated female rats were reported to be 81% and 100% that of control animals;   the corresponding figures for treated males were 94% and 100%. Animals that died before day 100 on test were excluded from evaluation.   Of treated females, 24/36 (67%) developed tumours: 9 breast tumours, 6 lung tumours, 2 brain tumours, 1 liver, 1 bladder and 1 ovary tumour were recorded.   In the control group, only 1 lung tumour in 181 animals was reported.   Of treated male rats, 30/40 (75%)

developed tumours; 14 lung tumours, 3 subcutaneous tumours, 2 pancreatic tumours and 2 prostatic tumours were recorded (Weisburger, 1977). [The Working Group considered that the inadequate reporting of certain items, such as survival times, the amalgamation of various experimental groups and tumour types, as well as the lack of age-adjustment in the analyses precluded a complete evaluation of this study.]

In a lifetime experiment with Sprague-Dawley rats, still in progress at the time of reporting, groups of 20 male and 20 female rats were injected intraperitoneally once a week for 52 weeks with 0.6 ml of solvent or with 0.6 ml of solvent containing either 0.2 or 1.0 mg/kg bw BCNU. The solvent was composed of 25% Cremophor EL (a surfactant based on castor oil), 25% ethanol and 50% physiological saline. The mean survival times were 803, 703 and 359 days in the solvent controls, in the group given the low dose of BCNU, and in the group given the high dose, respectively. Tumours developed in 8 solvent-treated animals (23% of the animals that were alive when the first animal died with a malignant tumour, i.e., at day 237), 15 (45%) animals given the low dose of BCNU and 12 (46%) animals given the high dose. The incidences of malignant tumours in the peritoneal cavity [histology unspecified] were 2 [5%] in controls, 5 [15%] in the low-dose group, and 10 [38%] in the high-dose group (Schmähl & Habs, 1978).

(d) Intravenous administration

Rat: BCNU was included in a chronic toxicity and carcinogenicity study on cyto-static *N*-nitroso(2-chloroethyl)ureas, still in progress at the time of reporting. Groups of 30 male Wistar rats (age unspecified) received i.v. injections every 6 weeks of 9.5, 19.0, 38.0 or 75.0 mg/m^2 BCNU (1,2,4 or 8 mg/kg bw) dissolved in Cremophor EL (a surfactant based on castor oil), ethanol and water (1.5:1.5:20 vol/vol). Controls consisted of 120 animals that received the same amount of solvent. Treatment was discontinued when severe lethal toxicity became apparent, i.e., after 4 applications of the highest dose or after 10 applications of any of the other three doses. All animals were observed for life. Median survival times after the start of treatment were 621 days for controls, 568 days for the group treated with 9.5 mg/m^2 (1.0 mg/kg bw), 314 days for the group treated with 19 mg/m^2 (2 mg/kg bw), 263 days for the group treated with 38 mg/m^2 (4 mg/kg bw) and 164 days for the group treated with 75 mg/m^2 (8 mg/kg bw). Malignant tumours occurred in 8% (10/120) of solvent controls and in 27% of animals treated with the highest dose of BCNU. Of the latter group, 23% of the animals had malignant lung tumours. No clear-cut result was reported for the lower dose groups. It was stated that histopathological exami-nations had not been completed and that the results were thus preliminary (Eisenbrand & Habs, 1980; Eisenbrand *et al.*, 1981). [The Working Group was unable to use this limited information for further evaluation.] In a further report on the same study, 5 adenocarci-nomas of the lung were described in the highest dose group; this incidence was signif-icantly different from 0/120 in controls (Habs, 1980).

(e)   Administration with other agents

Mouse: The influence of BCNU on ultra-violet-induced carcinogenesis was examined on the skin of hairless mice. Thus, 145 female Uscd:(HR) hairless mice, 3-4 months old, were divided into 4 groups. One group of 40 mice received a single weekly application of 0.5 mg BCNU in 0.1 ml acetone solution and a thrice weekly administration of ultra-violet B (UV) energy (280-320 nm; 1.25×10^3 mJ/cm^2) to the posterior parts of their backs for the duration of the study. A second group of 36 mice received only the acetone applications and UV exposures. The third group [described above in (a)] received BCNU alone, and the last acetone alone. The first tumour greater than 4 mm^3 was recorded after 9 weeks in the group treated with BCNU plus UV, and by 10 weeks in the group treated with UV alone. All survivors in the group that received BCNU plus UV and 94% of those in the group that received UV developed skin tumours at the site of application. A life-table analysis of the occurrence of tumours larger than 4, 50 or 100 mm^2 was made. For all three sizes, the time to tumour appearance was significantly lower in the group that received BCNU in addition to UV exposure (Epstein, 1979).

3.2 Other relevant biological data

(a)   Experimental systems

Toxic effects

The LD_{50} of BCNU in rats after a single oral dose in corn oil was 30 mg/kg bw over a 30-day observation period, with no significant difference between the sexes. In male mice, the LD_{50} of BCNU was 19 mg/kg bw by oral administration under the same conditions and with no significant difference between the sexes. LD_{50} values were similar when the drug was given intraperitoneally or subcutaneously (Thompson & Larson, 1972). In dogs, the single oral lethal dose of BCNU was 5 mg/kg bw (Oliverio, 1973).

Weekly i.p. treatment of male rats for 9 weeks resulted in suppression of weight gain at dose levels of 4 and 8 mg/kg bw per week and 70% mortality at 8 mg/kg bw per week (Thompson *et al.*, 1974).

A characteristic feature of the antitumour nitrosoureas is their delayed bone-marrow toxicity (Young *et al.*, 1971). In dogs, severe bone-marrow hypoplasia occurred with high doses, with delayed, reversible thrombocytopenia. The other major toxicities observed were cardiopulmonary (pulmonary oedema, myocardial infarction and pericardial haemorrhage), intestinal mucosal damage with haemorrhaging, renal toxicity and delayed hepatotoxicity. Similar toxicity was seen in monkeys, except that cardiopulmonary toxicity did not occur (Oliverio, 1973). In rats and mice, doses well tolerated in a 30-day test caused deaths as late as 100 days after treatment; for example, in one experiment in rats all BCNU doses above the LD_1 (10 mg/kg bw) ultimately caused 100% mortality when the observation time was extended beyond 30 days (Thompson & Larson, 1972). BCNU can also cause hepatotoxicity in rats, which may not be apparent until more than 60 days after dosing (Thompson & Larson, 1969). Delayed hepatotoxicity was also the factor that limited the dose that could be given to dogs (Oliverio, 1973).

Effects on reproduction and prenatal toxicity

Weekly i.p. administration of 4 or 8 mg/kg BCNU for 9 weeks produced a decline in fertility in male rats. When treated males were mated with untreated females, the numbers of implantations and viable fetuses on day 20 of gestation were significantly decreased and the resorption rate increased. This effect in males was reversible within 48 days (Thompson *et al.*, 1974).

BCNU was highly teratogenic when given to pregnant Sprague-Dawley rats in i.p. doses of 1, 2 or 4 mg/kg bw per day during various 4-day periods of organogenesis or 1.5 mg/kg bw per day throughout organogenesis (days 6 - 15 of pregnancy). The principal period of sensitivity was on days 6 - 9 of pregnancy; thoracoabdominal closure defects and eye and central nervous system defects occurred most frequently. Treatment of rabbits with i.v. doses of 0.5 - 4 mg/kg bw once daily on days 6 - 18 caused no teratogenic effects, but growth retardation, abortion and death of some mother animals were observed (Thompson *et al.*, 1974).

When 10 mg/kg bw BCNU were given intravenously to BD IX rats during the last quarter of pregnancy, the offspring died within 4 months. This effect was not seen with doses of 2.5 or 5 mg/kg bw (Weiss *et al.*, 1973).

Absorption, distribution, excretion and metabolism

BCNU undergoes spontaneous decomposition under physiological conditions to release both alkylating and carbamoylating entities (Schein *et al.*, 1978). A scheme for the degradation of 2-chloroethyl-nitrosoureas leading to alkylating intermediates (Reed *et al.*, 1975) and carbamoylation of proteins (Connors & Hare, 1974) has been formulated.

Some 40 minutes after injection, BCNU is no longer an effective antitumour agent (Connors & Hare, 1975), and a few minutes after administration no unchanged BCNU can be detected in plasma (Loo *et al.*, 1966). Following its i.p. or s.c. injection or oral adminis-tration, BCNU was rapidly distributed to most tissues, including brain and cerebrospinal fluid. Excretion was primarily in the urine; it was most rapid in mice (80% of the dose excreted in 24 hours) and less rapid in monkeys and dogs (Loo *et al.*, 1966; DeVita *et al.*, 1967; Levin *et al.*, 1978a).

In addition to chemical decomposition, BCNU may be denitrosated enzymically to its corresponding urea (Hill *et al.*, 1975); it is also a substrate for glutathione S-transferases (Hill, 1976). Following injection to mice, BCNU significantly decreased the glutathione concentration of liver but not lung (McConnell *et al.*, 1979). It is thought that alkylating entities, particularly chloroethyl carbonium ions, are responsible for most of the anti-tumour effects of the antitumour nitrosoureas, since analogues with negligible carbamoylating but good alkylating activity have the same antitumour effects as BCNU (Schein *et al.*, 1978). BCNU binds extensively to proteins, also forming alkylated and carbamoylated products (Bowdon & Wheeler, 1971). It also reacts with a variety of nucleosides and nucleic acids to form not only monofunctionally alkylated products, such as 3-hydroxyethyldeoxycytidine, $3,N^4$-ethanocytidine-monophosphate and 7-amino-ethylguanine, but also DNA cross-links (Ludlum *et al.*, 1975; Kohn, 1977; Gombar *et al.*, 1980).

Effects on intermediary metabolism

BCNU decreases transglutaminase activity in the liver and spleen of mice (Sipka *et al.*, 1979).

Mutagenicity and other short-term tests

BCNU was mutagenic in *Salmonella typhimurium* strains *his* G46 (Zimmer & Bhuyan, 1976), TA1535 and TA100 (Matheson *et al.*, 1978; Franza *et al.*, 1980). It induced sex-linked recessive lethals in spermatozoa of *Drosophila melanogaster* (Kortselius, 1978) and mutations in the mouse lymphoma line L5178Y (Matheson *et al.*, 1978). BCNU also induced mutation at the hypoxanthine-guanine phosphoribosyltransferase locus in V79 Chinese hamster cells (Bradley *et al.*, 1980).

BCNU caused increases in chromosomal aberrations in a mouse fibroblast line *in vitro*. It also produced significant increases in chromatid aberrations and micronuclei formation in bone-marrow cells of CBA male mice after single i.p. injections of 9 and 27 mg/kg bw (Tates *et al.*, 1977).

(b) Humans

Toxic effects

A late onset of bone-marrow depression is characteristic of the nitrosoureas, including BCNU. Thrombocytopenia develops 4 weeks and leucopenia 6 weeks after a single i.v. dose of 100-200 mg/m^2 (Wasserman, 1976). Toxicity is dose-related and cumulative and is aggravated by prior X-irradiation or cytotoxic chemotherapy. Nausea and vomiting are almost universal within two hours of drug administration; diarrhoea also occurs, but to a lesser degree and less often (25%). Local toxicity at injection sites consists of transient burning and redness; thrombophlebitis is infrequent (Young *et al.*, 1971; Ramirez *et al.*, 1972). Stomatitis, anorexia and alopecia occur rarely.

Recently, however, dose-related pulmonary toxicity has been noted, the incidence of which has increased since the first report (Holoye *et al.*, 1976). Ten cases were seen by Durant *et al.* (1979), although all but one had also received other drugs (bleomycin, vincristine, procarbazine or cyclophosphamide) or radiation (5 patients), which might also be implicated in the pathogenesis of the disease. Seven further patients who were exposed only to BCNU were subsequently found to have iatrogenic pulmonary disease. Doses of over 1 g/m^2 had been given to all of these patients; one, a child with a medulloblastoma, had no evidence of the tumour at autopsy. Death was due to diffuse pulmonary fibrosis typical of 'bleomycin' or 'busulphan lung', which had been extremely insidious in onset. Most reports agree that the only early sign is impaired diffusion capacity in the lungs, followed by symptoms of cough, dyspnoea and late radiological changes (Bailey *et al.*, 1978; Selker *et al.*, 1978; Melato & Tuveri, 1980).

In a study of 93 patients given BCNU as treatment for malignant glioma, 20% developed symptomatic pulmonary toxicity. Retrospective analysis of risk factors indicated a cumulative dose effect. Pre-existing pulmonary disease, older age and severity of myelosuppression also predisposed to lung toxicity. Administration of steroids did not have a protective effect (Aronin *et al.*, 1980).

In 26% of one series of patients, reversible alterations in liver function tests were reported (DeVita *et al.*, 1965). It was reported in an abstract that when high doses of BCNU (up to 1.4 g/m^2) were given before autologous bone-marrow infusion, severe liver toxicity, which limited the dose that could be given, was seen in 1 out of 4 patients (Takvorian *et al.*, 1980).

A single case report of neuroretinitis concerned a patient given both BCNU and procarbazine (Lennan & Taylor, 1978).

Effects on reproduction and prenatal toxicity

No data were available to the Working Group.

Absorption, distribution, excretion and metabolism

Until 1978, only pharmacokinetic data from one radiolabelling study were available (DeVita *et al.*, 1967). Chemical ionization-mass spectrometry has enabled measurement of BCNU without radioisotope labelling (Levin *et al.*, 1978b). This indicated that BCNU was absorbed very quickly from the gut and was metabolized even more rapidly when it reached the plasma. Peak metabolite levels were seen within 6 hours of oral administration (Oliverio, 1976), and their distribution was widespread to brain, liver, kidney, lungs, gut, bone marrow and lymphoid tissue. Cerebrospinal fluid contains BCNU metabolites within minutes of i.v. injection due to the lipid solubility of the drug. Plasma levels of isotope had a half-life of 34 hours after oral administration and 67 hours after i.v. injection. Urinary excretion did not vary with the route of administration, and 60% of the isotope was usually recovered by 4 days; the remainder was not accounted for. Excretion in man is similar to that in monkeys but considerably slower than in mice (DeVita *et al.*, 1967). Degradation *in vitro* in patients' serum indicated catalysis by a heat-labile macromolecule and impairment of degradation by high serum lipid levels (Levin *et al.*, 1978b).

At therapeutic doses, BCNU almost completely inhibits glutathione reductase in red cells and platelets (Benöhr & Waller, 1979).

Mutagenicity and chromosomal effects

No data were available to the Working Group.

3.3 Case reports and epidemiological studies of carcinogenicity in humans

There is no case report of cancer developing in patients treated with BCNU alone. Acute nonlymphocytic leukaemia after administration of BCNU in combination with other drugs or with radiation has been reported in 7 patients: 3 with multiple myeloma (Mills *et al.*, 1971; Rosner & Grünwald, 1974; Preisler & Lyman, 1977), 1 with Hodgkin's disease (Foucar *et al.*, 1979), 1 with non-Hodgkin's lymphoma (Zarrabi *et al.*, 1979) and 2 with malignant brain tumours (Cohen *et al.*, 1976; Vogl, 1978). One patient developed cancer of the pancreas after receiving BCNU with other drugs for treatment of non-Hodgkin's lymphoma (Jochimsen *et al.*, 1976), and one developed cancer of the floor of the mouth after therapy with a combination including BCNU for multiple myeloma (Penn, 1976).

In an abstract, two cases of acute nonlymphocytic leukaemia were reported among 76 cases of Hodgkin's disease assigned randomly to a combination regimen of BCNU, vincristine, procarbazine and chlorambucil. The ratio of observed to expected leukaemia cases in this group was 250 (Pajak *et al.*, 1979).

There has been no epidemiological study evaluating BCNU alone. In a follow-up study of 364 patients with multiple myeloma, more than 239 received BCNU and all received melphalan, a known human leukaemogen (see IARC, 1975). Fourteen cases of acute nonlymphocytic leukaemia were observed, compared with 0.07 cases expected (relative risk = 214) (Bergsagel *et al.*, 1979). [The number of patients who received BCNU was not specified.]

4. SUMMARY OF DATA REPORTED AND EVALUATION

4.1 Experimental data

BCNU is carcinogenic in rats, producing tumours of the lung after intraperitoneal or intravenous administration, and intra-abdominal tumours after intraperitoneal adminis-tration. Tests in mice by intraperitoneal administration and skin application and in rats by oral administration could not be evaluated.

When tested in mice by skin application together with ultra-violet B irradiation, BCNU caused an earlier appearance of skin tumours.

BCNU is embryo- and fetolethal in rats and rabbits at doses nontoxic to the mother and can induce a variety of severe teratogenic effects in rats.

BCNU is mutagenic in bacteria, *Drosophila melanogaster* and mammalian cells. It also produces chromosomal aberrations in mammalian cells both in cell culture and *in vivo*.

4.2 Human data

BCNU has had limited use since the mid-1960s in the treatment of neoplastic diseases.

No data were available to evaluate the teratogenic potential or the mutagenicity or chromosomal effects of BCNU in humans.

BCNU has been associated in case reports with the development of acute nonlympho-cytic leukaemia following treatment of primary malignant diseases. In all such cases, BCNU was administered with other anticancer therapies known or suspected of being carcinogenic. No epidemiological study was available.

4.3 Evaluation

There is *sufficient evidence*[1] for the carcinogenicity of BCNU in rats. The data from studies in humans are inadequate to evaluate the carcinogenicity of BCNU in man.

This chemical should be regarded for practical purposes as if it presented a carcinogenic risk to humans.

---

[1] See preamble, p. 18.

5. REFERENCES

Aronin, P.A., Mahaley, M.S., Jr, Rudnick, S.A., Dudka, L., Donohue, J.F., Selker, R.G. & Moore, P. (1980) Prediction of BCNU pulmonary toxicity in patients with malignant gliomas. An assessment of risk factors. *New Engl. J. Med., 303,* 183-188

Bailey, C.C., Marsden, H.B. & Morris Jones, P.H. (1978) Fatal pulmonary fibrosis following 1,3-bis(2-chloroethyl)-1-nitrosourea (BCNU) therapy. *Cancer, 42,* 74-76

Baker, C.E., Jr, ed. (1980) *Physicians' Desk Reference,* 34th ed., Oradell, NJ, Medical Economics Co., pp. 705-706

Bartošek, I., Daniel, S. & Sýkora, S. (1978) Differential pulse polarographic determination of submicrogram quantities of carmustine and related compounds in biological samples. *J. pharm. Sci., 67,* 1160-1163

Benöhr, H.C. & Waller, H.D. (1979) Influence of BCNU on glutathione metabolism of human blood cells (Ger.). *Klin. Wochenschr., 57,* 845-850

Bergsagel, D.E., Bailey, A.J., Langley, G.R., MacDonald, R.N., White, D.F. & Miller, A.B. (1979) The chemotherapy of plasma-cell myeloma and the incidence of acute leukemia. *New Engl. J. Med., 301,* 743-748

Bowdon, B.J. & Wheeler, G.P. (1971) Reaction of 1,3-bis(2-chloroethyl)-1-nitrosourea (BCNU) with protein (Abstract no. 268). *Proc. Am. Assoc. Cancer Res., 12,* 67

Bradley, M.O., Sharkey, N.A., Kohn, K.W. & Layard, M.W. (1980) Mutagenicity and cytotoxicity of various nitrosoureas in V-79 Chinese hamster cells. *Cancer Res., 40,* 2719-2725

Cohen, R.J., Wiernik, P.H. & Walker, M.D. (1976) Acute nonlymphocytic leukemia associated with nitrosourea chemotherapy: report of two cases. *Cancer Treat. Rep., 60,* 1257-1261

Connors, T.A. & Hare, J.R. (1974) The binding of ^{14}C-labelled 1-(2-chloroethyl)-3-cyclohexyl-1-nitrosourea (CCNU) to macromolecules of sensitive and resistant tumours. *Br. J. Cancer, 30,* 477-480

Connors, T.A. & Hare, J.R. (1975) Studies of the mechanisms of action of the tumour-inhibitory nitrosoureas. *Biochem. Pharmacol., 24,* 2133-2140

DeVita, V.T., Carbone, P.P, Owens, A.H., Jr, Gold, G.L., Krant, M.J. & Edmonson, J. (1965) Clinical trials with 1,3-bis(2-chloroethyl)-1-nitrosourea, NSC - 409962. *Cancer Res., 25,* 1876-1881

DeVita, V.T., Denham, C., Davidson, J.D. & Oliverio, V.T. (1967) The physiological disposition of the carcinostatic 1,3-bis(2-chloroethyl)-1-nitrosourea (BCNU) in man and animals. *Clin. pharmacol. Ther., 8,* 566-577

Durant, J.R., Norgard, M.J., Murad, T.M., Bartolucci, A.A. & Langford, K.H. (1979) Pulmonary toxicity associated with bischloroethyl nitrosourea (BCNU). *Ann. intern. Med., 90,* 191-194

Eisenbrand, G. & Habs, M. (1980) *Chronic toxicity and carcinogenicity of cytostatic N-nitroso(2-chloro-ethyl)ureas after repeated intravenous application to rats.* In: Holmstedt, B., Lauwerys, R., Mercier, M. & Roberfroid, M., eds, *Mechanisms of Toxicity and Hazard Evaluation,* Amsterdam, Elsevier/North-Holland Biomedical Press, pp. 273-278

Eisenbrand, G., Habs, M., Zeller, W.J., Fiebig, H., Berger, M., Zelesny, O. & Schmähl, D. (1981) *New nitrosoureas - therapeutic and long-term toxic effects of selected compounds in comparison to selected drugs.* In: Imbach, J.L., Serrou, B. & Schein, P., eds, *Proceedings of an International Symposium on Nitrosoureas in Cancer Treatment, Montpellier,* Amsterdam, Elsevier (in press)

Epstein, J.H. (1979) Stimulation of ultraviolet-induced carcinogenesis by 1,3-bis(2-chloroethyl)-1-nitroso-urea. *Cancer Res., 39,* 408-410

Foucar, K., McKenna, R.W., Bloomfield, C.D., Bowers, T.K. & Brunning, R.D. (1979) Therapy-related leukemia. A panmyelosis. *Cancer, 43,* 1285-1296

Franza, B.R., Jr, Oeschger, N.S., Oeschger, M.P. & Schein, P.S. (1980) Mutagenic activity of nitroso-urea antitumor agents. *J. natl Cancer Inst., 65,* 149-154

Gombar, C.T., Tong, W.P. & Ludlum, D.B. (1980) Mechanism of action of the nitrosoureas. IV. Reactions of bis-chloroethyl nitrosourea and chloroethyl cyclohexyl nitrosourea with deoxyribonucleic acid. *Biochem. Pharmacol., 29,* 2639-2643

Griswold, D.P., Casey, A.E., Weisburger, E.K., Weisburger, J.H. & Schabel, F.M., Jr (1966) On the carcinogenicity of a single intragastric dose of hydrocarbons, nitrosamines, aromatic amines, dyes, coumarins, and miscellaneous chemicals in female Sprague-Dawley rats. *Cancer Res., 26,* 619-625

Habs, M. (1980) *Experimentelle Untersuchungen zur Cancerogenese Wirkung Zytostatischer Arzneimittel (Experimental Studies on the Carcinogenic Effect of Cytostatic Drugs),* Thesis, Medical Faculty of Heidelberg University

Hill, D.L. (1976) *N,N'*-Bis(2-chloroethyl)-*N*-nitrosourea (BCNU), a substrate for glutathione (GSH) S-transferase (Abstract no. 206). *Proc. Am. Assoc. Cancer Res., 17,* 52

Hill, D.L., Kirk, M.C. & Struck, R.F. (1975) Microsomal metabolism of nitrosoureas. *Cancer Res., 35,* 296-301

Holoye, P.Y., Jenkins, D.E. & Greenberg, S.D. (1976) Pulmonary toxicity in long-term administration of BCNU. *Cancer Treat. Rep., 60,* 1691-1694

Hunt, D.E. & Pittillo, R.F. (1966) *Antifungal action of 1,3-bis(2-chloroethyl)-1-nitrosourea.* In: Hobby, G.L., ed., *Antimicrobial Agents and Chemotherapy - 1965,* Vol. 5, Washington DC, American Society for Microbiology, pp. 710-716

IARC (1975) *IARC Monographs on the Evaluation of Carcinogenic Risk of Chemicals to Man,* Vol. 9, *Some aziridines, N-, S- & O- mustards and selenium,* Lyon, pp. 167-180

Jochimsen, P.R., Pearlman, N.W. & Lawton, R.L. (1976) Pancreatic carcinoma as a sequel to therapy of lymphoma. *J. surg. Oncol., 8,* 461-464

Johnston, T.P., McCaleb, G.S. & Montgomery, J.A. (1963) The synthesis of antineoplastic agents. XXXII. *N*-Nitrosoureas. I. *J. med. Chem., 6,* 669-681

Kohn, K.W. (1977) Interstrand cross-linking of DNA by 1,3-bis(2-chloroethyl)-1-nitrosourea and other 1-(2-haloethyl)-1-nitrosoureas. *Cancer Res., 37,* 1450-1454

Kortselius, M.J.H. (1978) Mutagenicity of BCNU and related chloroethylnitrosoureas in *Drosophila. Mutat. Res., 57,* 297-305

Lennan, R.M. & Taylor, H.R. (1978) Optic neuroretinitis in association with BCNU and procarbazine therapy. *Med. pediatr. Oncol., 4,* 43-48

Levin, V.A., Kabra, P.A. & Freedman-Dove, M.A. (1978a) Relationship of 1,3-bis(2-chloroethyl)-1-nitrosourea (BCNU) and 1-(2-chloroethyl)-3-cyclohexyl-1-nitrosourea (CCNU) pharmacokinetics of uptake, distribution, and tissue/plasma partitioning in rat organs and intracerebral tumors. *Cancer Chemother. Pharmacol., 1,* 233-242

Levin, V.A., Hoffman, W. & Weinkam, R.J. (1978b) Pharmacokinetics of BCNU in man: a preliminary study of 20 patients. *Cancer Treat. Rep., 62,* 1305-1312

Loo, T.L., Dion, R.L., Dixon, R.L. & Rall, D.P. (1966) The antitumor agent, 1,3-bis(2-chloroethyl)-1-nitrosourea. *J. pharm. Sci., 55,* 492-497

Ludlum, D.B., Kramer, B.S., Wang, J. & Fenselan, C. (1975) Reaction of 1,3-bis(2-chloroethyl)-1-nitrosourea with synthetic polynucleotides. *Biochemistry (NY), 14,* 5480-5485

Matheson, D., Brusick, D. & Carrano, R. (1978) Comparison of the relative mutagenic activity for eight antineoplastic drugs in the Ames *Salmonella*/microsome and TK$^{+/-}$ mouse lymphoma assays. *Drug chem. Toxicol., 1,* 277-304

McConnell, W.R., Kari, P. & Hill, D.L. (1979) Reduction of glutathione levels in livers of mice treated with *N,N'*-bis(2-chloroethyl)-*N*-nitrosourea. *Cancer Chemother. Pharmacol., 2,* 221-223

Melato, M. & Tuveri, G. (1980) Pulmonary fibrosis following low-dose 1,3-bis(2-chloroethyl)-1-nitrosourea (BCNU) therapy. *Cancer, 45,* 1311-1314

Mills, R.C., Cornwell, G.G., III & McIntyre, O.R. (1971) Remission of leukemia associated with multiple myeloma. *New Engl. J. Med., 285,* 920-921

Oliverio, V.T. (1973) Toxicology and pharmacology of the nitrosoureas. *Cancer Chemother. Rep., Part 3, 4,* 13-20

Oliverio, V.T. (1976) Pharmacology of the nitrosoureas: an overview. *Cancer Treat. Rep., 60,* 703-707

Pajak, T.F., Nissen, N.I., Stutzman, L., Hoogstraten, B., Cooper, M.R., Glowienka, L.P., Glidewell, O. & Glicksman, A. (1979) Acute myeloid leukemia (AML) occurring during complete remission (CR) in Hodgkin's disease (Abstract no. C-425). *Proc. Am. Soc. clin. Oncol., 20,* 394

Penn, I. (1976) Second malignant neoplasms associated with immunosuppressive medications. *Cancer, 37,* 1024-1032

Pittillo, R.F., Narkates, A.J. & Burns, J. (1964) Microbiological evaluation of 1,3-bis(2-chloroethyl)-1-nitrosourea. *Cancer Res., 24,* 1222-1228

Preisler, H.D. & Lyman, G.H. (1977) Acute myelogenous leukemia subsequent to therapy for a different neoplasm: clinical features and responses to therapy. *Am. J. Hematol., 3,* 209-218

Ramirez, G., Wilson, W., Grage, T. & Hill, G. (1972) Phase II evaluation of 1,3-bis(2-chloroethyl)-1-nitrosourea (BCNU; NSC-409962) in patients with solid tumors. *Cancer Chemother. Rep., 56,* 787-790

Reed, D.J., May, H.E., Boose, R.B., Gregory, K.M. & Beilstein, M.A. (1975) 2-Chloroethanol formation as evidence for a 2-chloroethyl alkylating intermediate during chemical degradation of 1-(2-chloroethyl)-3-cyclohexyl-1-nitrosourea and 1-(2-chloroethyl)-3-(*trans*-4-methylcyclohexyl)-1-nitrosourea. *Cancer Res., 35,* 568-576

Rosner, F. & Grünwald, H. (1974) Multiple myeloma terminating in acute leukemia. Report of 12 cases and review of the literature. *Am. J. Med., 57,* 927-939

Schein, P.S., Heal, J., Green, D. & Woolley, P.V. (1978) Pharmacology of nitrosourea antitumor agents. *Fundam. Cancer Chemother. Antibiot. Chemother., 23,* 64-75

Schmähl, D. & Habs, M. (1978) Experimental carcinogenesis of antitumour drugs. *Cancer Treat. Rev., 5,* 175-184

Selker, R.G., Jacobs, S.A. & Moore, P. (1978) Interstitial pulmonary fibrosis as a complication of 1,3-bis(2-chloroethyl)-1-nitrosourea (BCNU) therapy (Abstract no. C-107). *Proc. Am. Soc. clin. Oncol., 19,* 333

Sidwell, R.W., Dixon, G.J., Sellers, S.M. & Schabel, F.M., Jr (1965) *In vivo* antiviral activity of 1,3-bis(2-chloroethyl)-1-nitrosourea. *Appl. Microbiol. 13,* 579-589

Sipka, S., Laki, K. & Csák, É. (1979) Inhibition of transglutaminase *in vivo* and *in vitro* by BCNU (Abstract). *Acta physiol. acad. sci. hung., 53,* 210

Takvorian, T., Parker, L.M., Hochberg, F.H., Zervas, N.P., Frei, E. & Canellos, G.P. (1980) Single high doses of BCNU with autologous bone marrow (ABM): a phase I study (Abstract no. C-88). *Proc. Am. Soc. clin. Oncol., 21,* 341

Tates, A.D., Natarajan, A.T., De Vogel, N. & Meijers, M. (1977) A correlative study on the genetic damage induced by chemical mutagens in bone marrow and spermatogonia of mice. III. 1,3-Bis-(2-chloroethyl)-3-nitrosourea (BCNU). *Mutat. Res., 44,* 87-95

Thompson, G.R. & Larson, R.E. (1969) The hepatotoxicity of 1,3-bis(2-chloroethyl)-1-nitrosourea (BCNU) in rats. *J. Pharmacol. exp. Ther., 166,* 104-112

Thompson, G.R. & Larson, R.E. (1972) A toxicologic comparison of the potency and activity of 1,3-bis(2-chloroethyl)-1-nitrosourea (BCNU) and 1-(2-chloroethyl)-3-cyclohexyl-1-nitrosourea (CCNU) in mice and rats. *Toxicol. appl. Pharmacol., 21,* 405-413

Thompson, D.J., Molello, J.A., Strebing, R.J., Dyke, I.L. & Robinson, V.B. (1974) Reproduction and teratology studies with oncolytic agents in the rat and rabbit. I. 1,3-Bis(2-chloroethyl)-1-nitrosourea (BCNU). *Toxicol. appl. Pharmacol., 30,* 422-439

Vogl, S.E. (1978) Acute leukemia complicating treatment of glioblastoma multiforme. *Cancer, 41,* 333-336

Wade, A., ed. (1977) *Martindale, The Extra Pharmacopoeia,* 27th ed., London, The Pharmaceutical Press, pp. 130-131

Wasserman, T.H. (1976) The nitrosoureas: an outline of clinical schedules and toxic effects. *Cancer Treat. Rep., 60,* 709-711

Weinkam, R.J., Wen, J.H.C., Furst, D.E. & Levin, V.A. (1978) Analysis for 1,3-bis(2-chloroethyl)-1-nitrosourea by chemical ionization mass spectrometry. *Clin. Chem., 24,* 45-49

Weisburger, E.K. (1977) Bioassay program for carcinogenic hazards of cancer chemotherapeutic agents. *Cancer, 40,* 1935-1951

Weiss, E. de C., Cravioto, H., Weiss, J.F. & Ransohoff, J. (1973) Pathologic effects in rats surviving prenatal and neonatal administration of 1,3-bis(2-chloroethyl)-1-nitrosourea. *J. natl Cancer Inst., 51,* 1363-1366

Windholz, M., ed. (1976) *The Merck Index,* 9th ed., Rahway, NJ, Merck & Co., p. 235

Young, R.C., DeVita, V.T., Jr, Serpick, A.A. & Canellos, G.P. (1971) Treatment of advanced Hodgkin's disease with [1,3-bis(2-chloroethyl)-1-nitrosourea] BCNU. *New Engl. J. Med., 285,* 475-479

Zarrabi, M.H., Rosner, F. & Bennett, J.M. (1979) Non-Hodgkin's lymphoma and acute myeloblastic leukemia. A report of 12 cases and review of the literature. *Cancer, 44,* 1070-1080

Zimmer, D.M. & Bhuyan, B.K. (1976) Mutagenicity of streptozotocin and several other nitrosourea compounds in *Salmonella typhimurium. Mutat. Res., 40,* 281-288

BLEOMYCINS
(sulphates and hydrochlorides)

1. CHEMICAL AND PHYSICAL DATA

BLEOMYCIN[1]

1.1 Synonyms and trade names

Chem. Abstr. Services Reg. No.: 11056-06-7

Chem. Abstr. Name and IUPAC Systematic Name: Bleomycin

Trade names: Bleo; Bleomycins; NSC-125066

1.2 Structural and molecular formulae[2] and molecular weights

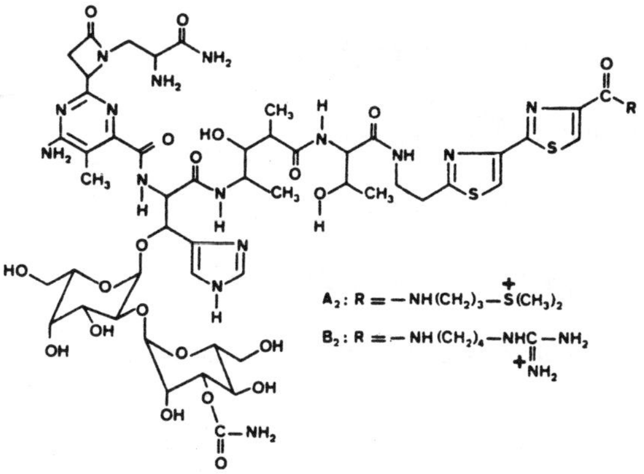

A$_2$: R = —NH(CH$_2$)$_3$—S$^+$(CH$_3$)$_2$
B$_2$: R = —NH(CH$_2$)$_4$—NHC(=$^+$NH$_2$)—NH$_2$

(From Crooke & Bradner, 1976)

$A_2 = C_{55}H_{84}N_{17}O_{21}S_3$ Mol. wts: A_2 = 1415.6

$B_2 = C_{55}H_{84}N_{20}O_{21}S_2$ B_2 = 1425.5

---

[1] 'Bleomycin' is the generic name for a mixture of antineoplastic antibiotics including bleomycins A_2 and B_2.

[2] Two recent articles (Burger *et al.*, 1981; Tsukayama *et al.*, 1981) have proposed a slightly different structural formula, in which the lactam ring in the upper left-hand corner is replaced by an amide group.

Thus, becomes

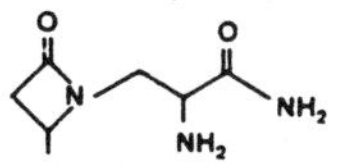

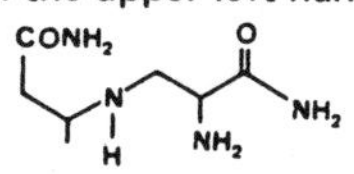

1.3 Chemical and physical properties of the pure substances

(a) *Description:* Colourless or yellowish powder (Windholz, 1976)

(b) *Optical rotation:* $[\alpha]_D^{20} = +12.5°$ to $+16°$ (0.5% solution in water) (Rosenbaum & Carter, 1970)

(c) *Spectroscopy data:* λ_{max} 244-248 nm, $A_1^1 = 121\text{-}148$; 289-294 nm, $A_1^1 = 102\text{-}121.5$. Infra-red spectra have been tabulated (Rosenbaum & Carter, 1970).

(d) *Solubility:* Very soluble in water and methanol; slightly soluble in ethanol; practically insoluble in acetone, ethyl acetate, butyl acetate and diethyl ether (Windholz, 1976)

BLEOMYCIN SULPHATES

1.1 Synonyms and trade names

Chem. Abstr. Services Reg. No: 9041-93-4

Chem. Abstr. Name: Bleomycin, sulfate (salt)

IUPAC Systematic Name: Bleomycin sulfate

Trade names: Blenoxane; Bleocin; Bléomycine; Blexane

1.2 Structural and molecular formulae and molecular weights

$\cdot \, H_2SO_4$

$A_2: R = -NH(CH_2)_3 - \overset{+}{S}(CH_3)_2$

$B_2: R = -NH(CH_2)_4 - NH\overset{\|}{C} - NH_2$
$\qquad\qquad\qquad\qquad \overset{+}{N}H_2$

$A_2 = C_{55}H_{84}N_{17}O_{21}S_3 \cdot H_2SO_4$

$B_2 = C_{55}H_{84}N_{20}O_{21}S_2 \cdot H_2SO_4$

Mol. wts: $A_2 = 1513.6$

$B_2 = 1523.6$

1.3 Chemical and physical properties of the pure substances

From Wade (1977), unless otherwise specified

(a) *Description:* Yellowish-white powder

(b) *Solubility:* Very soluble in water

(c) *Stability:* Sterile powder is stable for 18 months (Baker, 1980).

BLEOMYCIN HYDROCHLORIDES

1.1 Synonyms and trade names

Chem. Abstr. Services Reg. No: 67763-87-5

Chem. Abstr. Name: Bleomycin, hydrochloride

IUPAC Systematic Name: Bleomycin hydrochloride

1.2 Structural and molecular formulae and molecular weight

$$A_2 = C_{55}H_{84}N_{17}O_{21}S_3 \cdot HCl$$
$$B_2 = C_{55}H_{84}N_{20}O_{21}S_2 \cdot HCl$$

Mol. wts: A_2 = 1452

B_2 = 1461

1.3 Chemical and physical properties of the pure substance

No data were available to the Working Group.

1.4 Technical products and impurities

Bleomycins are a group of related glycopeptides isolated from *Streptomyces verticillus* (Windholz, 1976). Most of the bleomycin used clinically is a mixture of bleomycin A_2 and B_2 with other fractions (e.g., B_4) present in small amounts (Sakai, 1978). Various national and international pharmacopoeias give specifications for the purity of bleomycin in pharmaceutical products. For example, bleomycin is available in the US as USP grade bleomycin sulphate measured as containing 90.0 - 120.0% of the labelled amount of bleomycin. Bleomycin sulphate has a potency of 1.5 - 2.0 bleomycin units per mg and contains 60 - 70% bleomycin A_2, 25 - 32% bleomycin B_2 and not more than 1% bleomycin B_4; not less than 90% of the total bleomycin content is bleomycin A_2 and B_2 (US Pharmacopeial Convention, Inc., 1980). Under US Food & Drug Administration (1978) regulations, bleomycin sulphate must meet the following requirements: be sterile and nonpyrogenic; pass a 'safety test'; contain no histamine or histamine-like substances; lose 6% max. on drying; produce an aqueous solution (10 units per ml) with pH 4.5 - 6.0; contain 0.1% max. copper; contain the various bleomycins as specified above; and pass an identity test. Bleomycin sulphate is also available as an injection containing 15 units per ampoule (Baker, 1980).

In the UK, bleomycin is available as bleomycin sulphate in injection ampoules containing the equivalent of 15 mg bleomycin (Wade, 1977).

In Japan, bleomycin is available as bleomycin hydrochloride injections and as an ointment containing 5 mg/g bleomycin hydrochloride.

2. PRODUCTION, USE, OCCURRENCE AND ANALYSIS

2.1 Production and use

(a) Production

Bleomycin was first isolated from substrains of *Streptomyces verticillus* in 1965 (Umezawa, 1966). It is produced from strain B80-Z2 when shake-cultured in a medium containing glucose, starch, soya bean meal, potassium phosphate, zinc sulphate and copper sulphate and subsequently fermented. Bleomycin is extracted from the aqueous portion of the cultured broth by adsorption on activated carbon or by using cation exchange resins (Umezawa *et al.*, 1966). Although *The US Pharmacopeia* indicates that synthetic bleomycin would meet its specifications, no evidence was found that bleomycin is produced commercially by chemical synthesis.

It has not been produced commercially in the US. Bleomycin sulphate is supplied by one company; however, the country where it is manufactured was not known, and no data were available on the quantities produced. No information was available on its production in Europe, although it is believed to be produced in Denmark.

In Japan, bleomycin hydrochloride was first produced commercially in 1969. In 1978, one Japanese company produced 4 kg bleomycin hydrochloride; there were no imports.

(b) Use

Bleomycin (as the sulphate or hydrochloride) is used in human medicine as an anti-neoplastic agent, either alone or in combination with other agents, in the treatment of squamous-cell carcinoma, Hodgkin's disease, non-Hodgkin's lymphoma and malignant neoplasms of the testis (Wade, 1977).

It is administered by subcutaneous, intramuscular, intravenous and intra-arterial injection. (In some countries the amount of bleomycin is expressed as units, which are equal to the previously used milligram of activity.) The usual dose is 15 - 60 mg (units)/m^2 body-surface area weekly in divided doses, or 10 - 20 mg (units)/m^2 body-surface area once or twice weekly to a total dose of 300 mg (units) (Wade, 1977). For some indications, and because of its short half-life in the body (mean value, 115 minutes) (Prestayko & Crooke, 1978), bleomycin is given as a continuous infusion over a 5 - 7 - day period for a total dose of 40 mg (units) per day or approximately 300 mg (units) per course. In Hodgkin's disease, a maintenance dose of 1 mg (unit) daily or 5 mg (units) weekly is given intramuscularly or intravenously. Because of toxicity, the total dose received by a patient is usually limited to 400 mg (units).

2.2 Occurrence

Bleomycin is produced only by *Streptomyces verticillus* (Pietsch, 1975).

2.3 Analysis

Typical methods for the analysis of bleomycin in formulations are summarized in Table 1.

Table 1. Methods for the analysis of bleomycin

Sample matrix	Sample preparation	Assay procedure[a]	Sensitivity or limit of detection	Reference
Formulations	Dissolve in distilled water; filter; add to heptane-sulphonic acid in aqueous methanol	HPLC-UV	10 pmol	Sakai (1978)
	Add to solution of ammonium formate in methanol	HPLC-UV	not given	Williams (1977)
Plasma, urine	Incubate with borate buffer, antiserum and [^{125}I] bleomycin	RIA	8 ng/l	Teale *et al.* (1977)
Serum, urine	Incubate with phosphate buffer, antiserum and [^{57}Co] bleomycin	RIA	25 μg/l	Elson *et al.* (1977, 1978)
Blood, urine, tissue	Place sample on agar plate containing *Bacillus subtilis*; incubate	MA	1 mg/l	Ohnuma *et al.* (1974)

[a]Abbreviations: HPLC-UV, high-performance liquid chromatography with ultra-violet spectrometry; RIA, radioimmunoassay; MA, microbiological assay

3. BIOLOGICAL DATA RELEVANT TO THE EVALUATION
OF CARCINOGENIC RISK TO HUMANS

3.1 Carcinogenicity studies in animals

Two studies were reviewed, one in mice treated by s.c. or i.m. injection (Pomeroy, 1979) and the other in rats given bleomycin transplacentally (Llombart, 1976). [Neither of the experiments could be evaluated because of incomplete reporting.]

3.2 Other relevant biological data

(a) Experimental systems

The pharmacokinetics, pharmacology, toxicology and mechanisms of action of bleomycin have been reviewed (Crooke & Bradner, 1976).

Toxic effects

In mice, the lethal single i.p. dose of bleomycin A (potency, 752 μg/mg) was approximately 200 mg/kg bw (Ichikawa *et al.*, 1967). In rabbits, the i.v. LD_{50} of bleomycin A complex (potency, 337 μg/mg) was 150-200 mg/kg bw. A single injection of 50 mg/kg bw to dogs was lethal after 12-14 days (Ishizuka *et al.*, 1967).

The i.p. LD_{50} for young mice was 15 mg/kg bw daily for 14 days; in older mice bleomycin was somewhat more toxic. The main signs of toxicity were bad hair condition, nail deformations and salivation (Ichikawa *et al.*, 1967).

I.p. administration to mice of 0.1 - 0.5 mg bleomycin twice weekly for 8 weeks was lethal to 50% of animals. It also produced pulmonary fibrosis after 4 weeks. The earliest changes, observed 2 weeks after the start of injections, involved the endothelium of pulmonary arteries and veins. Capillary endothelial blebbing and interstitial oedema were observed after 4 weeks, when multifocal necrosis of type 1 alveolar epithelial cells was accompanied by fibrinous exudation into the alveoli. The process of repair was characterized by proliferation and metaplasia of type 2 epithelial cells, fibroblastic organization of alveolar fibrin and fibrosis of the interstitium within 8 - 12 weeks (Adamson & Bowden, 1974).

The main signs of toxicity in dogs were loss of appetite, increased serum glutamic-oxaloacetic transaminase and glutamic-pyruvic transaminase levels, jaundice and leuco-cytosis. I.v. injection to dogs of 5 - 10 mg/kg bw every 4 days did not impair liver or kidney function or lead to weight loss (Ishizuka *et al.*, 1967).

Dogs that received 0.625 - 5 mg/kg bw bleomycin intravenously every fourth day for 11 treatments or 0.625 mg/kg bw for 31 treatments, and monkeys that received 1 - 8 mg/kg bw bleomycin intravenously every fourth day for 11 treatments, developed pyrexia, footpad ulceration, dermatitis, alopecia and pulmonary lesions. Macroscopic pulmonary changes were seen in all animals killed 70 or more days after the onset of treatment. All dogs also showed microscopic evidence of a focal and confluent inter-stitial pneumonia and interstitial fibrosis with marked hyperplasia of type II pneumo-cytes. In dogs, skin ulceration occurred only on footpads and tail tips; while in monkeys the neck, elbows, cubital fossae and palmar and plantar surfaces of the hands and feet were affected. Microscopic changes at pressure and friction sites included ulceration, focal necrosis, subacute inflammation, haemorrhage, oedema and occasional foreign body granulomas. Atrophy of sweat glands and of the pilosebaceous apparatus was also observed. Depression of serum zinc concentrations correlated with the onset of skin lesions and suggested that zinc deficiency played a role in the pathogenesis of the lesions (Fleischman et al., 1971; Baker *et al.*, 1973).

Bleomycin selectively inhibits incorporation of thymidine into DNA of mammalian cells (Umezawa *et al.*, 1967) and causes DNA fragmentation at doses as low as 0.1-1.0 µg/ml (Terasima *et al.*, 1970). It also causes single strand scission of DNA and poly-nucleotides (Umezawa, 1974).

Effects on reproduction and prenatal toxicity

No data were available to the Working Group.

Absorption, distribution, excretion and metabolism

The plasma concentration of bleomycin in rabbits, as measured in a *Bacillus subtilis* assay, was found to decrease in a biphasic manner after i.m. injection of 15 mg/kg bw. The half-life of the first phase was approximately one hour and that of the second phase 10 hours; 40-70% of the dose was excreted within 20 hours. One hour after injection, the highest concentration of drug was found in kidney and serum; smaller amounts were found in spleen, skin, lymph nodes and lung. No drug was detected in liver, stomach or brain at any time after injection. In dogs injected into the submucosa of the cheek, 60% of the drug was excreted in the urine within 6 hours (Abe *et al.*, 1976).

After i.v. or s.c. injection of [57]Co-bleomycin to mice, more than 70% of the radio-active dose was eliminated from the body within 3 hours and more than 90% within 12 hours. No difference was detected between tumour-bearing mice and controls. Three hours after i.v. or intratumoral injection, 60% of the injected dose was found in the kid-neys, 30% in the lymph nodes and less than 20% in the other major organs (Bier *et al.*, 1979). In another study, no major difference was found in the [57]Co-bleomycin distri-bution between liver and kidney when doses of 0.3-30 mg/kg bw were given intra-venously, but the concentrations in skin and brain were at least one order of magnitude lower (Robert *et al.*, 1973).

In rats given 1 mg/kg bw bleomycin intraperitoneally, a peak serum level of 0.7 µg/ml was reached in 54 minutes, as measured by radioimmunoassay; bleomycin was eliminated with a half-life of 32 minutes. No change in half-life was observed when rats were pretreated with phenobarbital. I.p. administration of 0.2 g/kg bw Probenecid, a drug which affects the renal handling of a number of organic compounds that are actively transported by the renal tubules, 20 minutes prior to bleomycin administration increased the half-life two-fold. Investigation of the tissue distribution of [57]Co-bleomycin 2 hours after i.p. administration of 1 mg/kg bw revealed about 10-fold higher concentrations in the kidneys when compared with liver, lung and spleen, and even lower concentrations in heart and thymus. Similar results were obtained with unlabelled bleomycin, detected by radioimmunoassay (Tom & Montgomery, 1979). The [57]Co label has been shown to remain essentially bound to the drug and to be excreted in that form (Rapin *et al.*, 1973).

In rabbits, liver, spleen and digestive organs were very effective in deactivating bleomycin, as measured by the *B. subtilis* bioassay. Toxic effects of bleomycin occur predominantly in organs such as skin and lung where inactivation is weak (Fujita, 1971). The selective effect of bleomycin on squamous-cell carcinoma is thought to be due to the low concentration of inactivating enzyme in the tumour. Inactivation results from cleavage of the amide from the β-aminoalanine moiety of bleomycin (Umezawa, 1974).

Mutagenicity and other short-term tests

The genetic toxicology of bleomycin has been reviewed by Vig & Lewis (1978).

Bleomycin was not mutagenic in *Salmonella typhimurium* tester strains TA1535, TA1537, TA98 and TA100 when tested in the presence or absence of a rat liver metabolic activation system (Benedict *et al.*, 1977a). However, it was both mutagenic and induced mitotic recombination in *Saccharomyces cerevisiae* (Moore, 1978) and induced recessive sex-linked lethal mutations in *Drosophila melanogaster* (Traut, 1980).

Concentration-dependent increases in chromosomal aberrations have been reported following bleomycin treatment in various mammalian cells in culture, including a human cervical carcinoma line (HeLa), human lymphoblasts (CCRF-CEM), mouse fibroblasts (Paika & Krishan, 1973) and human lymphocytes (Ohama & Kadotani, 1970; Promchainant, 1975; Dresp *et al.*, 1978). The drug also produced increases in sister chromatid exchanges and chromosomal aberrations in Chinese hamster fibroblasts (Perry & Evans, 1975), in a transformed Syrian hamster cell line (Benedict *et al.*, 1977b; Banerjee & Benedict, 1979) and in normal and abnormal human lymphoid cell lines (Shiraishi & Sandberg, 1979).

Bleomycin also produced a dose-dependent increase in morphological transformation in the mouse C3H/10T½ clone 8 cell line at concentrations achieved in human plasma (Benedict *et al.*, 1977b). Such transformed cells have been shown to produce malignant tumours when injected into immunosuppressed syngeneic mice (Reznikoff *et al.*, 1973; Jones *et al.*, 1976).

(b) Humans

Toxic effects

The principal toxicity of bleomycin is diffuse interstitial pneumonitis. In a review summarizing the results from several studies, the incidence of pulmonary toxicity was found to be about 11% (fatal in 1%) (Comis, 1978). A dose relationship has been observed, except in young children and elderly patients in whom toxicity can occur after a single dose. The recommended total dose is 330 - 400 mg, unless other risk factors prevail: these include previous X-irradiation to the chest area, pre-existing lung disease (e.g., chronic bronchitis, emphysema, interstitial pneumonitis) and exposure to hyperbaric oxygen (Goldiner et al., 1977; Comis, 1978).

Mucocutaneous toxicity is the other important toxic effect of bleomycin. This effect takes the form of pigmentation, striae, blistering, inflammation of mucous membranes and hyperkeratosis and alopecia. It is reversible, and only the inflammatory response may limit the therapeutic dose which can be given (Blum et al., 1973; Cvitkovic et al., 1974).

Rarely, cardiorespiratory failure has been noted, distinct from anaphylaxis. This response was first reported in lymphoma patients (Blum et al., 1973), but was noted recently (as reported in an abstract) in 6/35 terminal patients with a variety of malignancies given intracavitary bleomycin as a treatment for pleural or peritoneal effusion (Stuart et al., 1980).

Further toxicities of bleomycin consist of abdominal pain, fever, occasional shivering, headache, nausea and vomiting (Blum et al., 1973).

Effects on reproduction and prenatal toxicity

No relevant data were available to the Working Group.

Absorption, distribution, excretion and metabolism

Bleomycin has been measured in plasma and urine by radioimmunoassay, although it was not clear which bleomycin was used as the antigen. Systemic absorption of bleomycin was reported to be 40% or 80% of the dose, following intrapleural or intraperitoneal administration, respectively (Alberts et al., 1978). The pharmacokinetics of large, single i.m. or i.v. injections are almost identical. Bleomycin has a short half-life: mean value, 115 minutes. As it is excreted in urine (50% in 4 hours and > 70% by 24 hours), in patients with a creatinine clearance of less than 25-35 ml/min it has an exponentially rising half-life. Renal clearance is probably not the only route of elimination of bleomycin, and it may be partly metabolized (Prestayko & Crooke, 1978).

Mutagenicity and chromosomal effects

A significant increase in the number of chromosomal aberrations was observed in bone-marrow cells (Bornstein et al., 1971) and in peripheral lymphocytes of patients treated with bleomycin only (total cumulative i.v. doses ranging from 30-80 mg per patient) (Dresp et al., 1978).

3.3 Case reports and epidemiological studies of carcinogenicity in humans

No case report or epidemiological study of cancer occurring in patients treated with bleomycin alone was available to the Working Group.

Fifteen patients with malignant lymphoma (10 with Hodgkin's disease and 5 with non-Hodgkin's lymphoma) developed second malignant neoplasms following treatment with chemotherapy regimens containing bleomycin. Acute non-lymphocytic leukaemia developed in 10 of these patients (Bonadonna et al., 1973; Sahakian et al., 1974; Canellos, 1975; Rosner & Grünwald, 1975; Cavalli et al., 1977; Zarrabi et al., 1979; Valagussa et al., 1980), a preleukaemic syndrome in 1 (Collins et al., 1977), and cutaneous malignant melanoma in the remaining patient (Bonadonna et al., 1973). All 15 received bleomycin in combination with multiple other cytotoxic agents, and 12 also received radiation therapy.

In a retrospective cohort study of 764 patients with Hodgkin's disease given several different combinations of chemotherapy and radiation (Valagussa et al., 1980), 55 patients were followed for a median of 45 months after receiving a regimen consisting of bleomycin, dacarbazine, adriamycin and vinblastine sulphate. No second malignancies were observed in this subgroup.

4. SUMMARY OF DATA REPORTED AND EVALUATION

4.1 Experimental data

No adequate study on the carcinogenicity of bleomycins in experimental animals was available to the Working Group.

No data were available to evaluate the teratogenic potential of bleomycin in animals. It is mutagenic in yeast and in *Drosophila melangaster*. It induces chromosomal changes and increases in sister chromatid exchanges in various mammalian cells in culture. The drug also induced neoplastic transformation in a mouse cell line.

4.2 Human data

Bleomycin sulphate or hydrochloride has been used since the early 1970s, mainly in the treatment of Hodgkin's and non-Hodgkin's lymphoma, squamous-cell carcinoma at various sites and testicular malignancies.

No data were available to evaluate the teratogenic potential of bleomycin in humans. Chromosomal changes were seen in bone-marrow cells and peripheral lymphocytes of patients treated with bleomycin alone. No data were available to evaluate its mutagenic potential in humans.

The development of acute nonlymphocytic leukaemia following the administration of bleomycin with multiple other cytotoxic agents has been described in patients with Hodgkin's disease or non-Hodgkin's lymphoma. In a small epidemiological study of short duration, no excess of subsequent neoplasms was observed in patients treated with a regimen consisting of bleomycin, adriamycin, vinblastine and dacarbazine.

4.3 Evaluation

The available data from studies in experimental animals and in humans were inadequate to evaluate the carcinogenicity of bleomycins to man.

5. REFERENCES

Abe, F., Tsubosaki, M., Tanaka, T., Kato, Y., Yoshioka, O. & Matsuda, A. (1976) Studies on absorption, excretion and organ distribution of bleomycin oil suspension (Jpn.). *Jpn. J. Antiobiot., 29,* 826-833

Adamson, I.Y.R. & Bowden, D.H. (1974) The pathogenesis of bleomycin-induced pulmonary fibrosis in mice. *J. Pathol., 77,* 185-197

Alberts, D., Chen, H.-S., Liu, R., Chen, J., Mayersohn, M., Perrier, D., Moon, T., Gross,J., Broughton, A. & Salmon, S. (1978) Systemic absorption of bleomycin (BLEO) after intracavitary (IC) administration (Abstract. no. 305). *Proc. Am. Assoc. Cancer Res., 19,* 77

Baker, C.E., Jr, ed. (1980) *Physicians' Desk Reference,* 34th ed., Oradell, NJ, Medical Economics Co., pp. 706-707

Baker, J.R., Fleischman, R.W., Thompson, G.R., Schaeppi, U., Ilievski, V., Cooney, D.A. & Davis, R.D. (1973) Pathological effects of bleomycin on the skin of dogs and monkeys. *Toxicol. appl. Pharmacol., 25,,* 190-200

Banerjee, A. & Benedict, W.F. (1979) Production of sister chromatid exchanges by various cancer chemotherapeutic agents. *Cancer Res., 39,* 797-799

Benedict, W.F., Baker, M.S., Haroun, L., Choi, E. & Ames, B.N. (1977a) Mutagenicity of cancer chemotherapeutic agents in the *Salmonella*/microsome test. *Cancer Res., 37,* 2209-2213

Benedict, W.F., Banerjee, A., Gardner, A. & Jones, P.A. (1977b) Induction of morphological transformation in mouse C3H/10T½ clone 8 cells and chromosomal damage in hamster A(T$_1$)Cl-3 cells by cancer chemotherapeutic agents. *Cancer Res., 37,* 2202-2208

Bier, J., Benders, P., Wenzel, M. & Bitter, K. (1979) Kinetics of [57]Co-bleomycin in mice after intravenous, subcutaneous and intratumoral injection. *Cancer, 44,* 1194-1200

Blum, R.H., Carter, S.K. & Agre, K. (1973) A clinical review of bleomycin - a new antineoplastic agent. *Cancer, 31,* 903-914

Bonadonna, G., De Lena, M., Banfi, A. & Lattuada, A. (1973) Secondary neoplasms in malignant lymphomas after intensive therapy. *New Engl. J. Med., 288,* 1242-1243

Bornstein, R.S., Hungerford, D.A., Haller, G., Engstrom, P.F. & Yarbro, J.W. (1971) Cytogenetic effects of bleomycin therapy in man. *Cancer Res., 31,* 2004-2007

Burger, R.M., Peisach, J. & Horwitz, S.B. (1981) Mechanism of bleomycin action: *in vitro* studies. *Life Sci., 28,* 715-727

Canellos, G.P. (1975) Second malignancies complicating Hodgkin's disease in remission. *Lancet, i,* 1294

Cavalli, F., Gerber, A., Mosimann, W., Sonntag, R.W. & Tschopp, L. (1977) Acute myeloid leukaemia in the course of Hodgkin's disease (Ger.). *Dtsch. med. Wochenschr., 102,* 1019-1024

Collins, A.J., Bloomfield, C.D., Peterson, B.A. & McKenna, R.W. (1977) Acute nonlymphocytic leukemia in patients with nodular lymphoma. *Cancer, 40,* 1748-1754

Comis, R.L. (1978) *Bleomycin pulmonary toxicity.* In: Carter, S.K., Crooke, S.T. & Umezawa, H., eds, *Bleomycin. Current Status and New Developments,* New York, Academic Press, pp. 279-291

Crooke, S.T. & Bradner, W.T. (1976) Bleomycin, a review. *J. Med., 7,* 333-427

Cvitkovic, E., Currie, V., Ochoa, M., Pride, G. & Krakoff, I.H. (1974) Continuous intravenous infusion of bleomycin in squamous cancer (Abstract no. 780). *Proc. Am. Soc. clin. Oncol., 15,* 179

Dresp, J., Schmid, E. & Bauchinger, M. (1978) The cytogenetic effect of bleomycin on human peripheral lymphocytes *in vitro* and *in vivo. Mutat. Res., 56,* 341-353

Elson, M.K., Oken, M.M. & Shafer, R.B. (1977) A radioimmunoassay for bleomycin. *J. nucl. Med., 18,* 296-299

Elson, M.K., Oken, M.M., Shafer, R.B., Broughton, A., Strong, J., Braun, C.T. & Crooke, S.T. (1978) Comparison of two radioimmunoassays and a microbiologic assay for bleomycin. *Med. pediatr. Oncol., 5,* 213-218

Fleischman, R.W., Baker, J.R., Thompson, G.R., Schaeppi, U.H., Illievski, V.R., Cooney, D.A. & Davis, R.D. (1971) Bleomycin-induced interstitial pneumonia in dogs. *Thorax, 26,* 675-682

Fujita, H. (1971) Comparative studies on the blood level, tissue distribution, excretion and inactivation of anticancer drugs. *Jpn. J. clin. Oncol., 12,* 151-162

Goldiner, P.L., Howland, W.S. & Carlon, G.C. (1977) Severe oxygen toxicity in patients with bleomycin lung (Abstract no. 355). *Intensive Care Med., 3,* 190

Ichikawa, T., Matsuda, A., Miyamoto, K., Tsubosaki, M., Kaihara, T., Sakamoto, K. & Umezawa, H. (1967) Biological studies on bleomycin A. *J. Antibiot., Ser. A, 20,* 149-155

Ishizuka, M., Takayama, H., Takeuchi, T. & Umezawa, H. (1967) Activity and toxicity of bleomycin. *J. Antibiot., Ser. A, 20,* 15-24

Jones, P.A., Benedict, W.F., Baker, M.S., Mondal, S., Rapp, U. & Heidelberger, C. (1976) Oncogenic transformation of C3H/10T½ clone 8 mouse embryo cells by halogenated pyrimidine nucleosides. *Cancer Res., 36,* 101-107

Llombart, A. (1976) Tumoral drugs as possible blastogenic agents. The problem of anti-blastic medication. *Österr. Z. Onkol., 3,* 72-76

Moore, C.W. (1978) Bleomycin-induced mutation and recombination of *Saccharomyces cerevisiae*. *Mutat. Res., 58,* 41-49

Ohama, K. & Kadotani, T. (1970) Cytologic effects of bleomycin on cultured human leucocytes. *Jpn. J. Hum. Genet., 14,* 293-297

Ohnuma, T., Holland, J.F., Masuda, H., Waligunda, J.A. & Goldberg, G.A. (1974) Microbiological assay of bleomycin: inactivation, tissue distribution, and clearance. *Cancer, 33,* 1230-1238

Paika, K.D. & Krishan, A. (1973) Bleomycin-induced chromosomal aberrations in cultured mammalian cells. *Cancer Res., 33,* 961-965

Perry, P. & Evans, H.J. (1975) Cytological detection of mutagen-carcinogen exposure by sister chromatid exchange. *Nature, 258,* 121-125

Pietsch, P. (1975) *Phleomycin and bleomycin.* In: Sartorelli, A.C. & Johns, D.G., eds, *Antineoplastic and Immunosuppressive Agents,* Part II, New York, Springer, pp. 850-876

Pomeroy, T.C. (1979) Carcinogenesis effects of combined treatment: immunologic factors. *Front. Radiat. Ther. Oncol., 13,* 194-214

Prestayko, A.W. & Crooke, S.T. (1978) *Clinical pharmacology of bleomycin.* In: Carter, S.K., Crooke, S.T. & Umezawa, H., eds, *Bleomycins. Current Status and New Developments,* New York, Academic Press, pp. 117-130

Promchainant, C. (1975) Cytogenetic effect of bleomycin on human leukocytes *in vitro. Mutat. Res., 28,* 107-112

Rapin, J., Renault, H., Robert, J., Rudler, M. & Nouel, J.-P. (1973) Metabolism of bleomycin labelled with a divalent cation. II.   Study of urinary metabolites in rats and a comparison of the tissue excretion of the cation alone or chelated with bleomycin (Fr.). *Thérapie, 28,* 941-949

Reznikoff, C.A., Bertram, J.S., Brankow, D.W. & Heidelberger, C. (1973) Quantitative and qualitative studies of chemical transformation of cloned C3H mouse embryo cells sensitive to postconfluence inhibition of cell division. *Cancer Res., 33,* 3239-3249

Robert, J., Renault, H., Rapin, J., Rudler, M. & Nouel, J.-P. (1973) Metabolism of bleomycin labelled with cobalt 57 in the mouse. I.   Distribution and kinetics (Fr.). *Thérapie, 28,* 933-940

Rosenbaum, C. & Carter, S.K. (1970)   *Bleomycin (NSC 125066, 'Bleo', BLM) Clinical Brochure, Chemotherapy,* Bethesda, MD, National Cancer Institute

Rosner, F. & Grünwald, H. (1975) Hodgkin's disease and acute leukemia.   Report of eight cases and review of the literature. *Am. J. Med., 58,* 339-353

Sakai, T.T. (1978) Paired-ion high-performance liquid chromatography of bleomycins. *J. Chromatogr., 161,* 389-392

Sahakian, G.J., Al-Mondhiry, H., Lacher, M.J. & Connolly, C.E. (1974) Acute leukemia in Hodgkin's disease. *Cancer, 33,* 1369-1375

Shiraishi, Y. & Sandberg, A.A. (1979) Effects of various chemical agents on sister chromatid exchanges, chromosome aberrations, and DNA repair in normal and abnormal human lymphoid cell lines. *J. natl Cancer Inst., 62,* 27-35

Stuart, J.F.B., Trotter, J.M., McVie, J.G. & Calman, K.C. (1980) Bleomycin drug monitoring in the management of malignant effusions. *Br. J. Cancer, 42,* 193

Teale, J.D., Clough, J.M. & Marks, V. (1977) Radioimmunoassay of bleomycin in plasma and urine. *Br. J. Cancer, 35,* 822-827

Terasima, T., Yasukawa, M. & Umezawa, H. (1970) Breaks and rejoining of DNA in cultured mammalian cells treated with bleomycin. *Gann, 61,* 513-516

Tom, W.-M. & Montgomery, M.R. (1979) Disposition of the pulmonary toxin, bleomycin. *Drug Metab. Disposition, 7,* 90-93

Traut, H. (1980) Mutagenic effects of bleomycin in *Drosophila melanogaster. Environ. Mutagenesis, 2,* 89-96

Tsukayama, M., Randall, C.R., Santillo, F.S. & Dabrowiak, J.C. (1981) Transition-metal binding site of bleomycin. Cobalt (III) bleomycin. *J. Am. chem. Soc., 103,* 458-461

Umezawa, H. (1966) *Bleomycin and other antitumor antibiotics of high molecular weight.* In: Hobby, G.L., ed., *Antimicrobial Agents and Chemotherapy - 1965,* Ann Arbor, MI, American Society for Microbiology, pp. 1079-1985

Umezawa, H. (1974) Chemistry and mechanism of action of bleomycin. *Fed. Proc., 33,* 2296-2302

Umezawa, H., Maeda, K., Takeuchi, T. & Okami, Y. (1966) New antibiotics, bleomycin A and B. *J. Antibiot., Ser. A, 29,* 200-209

Umezawa, H., Ishizuka, M., Maeda, K. & Takeuchi, T. (1967) Studies on bleomycin. *Cancer, 20,* 891-895

US Food & Drug Administration (1978) Food and drugs. *US Code Fed. Regul., Title 21,* part 450.10a, pp. 651-654

US Pharmacopeial Convention, Inc. (1980) *The US Pharmacopeia,* 20th rev., Rockville, MD, pp. 93-94

Valagussa, P., Santoro, A., Kenda, R., Fossati Bellani, F., Franchi, F., Banfi, A., Rilke, F. & Bonaddona, G. (1980) Second malignancies in Hodgkin's disease: a complication of certain forms of treatment. *Br. med. J., i,* 216-219

Vig, B.K. & Lewis, R. (1978) Genetic toxicology of bleomycin. *Mutat. Res., 55,* 121-145

Wade, A., ed. (1977) *Martindale, The Extra Pharmacopoeia,* 27th ed., London, The Pharmaceutical Press, pp. 127-129

Williams, C.R. (1977) High-performance liquid chromatography of bleomycins. *Proc. anal. Div. chem. Soc., 14,* 242-244

Windholz, M., ed. (1976) *The Merck Index,* 9th ed., Rahway, NJ, Merck & Co., p. 171

Zarrabi, M.H., Rosner, F. & Bennett, J.M. (1979) Non-Hodgkin's lymphoma and acute myeloblastic leukemia. A report of 12 cases and review of the literature. *Cancer, 44,* 1070-1080

This substance was considered by a previous Working Group, in April 1975 (IARC, 1975a). Since that time new data have become available, and these have been incorporated into the monograph and taken into consideration in the present evaluation.

1. CHEMICAL AND PHYSICAL DATA

1.1 Synonyms and trade names

Chem. Abstr. Services Reg. No.: 305-03-3

Chem. Abstr. Name: Benzenebutanoic acid, 4-[bis(2-chloroethyl)amino] -

IUPAC Systematic Name: 4- $\left\{ p\text{-}[\text{Bis(2-chloroethyl)amino] phenyl} \right\}$ butyric acid

Synonyms: 4-[*para*-Bis(2-chloroethyl)aminophenyl] butyric acid; 4-[*para*-bis(β-chloroethyl)aminophenyl] butyric acid; γ-[*para*-bis(2-chloroethyl)aminophenyl] - butyric acid; chlorbutinum; chloroambucil; γ-[*para*-di(2-chloroethyl)aminophenyl] - butyric acid; *para*-[di(2-chloroethyl)aminophenyl] butyric acid; *para*-(*N,N*-di-2-chloroethyl)aminophenyl butyric acid; *N,N*-di-2-chloroethyl-γ-*para*-aminophenyl-butyric acid; *para*-*N,N*-di(β-chloroethyl)aminophenylbutyric acid; phenylbutyric acid nitrogen mustard

Trade names: Ambochlorin; Amboclorin; CB 1348; Chloroaminophen; Chloramino-phène; Chlorbutin; Chlorobutin; Chlorobutine; Ecloril; Elcoril; Leukeran; Leukersan; Leukoran; Linfolizin; Linfolysin; Lympholysin; NSC-3088

1.2 Structural and molecular formulae and molecular weight

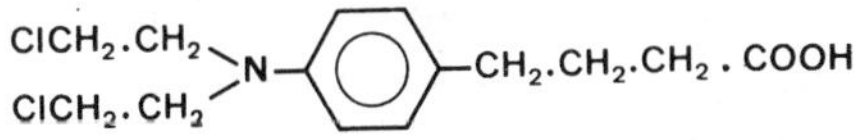

$C_{14}H_{19}Cl_2NO_2$

Mol. wt: 304.2

1.3   Chemical and physical properties of the pure substance

From Wade (1977) or Windholz (1976), unless otherwise specified

(a)   *Description:* A white crystalline powder with a slight odour

(b)   *Melting-point:* 64-66°C

(c)   *Spectroscopy data:* λ_{max} 258 nm, A_1^1 = 617 (in ethanol); 256 nm, A_1^1 = 517 (in water, pH ⩾ 7) (Linford, 1962)

(d)   *Solubility:* Very slightly soluble in water; soluble in ethanol (1 in 1.5), chloroform (1 in 2.5), acetone (1 in 2), diethyl ether and dilute solutions of alkali hydroxides

(e)   *Stability:* Sensitive to oxidation and moisture

1.4   Technical products and impurities

Various national and international pharmacopoeias give specifications for the purity of chlorambucil in pharmaceutical products. For example, chlorambucil is available in the US as a USP grade measured as containing 98.0 - 101.0% active ingredient on a dried basis, with 0.5% max. water content.   It is also available in tablets measured as containing 85.0 - 110.0% of the stated amount of chlorambucil (US Pharmacopeial Convention, Inc., 1980).

Chlorambucil is available in tablets containing 2 or 5 mg (Wade, 1977). No parenteral preparation is available.

2. PRODUCTION, USE, OCCURRENCE AND ANALYSIS

2.1   Production and use

(a)   *Production*

In the first reported method for preparing chlorambucil (Everett *et al.*, 1953), hydrogenation of the methyl or ethyl ester of 4-(*para*-nitrophenyl)butyric acid in the presence of a catalyst produced the *para*-amino analogue. Treatment of this with ethylene oxide [see IARC, 1976] followed by chlorination resulted in the 4-{*para*-[bis-2-(chloroethyl)-amino] phenyl}butyric acid ester, which was converted to the free acid by hydrolysis with hydrochloric acid.

Although chlorambucil has been formulated in the US since 1957, there are no US producers of the bulk chemical. US imports of chlorambucil through the principal US customs districts amounted to 48 kg in 1978 (US International Trade Commission, 1979).

The drug is believed to be produced by one company in Italy and one in the UK.

(b)   Use

Chlorambucil is used in human medicine as an antineoplastic agent, alone or in combination, for the treatment of Hodgkin's and non-Hodgkin's lymphomas, chronic lymphocytic leukaemia, Waldenström's macroglobulinaemia, Kaposi's disease and carcinomas, including those of the breast, lung, cervix, ovary and testis. It is also used as an immunosuppressive agent in the treatment of rheumatoid arthritis, systemic lupus erythematosus, acute and chronic glomerular nephritis, nephrotic syndrome, chronic active hepatitis, cold haemagglutinic disease, Wegener's granulomatosis and psoriasis (Harvey, 1975; Wade, 1977; Williams *et al.*, 1980).

Continuous and intermittent oral treatment schedules are employed. In the former, the daily dose is 0.1 - 0.2 mg/kg bw and is adjusted according to the response of the disease and bone marrow. In the latter case, it is common to give intermittent 2-week courses of 10 - 20 mg daily with rest periods of 2 - 4 weeks (McElwain *et al.*, 1977; Wade, 1977; Baker, 1980; Williams *et al.*, 1980).

2.2   Occurrence

Chlorambucil is not known to be produced in Nature.

2.3   Analysis

Typical methods for the analysis of chlorambucil in various matrices are summarized in Table 1.

Table 1. Methods for the analysis of chlorambucil

Sample matrix	Sample preparation	Assay procedure[a]	Limit of detection	Reference
Formulations	Dissolve in acetone; add water; titrate with sodium hydroxide	T	not given	US Pharmacopeial Convention, Inc. (1980)
Blood plasma	Centrifuge sample at 4°C; add ethyl acetate and mix well; freeze resulting emulsion and centrifuge at 4°C; remove and dry organic layer over anhydrous sodium sulphate; evaporate to dryness; redissolve residue in ethyl acetate	HPLC-UV	5 ng	Newell et al. (1979a)
	Dissolve in citric acid; add D_8-chlorambucil in acetone; add water; extract with chloroform:hexane (3:7); centrifuge; shake with phosphate and borate buffer solution; reextract; retain aqueous phase	GC-MS	8 ng/ml	Jakhammer et al. (1977)
Blood plasma and urine	Add D_8-chlorambucil and perchloric acid; extract with ethyl acetate:hexane (1:1); evaporate and derivatize with trimethylsilyl reagent	GC-MS	0.5 ng	Chang et al. (1980)

[a] Abbreviations: T, titrimetric analysis; HPLC-UV, high-performance liquid chromatography with ultra-violet detection; GC-MS, gas chromatography-mass spectrometry

3. BIOLOGICAL DATA RELEVANT TO THE EVALUATION OF CARCINOGENIC RISK TO HUMANS

3.1 Carcinogenicity studies in animals

(a)   Skin application

Mouse: A group of 25 S strain mice received 8 weekly skin applications of 0.1% chlorambucil in methanol and 2 of 0.05% (total dose, 2.7 mg). Thirty days after the start of the treatment the mice were painted with croton oil once weekly for 18 weeks. During the time that the treatments overlapped, chlorambucil and croton oil were applied alternately at 3-4 day intervals. Twenty control mice received 18 weekly applications of 0.17% croton oil. At the end of the treatment, 11/19 (58%) surviving mice had developed 30 skin papillomas (2.7 tumours/mouse), compared with 0/17 controls (P < 0.01). No malignant tumour developed in the 6 treated mice kept for longer periods (not specified) (Salaman & Roe, 1956). [The Working Group noted that no information was given on the time of appearance of the skin tumours.]

(b) Intraperitoneal administration

Mouse: Groups of 45-60 A/J mice of both sexes, 4-6 weeks old, received i.p. injections of chlorambucil in a 0.5% acacia solution or in a 0.1% tricaprylin solution 3 times a week for 4 weeks (total doses, 9.6, 37, 150 and 420/mg kg bw). At 39 weeks, the numbers of survivors were 38/45, 56/60, 47/60 and 30/60, and of these 18 (47%), 48 (86%), 45 (96%) and 30 (100%) had lung tumours (adenomas and adenocarcinomas), with 0.6, 1.6, 5.1 and 8.9 tumours per mouse, respectively. Of 173 male and 157 female controls that received the acacia vehicle only, 43% of male and 32% of female survivors developed lung tumours within 39 weeks, with 0.53 and 0.42 tumours per mouse; of 55 male and 53 females that received the tricaprylin only, 36% of male and 32% of female survivors developed lung tumours within 39 weeks, with 0.47 and 0.42 tumours per mouse (Shimkin *et al.*, 1966).

Two groups, each of 25 male and 25 female outbred Swiss-Webster-derived mice, 6 weeks of age, were given i.p. injections of 3 mg/kg bw (the maximally tolerated dose - MTD) or 1.5 mg/kg bw (0.5 MTD) chlorambucil 3 times weekly for 6 months. Animals that survived over 100 days were observed for up to 12 further months, at which time they were killed. The results reported had been combined for the two doses. Lung tumours occurred in 22/35 males and 20/28 females; tumours reported to be lymphosarcomas were found in 6/35 males and 4/28 females; and ovarian tumours were found in 10/28 females. These incidences were reported to be significantly different from those in controls: P < 0.001 for lung tumours in both males and females; P = 0.004 for lymphosarcomas in males and 0.012 in females; P < 0.001 for ovarian tumours in females. The spontaneous incidences of lung tumours were reported to be 10/101 in males and 21/153 in females; those of tumours of haematopoietic and lymphatic tissues, 3/101 in males and 3/153 in females; and that of ovarian tumours 6/153 in females (Weisburger *et al.*, 1975). [However, control animals were referred to as 'untreated' or 'treated with the vehicle only', and no precise indications were given as to the vehicle used or with which controls the treated animals were compared for tumour incidence. Therefore, the reported significance of the difference in tumour incidence between treated and control animals is difficult to evaluate. The Working Group considered that the inadequate reporting of other items, such as survival times, the amalgamation of various experimental groups and tumour types, as well as the lack of age adjustment in the analyses precluded a complete evaluation of this study.]

Rat: Two groups, each of 25 male and 25 female Sprague-Dawley-derived Charles River (CD) rats, 6 weeks of age, were given i.p. injections of 4.5 mg/kg bw (the maximally tolerated dose - MTD) or 2.2 mg/kg bw (0.5 MTD) chlorambucil 3 times weekly for 6 months. Animals that survived over 100 days were observed for 12 further months, at which time they were killed. The results reported had been combined for the two doses. Tumours reported to be lymphosarcomas, myelogenous leukaemia and reticulum-cell sarcomas occurred in 8/33 treated male animals. These incidences were reported to be significantly different from those in controls (P < 0.001). The spontaneous incidences of haemato-poietic and lymphatic tumours were 2/179 in males (2 disseminated myelocytic sarcomas) and 1/181 in females (1 disseminated lymphosarcoma) (Weisburger *et al.*, 1975). [However, control animals were referred to as 'untreated' or 'treated with the vehicle only', and no precise indication was given as to the vehicle used or with which controls the treated animals were compared for tumour incidence. Therefore, the reported significance of the difference in tumour incidence between treated and control animals is difficult to evaluate. The Working Group considered that the inadequate reporting of other items, such as survival times, the amalgamation of various experimental groups and tumour types, as well as the lack of age-adjustment in the analyses precluded a complete evaluation of this study.]

(c)   Effects of combinations

Mouse: In a further study, reported by Weisburger (1977), designed to test many anti-cancer drugs singly or in combination, two groups, each of 25 male and 25 female, weanling, pathogen-free outbred Swiss-Webster-derived mice were given i.p. injections 3 times weekly for 6 months of a drug combination consisting of individual doses of 1 mg/kg bw metho-trexate, 0.4 mg/kg bw chlorambucil and 0.02 mg/kg bw actinomycin D. Two other groups of animals were treated identically with one-half the individual doses, i.e., 0.5 mg/kg bw methotrexate, 0.2 mg/kg bw chlorambucil and 0.01 mg/kg bw actinomycin D. The animals were observed for 12 further months, at which time they were killed. It was indicated that generally the compounds were dissolved in physiological saline with the addition of 2% sodium bicarbonate, 2% ethanol, Tween 80, citric acid or sodium hydroxide as needed to stabilize or keep the compound in solution; the volume of vehicle used was 0.1 ml/10 g bw. The survival time in animals given the high doses was 47% that of controls in males and 91% in females; and in those given the low doses, it was 83% that of controls in males and 100% in females. The combined treatment was reported to cause the same tumour type as the individual drugs: tumours, which occurred mainly in the lung, were found in 4/9 males and 10/19 females given the high doses, and in 9/26 males and 10/22 females given the low doses. These incidences were reported, on average, to be less than those with chlorambucil or with actinomycin D alone, and the median latent period was longer. [The Working Group noted that the dose of chlorambucil used in the combination studies was much smaller than that used in the studies in which chlorambucil was given alone. No adequate controls were available].

Rat: In a further study, reported by Weisburger (1977), designed to test many anti-cancer drugs singly or in combination, two groups, each of 25 male and 25 female weanling, mycoplasma-free, outbred Sprague-Dawley rats (CD strain), were given i.p. injections 3 times weekly for 6 months of a drug combination consisting of individual doses of 0.6 mg/kg bw methotrexate, 0.48 mg/kg bw chlorambucil and 0.02 mg/kg bw actinomycin D. Other groups were treated identically with one-half the individual doses, i.e., 0.3 mg/kg bw metho-trexate, 0.24 mg/kg bw chlorambucil and 0.01 mg/kg bw actinomycin D, or with one-quarter the doses, i.e., 0.15 mg/kg bw methotrexate, 0.12 mg/kg bw chlorambucil and 0.005 mg/kg bw actinomycin D. The animals were observed for 12 further months, at which time they were killed. It was indicated that generally the compounds were dissolved in physiological saline with the addition of 2% sodium bicarbonate, 2% ethanol, Tween 80, citric acid or sodium hydroxide as needed to stabilize or keep the compound in solution; the volume of vehicle used was 0.25 mg/100 g bw. Because of high toxicity, no tumour was observed in animals of either sex given the highest dose or in males given the second level. Tumours were reported to be of the same type as those induced by the individual drugs; they occurred mainly in the mammary gland and were found in 7/12 females given the second dose level and in 9/24 males and 13/24 females given the lowest level. These incidences were reported to be less, on average, than those with chlorambucil or actinomycin D alone, and the median latent period was longer. [The Working Group noted that the dose of chlorambucil used in the combination studies was much smaller than that used in the studies in which chlorambucil was given alone. No adequate control was available].

3.2 Other relevant biological data

(a) Experimental systems

Toxic effects

The single i.p. LD_{50} for chlorambucil (free acid) given as a suspension in 0.5% carboxymethylcellulose to adult female Wistar rats was 23 mg/kg bw (Chaube *et al.*, 1967). In adult male Wistar rats bearing the Walker tumour, its i.p. LD_{50} when given as a single dose in arachis oil the day after tumour transplantation ranged from 17.8 to 28.0 mg/kg bw in a series of experiments (Rosenoer *et al.*, 1966). Hebborn *et al.* (1965) reported an i.p. LD_{50} of 28 mg/kg bw (single dose) and an i.m. LD_{50} (5 daily injections) of 10 mg/kg bw in adult Holzmann rats. I.v. administration of a single dose of 4 mg/kg bw to dogs caused severe leucopenia, vomiting and diarrhoea by the 7th day (Boyland *et al.*, 1961).

Phenylbutazone increased the cytotoxicity of chlorambucil to L1210 and P388 leukaemia cells *in vitro* by displacing alkylating agent bound to serum in the tissue culture medium. Such reduction in binding by phenylbutazone increased the toxicity of chlorambucil in mice (Schiffman *et al.*, 1978).

Effects on reproduction and prenatal toxicity

Repeated i.p. injections of the highest tolerated dose resulted in testicular atrophy and decreased spermatogenic activity in mice after 39 weeks (Shimkin *et al.*, 1966).

Chlorambucil was found to be teratogenic and embryolethal in rats in several studies when given as i.p. injections on days 11 - 14 of pregnancy at doses of 6 - 12 mg/kg bw. When given on day 11 or 12 of pregnancy the minimum fetal LD_{100} was estimated to be 18 mg/kg bw. A wide spectrum of abnormalities can be produced, including encephalocele, exencephaly, cleft palate and deformed appendages, paws and tails (Murphy *et al.*, 1958; Murphy, 1959; Chaube *et al.*, 1967; Soukup *et al.*, 1967; Chaube & Murphy, 1968).

Abnormalities of the limbs and of the urogenital tract induced by chlorambucil were studied in detail (macroscopically and microscopically) by i.p injections to Long-Evans rats of 9.5 mg/kg bw on day 14 of pregnancy or to Swiss mice of 5 - 6 mg/kg bw on days 11 - 12 of pregnancy. The defects appeared to result primarily from specific cell death and formation of aberrant cell types (Dellenbach & Gabriel-Robez, 1975; Sadler & Kochhar, 1975; Brummett & Johnson, 1979).

Abnormal development could also be induced *in vitro*, using an organ culture technique. When normal limb buds from 11-day-old mouse embryos (ICR/DUB) were cultured for 6 days in the presence of 0.5 - 2 µg/ml chlorambucil, cartilage abnormalities were found; the effect was dose-related. Abnormal cartilage development was also observed when limb buds from embryos were cultured for 24 hours after exposure *in vivo* to teratogenic doses of chlorambucil. The defects in limbs exposed *in vitro* were similar to those found after exposure *in vivo* (Sadler & Kochhar, 1975, 1976; Sadler, 1976).

Absorption, distribution, excretion and metabolism

After oral administration of 20 - 25 mg/kg bw ^{14}C-ring-labelled chlorambucil to rats, radioactivity was detected in most tissues within an hour; plasma, liver and kidney showed the highest concentrations of radioactivity. After i.v. administration of 5 mg/kg bw, plasma and kidney were most heavily labelled. By 24 hours after injection, the level of radioactivity had decreased in all tissues, although it was still detectable. The amount of radioactivity eliminated *via* the urine, faeces or expired air depended on the position at which the molecule was labelled (Godeneche *et al.*, 1975; Mitoma *et al.*, 1977).

When 8 mg/kg bw ^{3}H-chlorambucil were administered subcutaneously to Yoshida ascites sarcoma-bearing rats, the highest tritium concentration after 1 hour was found in the liver; that in the kidneys was 63% of the liver value. After 6 hours, the level of radioactivity in the liver had fallen by 52%, but that in the kidneys had increased by 25%. In the blood, radioactivity was associated mainly with the plasma, which was labelled maximally at 6 hours. After 24 hours, 60% of the administered activity was excreted in the urine, and less than 0.2% was found in the faeces (Hill & Riches, 1971).

Chlorambucil is extensively metabolized in rodents by monodechloroethylation and by β-oxidation, forming the phenylacetic acid derivative, which also has anticancer activity (Godeneche et al., 1975; McLean et al., 1976; Mitoma et al., 1977; Newell et al., 1978; Chang et al., 1980; McLean et al., 1980).

Chlorambucil binds covalently to proteins, mainly through carboxyl groups, both in vivo and in vitro (Stacey et al., 1958; Linford, 1962). Alkylation of DNA also occurs in vitro (Stacey et al., 1958). Incorporation of radioactivity into the DNA and RNA of sensitive and of resistant Yoshida ascites cells was maximal 12 and 6 hours, respectively, after s.c. injection of ^{3}H-chlorambucil into rats (Hill & Riches, 1971). This prolonged incorporation of label into the DNA and RNA in both tumourous and normal rat tissues has been confirmed in studies using tritiated chlorambucil. It has been suggested that this is due to the slow release of an alkylating moiety from an intracellular drug macromolecular complex (Tew & Taylor, 1978). Chlorambucil also causes polymerization of RNA (Brecher et al., 1979) and an increase in nuclear protein phosphorylation (Thraves et al., 1979).

Mutagenicity and other short-term tests

Chlorambucil induced point mutations in *Escherichia coli* Sd-4-73 (Szybalski, 1958), mitotic gene conversion in the diploid strain D4 of *Saccharomyces cerevisiae* (Zimmermann, 1971) and a dose-dependent increase in mutations in the haploid wild-type (RAD.REV) strain of *S. cerevisiae* (Ruhland et al., 1978).

Chromosomal aberrations of the chromatid type were also observed in short-term cultures of human peripheral lymphocytes following exposure to chlorambucil *in vitro* (Stevenson & Patel, 1973; Reeves & Margoles, 1974).

Increases in sister chromatid exchanges were observed when chlorambucil was added to human lymphocytes in cell cycle following phytohaemagglutinin stimulation (Raposa, 1978) or to human lymphocytes in G_0 prior to the addition of phytohaemagglutinin stimulation (Littlefield et al., 1979).

Chromosomal changes were found in direct preparations of rat embryos 6 - 30 hours after i.p. administration of 8 mg/kg bw chlorambucil on the 13th day of pregnancy (Soukup *et al.*, 1967).

(b)   Humans

Toxic effects

The toxic effects of chlorambucil described below occurred in patients receiving therapeutic doses, except where otherwise indicated.

Interstitial pulmonary fibrosis observed in 6 patients treated with chlorambucil was attributed to use of this drug (Rubio, 1972; Rose, 1975; Cole *et al.*, 1978). In the case described by Rose the lung disease regressed on discontinuation of the drug but recurred on resumption of treatment.

Myelosuppression was observed in 2/3 of an uncontrolled series of 495 patients treated with chlorambucil (dose unspecified) for rheumatoid arthritis. Viral, fungal and bacterial infections (attributed to immunosuppression) were observed in about 30% of patients. There was a low incidence of skin and gastrointestinal complaints (Deshayes *et al.*, 1971). Convulsions have been reported in 10 children treated with chlorambucil, two of whom accidentally received very large amounts (Green & Naiman, 1968; Williams *et al.*, 1978; Ammenti *et al.*, 1980).

Effects on reproduction and prenatal toxicity

Oligospermia, azoospermia and disappearance of testicular germinal cells have been observed in male patients treated with chlorambucil. These changes are dose-dependent; a minimum total dose of 400 mg was required to induce azoospermia. Although recovery from azoospermia was not documented, the oligospermia appeared to be reversible in cases in which the total dose had been less than 400 mg (Richter *et al.*, 1970).

A woman who received 10 mg/day chlorambucil for 6 weeks from 4.5 months of pregnancy, followed by six i.v. injections of 20 mg nitrogen mustard during the 5th, 6th and 7th months, had a normal infant (Smith *et al.*, 1958).

Another woman who became pregnant while receiving 6 mg/day chlorambucil, and who continued to receive it for another 2¼ months, had a therapeutic abortion at 3.5 months. The fetus had no left kidney or ureter (Shotton & Monie, 1963).

Absorption, distribution, excretion and metabolism

Chlorambucil is well absorbed from the human gastrointestinal tract. The areas under the plasma decay curve after i.v. or oral administration are similar; after oral administration, the plasma level declines with a half-life of approximately 2 hours (Newell *et al.*, 1979b). The phenylacetic acid derivative is produced in significant quantities by β-oxidation (Alberts *et al.*, 1979; Newell *et al.*, 1979b).

Mutagenicity and chromosomal effects

A small increase in chromatid-type chromosomal damage was found in bone-marrow biopsies from patients receiving chlorambucil for chronic lymphocytic leukaemia; the same effect was seen in peripheral blood lymphocytes from patients treated with chlorambucil for other conditions such as rheumatoid arthritis, lymphoid follicular reticulosis and disseminated lupus erythematosus (Stevenson & Patel, 1973). The accumulated dose given before analysis ranged from approximately 0.08 - 2.5 g. A similar small increase in chromatid gaps was seen in the peripheral lymphocytes of patients treated with chlorambucil for uveitis following a total dose of between 0.065 and 2.9 g (Reeves *et al.*, 1975). The significance of these chromosomal findings is, however, questionable.

3.3 Case reports and epidemiological studies of carcinogenicity in humans

At least 34 cases of cancer have been reported following chlorambucil therapy for non-malignant diseases, mainly rheumatoid arthritis, collagen diseases, glomerulonephritis and multiple sclerosis. Thirty-one of these cases were acute leukaemias, and most were acute non-lymphocytic leukaemia. Twenty-three of the patients were reported to have received chlorambucil in the absence of other cytotoxic drugs (Deshayes *et al.*, 1971; Videbaek, 1971; Laroche *et al.*, 1972; Sigwald *et al.*, 1973; Tulliez *et al.*, 1974; Lagrue *et al.*, 1975; Stachowiak *et al.*, 1976; Tchernia *et al.*, 1976; Westberg & Swolin, 1976; Bisson *et al.*, 1977; Blanc *et al.*, 1977; Carcassonne *et al.*, 1978; Fiere *et al.*, 1978; Mougeot-Martin *et al.*, 1978; Witz *et al.*, 1978; Lebranchu *et al.*, 1980); and 8 also received other cytotoxic drugs, radiation or both (Menkès *et al.*, 1975; Cazalis *et al.*, 1976; Tchernia *et al.*, 1976; Sheibani *et al.*, 1980). One patient with rheumatoid arthritis, who was also treated with phenylbutazone (see IARC, 1977), developed a lymphosarcoma of the small intestine (Zittoun *et al.*, 1972); one patient treated only with chlorambucil for autoimmune haemolytic anaemia developed a non-Hodgkin's lymphoma (Worlledge *et al.*, 1968); one patient with Wegener's granulomatosis, who also received other cytotoxic drugs, including cyclophosphamide, developed bladder cancer (Chasko *et al.*, 1980).

Following chlorambucil therapy for malignant diseases (mostly Hodgkin's disease, non-Hodgkin's lymphoma, chronic lymphocytic leukaemia, and ovarian cancer), 37 subsequent neoplasms have been reported, 35 of which were acute leukaemias (mainly acute non-lymphocytic leukaemia). In only 4 cases was chlorambucil the only therapy used (Castro *et al.*, 1973; Steigbigel *et al.*, 1974; Morrison & Yon, 1978; Kapadia *et al.*, 1980); the rest received other anticancer drugs and/or radiation (Gosselin *et al.*, 1970; McPhedran & Heath, 1970; Steinberg *et al.*, 1970; Catovsky & Galton, 1971; Poth *et al.*, 1971; Chan & McBride, 1972; Davis *et al.*, 1973; Gunz *et al.*, 1973; Rosner & Grünwald, 1974; Steigbigel *et al.*, 1974; Rosner & Grünwald, 1975; Ellman & Carey, 1976; Haque *et al.*, 1976; Sotrel *et al.*, 1976; Preisler & Lyman, 1977; Morrison & Yon, 1978; Casciato & Scott, 1979; Kaye *et al.*, 1979; Zarrabi *et al.*, 1979; Kapadia *et al.*, 1980). Two additional patients treated with chlorambucil and cyclophosphamide developed bladder cancers (Dale & Smith, 1974; Wall & Clausen, 1975).

Lerner (1978) reported that of 13 women with breast cancer treated with chlorambucil as adjuvant chemotherapy, 3 (23%), or possibly 4 (31%), developed acute myeloid leukaemia between 4 and 6 years after starting chlorambucil.

Lenoir *et al.* (1977) treated 300 infants with chlorambucil for glomerulonephritis over a 10-year period; of these 2 developed acute leukaemia and 1 a hypernephroma. One of the patients with leukaemia had also received nitrogen mustard (see IARC, 1975b).

Of 40 children with severe juvenile arthritis treated with chlorambucil and followed for up to 15 years, 3 (8%) developed acute nonlymphocytic leukaemia. No such case was reported among 160 other children with less severe juvenile arthritis not treated with chlorambucil (Buriot *et al.*, 1979).

Kahn *et al.* (1979) reported that among 1711 patients with nonmalignant diseases (mainly rheumatoid arthritis and collagen diseases) from 79 sources, who had received chlorambucil alone up to 13 years previously, 16 developed acute leukaemia. [Because the cases of leukaemia were diagnosed before the study was carried out, it is possible, however, that the occurrence of leukaemia may have influenced the participation of certain doctors in the survey and the identification of chlorambucil-treated patients.]

It was reported in an abstract that in a series of 802 patients with Hodgkin's disease in complete remission, 9 cases of acute nonlymphocytic leukaemia developed compared with 0.06 cases expected. Seven of the leukaemia cases occurred in 130 patients who initially received combination chemotherapy with one of several regimens (including procarbazine and BCNU), followed by long-term maintenance therapy with chlorambucil [0.014 cases expected]. Four of the 7 patients also received radiation therapy (Pajak *et al.*, 1979).

Reimer *et al.* (1977) studied 5455 women treated for ovarian cancer at centres in which alkylating agents were used regularly in therapy. Among these women, 13 developed acute nonlymphocytic leukaemia, whereas 0.62 were expected (relative risk, 21.0). Three of the 13 had received chlorambucil, 2 as the only treatment and 1 in combination with radiotherapy; but the proportion of the total group so treated was not specified. A separate study of 13,309 women with ovarian cancer (few of whom were treated with alkylating agents) showed 5 leukaemias compared with 6.9 expected, suggesting no increased risk of acute non-lymphocytic leukaemia in women with ovarian cancer in the absence of alkylating drugs.

Li *et al.* (1975) followed up 414 long-term survivors of childhood cancer for up to 20 years; 42 of these patients had been treated with chlorambucil as the only chemotherapeutic agent. Fifteen of the 414 children, all of whom had received radiation, subsequently developed new cancers, compared with 0.7 expected ($P < 0.001$); 12/13 solid tumours appeared at irradiated sites and were attributed by the authors to radiation. The authors did not attribute any of the cancer excess to chlorambucil therapy.

Kinlen *et al.* (1979, 1981) followed up 1349 non-transplant patients who had been treated with immunosuppressive drugs for nonmalignant diseases; 49 of these had received chlorambucil, and two of them developed cancers other than non-Hodgkin's lymphoma, skin cancer or bladder cancer.

No analytical epidemiological study referring to chlorambucil alone was available to the Working Group.

4. SUMMARY OF DATA REPORTED AND EVALUATION

4.1 Experimental data

Chlorambucil has been tested in mice and rats by intraperitoneal injection. It produced tumours of the lung in mice and probably produced tumours of the haemotopoietic system and ovary in mice and haematopoietic tumours in male rats. It was also tested in a two-stage skin carcinogenesis experiment in mice, in which it had an initiating effect.

Chlorambucil can induce teratogenic effects in several animal species and embryo-lethality at doses nontoxic to the mother. It has been shown to induce mutations in bacteria and yeast, and chromosomal aberrations in human lymphocytes in culture.

4.2 Human data

Chlorambucil has been used widely since the early 1960s, often for long periods, in the treatment of lymphomas, chronic leukaemias and certain solid tumours. It has also been used, to a lesser extent, in the treatment of rheumatoid arthritis, chronic glomerulonephritis and other nonmalignant diseases.

The available data are not sufficient to evaluate the teratogenic or mutagenic potential or chromosomal effects of chlorambucil in humans.

Although no well-controlled epidemiological study of chlorambucil alone was available to the Working Group, several highly suggestive descriptive studies and numerous case reports point to the increased occurrence of acute nonlymphocytic leukaemia in patients treated with chlorambucil.

4.3 Evaluation

There is *limited evidence*[1] for the carcinogenicity of chlorambucil in mice and rats. There is *limited evidence*[2] that it is carcinogenic in humans.[3]

The experimental and clinical evidence taken together indicate that chlorambucil is very likely to be a human carcinogen.

---

[1] See preamble, p. 19.

[2] See preamble, p. 17.

[3] Since the meeting of the Working Group, the Secretariat became aware of a new epidemiological study, which documents an excess incidence of acute leukaemia in patients treated with chlorambucil (Berk *et al.*, 1981). In a prospective, randomized clinical trial, 431 previously untreated patients with polycythemia vera were treated by phlebotomy alone, by phlebotomy plus chlorambucil or by phlebotomy plus radioactive phosphorus. The risk of acute leukaemia in patients given chlorambucil was 13 times that in patients treated by phlebotomy alone (P < 0.002). This study, in conjunction with the evaluation of the Working Group would provide *sufficient evidence* that chlorambucil is carcinogenic in humans.

5. REFERENCES

Alberts, D.S., Chang, S.Y., Chen, H.-S.G., Larcom, B.J. & Jones, S.E. (1979) Pharmacokinetics and metabolism of chlorambucil in man: a preliminary report. *Cancer Treat. Rev., 6,* 9-17

Ammenti, A., Reitter, B. & Müller-Wiefel, D.E. (1980) Chlorambucil neurotoxicity: report of two cases. *Helv. paediatr. Acta, 35,* 181-287

Baker, C.E., Jr, ed. (1980) *Physicians' Desk Reference,* 34th ed., Oradell, NJ, Medical Economics Co., p. 756

Berk, P.D., Goldberg, J.D., Silverstein, M.N., Weinfeld, A., Donovan, P.B., Ellis, J.T., Landaw, S.A., Laszlo, J., Najean, Y., Pisciotta, A.V. & Wasserman, L.R. (1981) Increased incidence of acute leukemia in polycythemia vera associated with chlorambucil therapy. *New Engl. J. Med., 304,* 441-447

Bisson, M., Galanaud, P. & Subtil, E. (1977) Acute myeloblastic leukaemia after immunosuppressive treatment (Fr.). *Nouv. Presse méd., 6,* 1980

Blanc, A.-P., Gastaut, J.-A., Dalivoust, P. & Carcassonne, Y. (1977) Malignant haemopathies occurring during immunosuppressive treatment. Four new observations (Fr.). *Nouv. Presse méd., 6,* 2503-2504, 2509

Boyland, E., Staunton, M.D. & Williams, K. (1961) Experimental regional administration (perfusion and infusion) of chlorambucil [*p*-*N,N*-di(β-chloroethyl)aminophenylbutyric acid]. *Br. J. Cancer, 15,* 498-510

Brecher, A.S., Hunsaker, W.R. & Vessey, K.B. (1979) Evidence for polymerisation of tRNA by chlorambucil (Abstract no. 6). *Fed. Proc., 38,* 225

Brummett, E.S. & Johnson, E.M. (1979) Morphological alterations in the developing fetal rat limb due to maternal injection of chlorambucil, *Teratology, 20,* 279-287

Buriot, D., Prieur, A.-M., Lebranchu, Y., Messerschmitt, J. & Griscelli, C. (1979) Acute leukaemia in three children treated with chlorambucil for juvenile rheumatoid arthritis (Fr.). *Arch. fr. Pédiatr., 36,* 592-598

Carcassonne, Y., Gastaut, J.A. & Blanc, A.P. (1978) Acute leukemia after prolonged immunosuppressive therapy for glomerulonephritis. *Cancer Treat. Rep., 62,* 1110-1111

Casciato, D.A. & Scott, J.L. (1979) Acute leukemia following prolonged cytotoxic agent therapy. *Medicine, 58,* 32-47

Castro, G.A.M., Church, A., Pechet, L. & Snyder, L.M. (1973) Leukemia after chemotherapy of Hodgkin's disease. *New Engl. J. Med., 289,* 103-104

Catovsky, D. & Galton, D.A.G. (1971) Myelomonocytic leukaemia supervening on chronic lymphocytic leukaemia. *Lancet, i,* 478-479

Cazalis, P., Caroit, M., Zittoun, R., Kahn, M.-F. & de Sèze, S. (1976) A particular risk in long-term immunosuppressive treatment: a case of acute myelomonocytic leukaemia after treatment with chlorambucil for severe rheumatoid polyarthritis (Fr.). *Rev. Rhum., 43,* 431-435

Chan, B.W.B. & McBride, J.A. (1972) Hodgkin's disease and leukemia. *Can. med. Assoc. J., 106,* 558-561

Chang, S.Y., Larcom, B.J., Alberts, D.S., Larsen, B., Walson, P.D. & Sipes, I.G. (1980) Mass spectrometry of chlorambucil, its degradation products, and its metabolites in biological samples. *J. pharm. Sci., 69,* 80-84

Chasko, S.B., Keuhnelian, J.G., Gutowski, W.T., III & Gray, G.F. (1980) Spindle cell cancer of bladder during cyclophosphamide therapy for Wegener's granulomatosis. *Am. J. surg. Pathol., 4,* 191-196

Chaube, S. & Murphy, M.L. (1968) *The teratogenic effects of the recent drugs active in cancer chemotherapy.* In: Woollam, D.H.M., ed., *Advances in Teratology,* Vol. 3, Plainfield, NJ, Logos Press, pp. 181-237

Chaube, S., Kury, G. & Murphy, M.L. (1967) Teratogenic effects of cyclophosphamide (NSC-26271) in the rat. *Cancer Chemother. Rep., 51,* 363-376

Cole, S.R., Myers, T.J. & Klatsky, A.U. (1978) Pulmonary disease with chlorambucil therapy. *Cancer, 41,* 455-459

Dale, G.A. & Smith, R.B. (1974) Transitional cell carcinoma of the bladder associated with cyclophosphamide. *J. Urol., 112,* 603-604

Davis, H.L., Jr, Prout, M.N., McKenna, P.J., Cole, D.R. & Korbitz, B.C. (1973) Acute leukemia complicating metastatic breast cancer. *Cancer, 31,* 543-546

Dellenbach, P. & Gabriel-Robez, O. (1975) Genito-urinary malformations. Experimental teratogenicity study with Chloraminophène (Fr.). *Rev. fr. Gynécol., 70,* 419-424

Deshayes, P., Rénier, J.-C., Bregeon, C. & Houdent, G. (1971) Incidents and accidents with immunosuppressive therapy for rheumatoid polyarthritis (Fr.). *Rev. Rhum., 38,* 797-806

Ellman, L. & Carey, R.W. (1976) Morphological discordance in acute leukemia. *Blood, 47,* 621-623

Everett, J.L., Roberts, J.J. & Ross, W.C.J. (1953) Aryl-2-halogenoalkylamines. XII. Some carboxylic derivatives of *N,N*-di-2-chloroethylaniline. *J. chem. Soc. (London),* 2386-2392

Fiere, D., Felman, P., Vu Van, H. & Coiffier, B. (1978) Acute myeloid leukaemia after administration of chlorambucil. Two cases. *Nouv. Presse méd., 7,* 756

Godeneche, D., Madelmont, J.C., Sauvezie, B. & Billaud, A. (1975) Study of the kinetics of the absorption, distribution and excretion of ^{14}C-labelled *N,N*-di-2-chloroethyl, 4-*p*-aminophenylbutyric acid (Chloraminophène) in the rat (Fr.). *Biochem. Pharmacol., 24,* 1303-1308

Gosselin, G., Neemeh, J., Long, L.A., Pretty, H. & Lefebvre, R. (1970) Appearance of acute myeloid leukaemia during the evolution of a lymphosarcoma (Fr.). *Union méd. Can., 99,* 866-870

Green, A.A. & Naiman, J.L. (1968) Chlorambucil poisoning. *Am. J. Dis. Child., 116,* 190-191

Gunz, F.W., Levi, J.A., Lind, D.E. & Vincent, P.C. (1973) Development of acute leukaemia in a patient with lymphosarcoma. *N.Z. med. J., 78,* 71-75

Haque, T., Lutcher, C., Faguet, G. & Talledo, O. (1976) Chemotherapy-associated acute myelogenous leukemia and ovarian carcinoma. *Am. J. med. Sci., 272,* 225-228

Harvey, S.C. (1975) *Antineoplastic and immunosuppressive drugs.* In: Osol, A., ed., *Remington's Pharmaceutical Sciences,* Easton, PA, Mack Publishing Co., p. 1076

Hebborn, P., Mishra, L.C., Dalton, C. & Williams, J.P.G. (1965) Dental lesions in rat induced by radiomimetic agents. *Arch. Pathol., 80,* 110-115

Hill, B.T. & Riches, P.G. (1971) The absorption, distribution and excretion of ^{3}H-chlorambucil in rats bearing the Yoshida ascites sarcoma. *Br. J. Cancer, 25,* 831-837

IARC (1975a) *IARC Monographs on the Evaluation of Carcinogenic Risk of Chemicals to Man,* Vol. 9, *Some aziridines,* N-, S- & O-*mustards and selenium,* Lyon, pp. 125-134

IARC (1975b) *IARC Monographs on the Evaluation of Carcinogenic Risk of Chemicals to Man,* Vol. 9, *Some aziridines,* N-, S- & O-*mustards and selenium,* Lyon, pp. 193-207

IARC (1976) *IARC Monographs on the Evaluation of Carcinogenic Risk of Chemicals to Man,* Vol. 11, *Cadmium, nickel, some epoxides, miscellaneous industrial chemicals and general considerations on volatile anaesthetics,* Lyon, pp. 157-167

IARC (1977) *IARC Monographs on the Evaluation of Carcinogenic Risk of Chemicals to Man,* Vol. 13, *Some Miscellaneous Pharmaceutical Substances,* Lyon, pp. 183-199

Jakhammer, T., Olsson, A. & Svensson, L. (1977) Mass fragmentographic determination of prednimustine and chlorambucil in plasma. *Acta pharm. seuc., 14,* 485-496

Kahn, M.F., Arlet, J., Bloch-Michel, H., Caroit, M., Chaouat, Y. & Renier, J.C. (1979) Acute leukaemias after treatment with cytotoxic agents in rheumatology: 19 observations among 2006 patients (Fr.). *Nouv. Presse méd., 8,* 1393-1397

Kapadia, S.B., Krause, J.R., Ellis, L.D., Pan, S.F. & Wald, N. (1980) Induced acute non-lymphocytic leukemia following long-term chemotherapy. A study of 20 cases. *Cancer, 45,* 1315-1321

Kaye, S.B., Juttner, C.A., Smith, I.E., Barrett, A., Austin, D.E., Peckham, M.J. & McElwain, T.J. (1979) Three years' experience with Ch1VPP (a combination of drugs of low toxicity) for the treatment of Hodgkin's disease. *Br. J. Cancer, 39,* 168-174

Kinlen, L.J., Sheil, A.G.R., Peto, J. & Doll, R. (1979) Collaborative United Kingdom-Australasian study of cancer in patients treated with immunosuppressive drugs. *Br. med. J., iv,* 1461-1466

Kinlen, L.J., Peto, J., Doll, R. & Sheil, A.G.R. (1981) Cancer in patients treated with immunosuppressive drugs. *Br. med. J., i,* 474

Lagrue, G., Bernard, D., Bariety, J., Druet, P. & Guenel, J. (1975) Treatment with chlorambucil and azathio-prine in cases of primary glomerulonephritis. Results of a controlled study (Fr.). *J. Urol. Nephrol., 9,* 655-672

Laroche, C., Caquet, R. & Remy, J.-M. (1972) Acute erythroleukaemia after treatment of a malignant exophthalmia with chlorambucil (Fr.). *Nouv. Presse méd., 1,* 3133

Lebranchu, Y., Drucker, J., Nivet, H., Rolland, J.C., Grenier, B., Lejars, O., Lamagnere, J.P. & Buriot, D. (1980) Acute monoblastic leukaemia in child receiving chlorambucil for juvenile rheumatoid arthritis. *Lancet, i,* 649

Lenoir, G., Guesry, P., Kleinknecht, C., Gagnadoux, M.-F. & Broyer, M. (1977) Extragonadal complications of chlorambucil in children (on the basis of 300 observations of treated glomerular nephropathies) (Fr.). *Arch. fr. Pédiatr., 34,* 798-807

Lerner, H.J. (1978) Acute myelogenous leukemia in patients receiving chlorambucil as long-term adjuvant chemotherapy for Stage II breast cancer. *Cancer Treat. Rep., 62,* 1135-1138

Li, F.P., Cassady, J.R. & Jaffe, N. (1975) Risk of second tumors in survivors of childhood cancer. *Cancer, 35,* 1230-1235

Linford, J.H. (1962) The recovery of free chlorambucil from solution in blood serum. *Biochem. Pharma-col., 11,* 693-706

Littlefield, L.G., Colyer, S.P., Sayer, A.M. & Dufrain, R.J. (1979) Sister-chromatid exchanges in human lymphocytes exposed during G_0 to four classes of DNA-damaging chemicals. *Mutat. Res., 67,* 259-269

McElwain, T.J., Toy, J., Smith, E., Peckham, M.J. & Austin, D.E. (1977) A combination of chlorambucil, vinblastine, procarbazine and prednisone for treatment of Hodgkin's disease. *Br. J. Cancer, 36,* 276-280

McLean, A., Newell, D. & Baker, G. (1976) The metabolism of chlorambucil. *Biochem. Pharmacol., 25,* 2331-2335

McLean, A., Newell, D., Baker, G. & Connors, T. (1980) The metabolism of chlorambucil. *Biochem. Pharmacol., 29,* 2039-2047

McPhedran, P. & Heath, C.W., Jr (1970) Acute leukemia occurring during chronic lymphocytic leukemia. *Blood, 35,* 7-11

Menkès, C.J., Lévy, J.P., Weill, B., Delrieu, F., Mathiot, C. & Delbarre, F. (1975) Acute megaloblastic leukaemia occurring after immunosuppressive treatment of rheumatoid polyarthritis (Fr.). *Nouv. Presse méd., 4,* 2869-2871

Mitoma, C., Onodera, T., Takegoshi, T. & Thomas, D.W. (1977) Metabolic disposition of chlorambucil in rats. *Xenobiotica, 7,* 205-220

Morrison, J. & Yon, J.L. (1978) Acute leukemia following chlorambucil therapy of advanced ovarian and fallopian tube carcinoma. *Gynecol. Oncol., 6,* 115-120

Mougeot-Martin, M., Krulik, M., Harousseau, J.-L., Audebert, A.-A., Chaouat, Y. & Debray, J. (1978) Acute leukaemias arising in a case of Behçet's disease and a case of multiple sclerosis treated with immuno-suppressors (Fr.). *Ann. Méd. intern. (Paris), 129,* 175-180

Murphy, M.L. (1959) A comparison of the teratogenic effects of five polyfunctional alkylating agents on the rat fetus. *Pediatrics, 23,* 231-244

Murphy, M.L., Del Moro, A. & Lacon, C. (1958) The comparative effects of five polyfunctional alkylating agents on the rat fetus, with additional notes on the chick embryo. *Ann. N.Y. Acad. Sci., 68,* 762-782

Newell, D.R., Hart, L.I. & Harrap, K.R. (1979a) Estimation of chlorambucil, phenyl acetic mustard and prednimustine in human plasma by high performance liquid chromatography. *J. Chromatogr., 164,* 114-119

Newell, D.R., Hart, L.I., Calvert, H., McElwain, T.J. & Harrap, K.R. (1979b) *The estimation of chlorambucil, phenyl acetic mustard and prednimustine in human plasma by high pressure liquid chromatography.* In: Hawk, G.L., ed., *Biological/Biomedical Applications of Liquid Chromatography,* Vol.2, New York, Basel, Marcel Dekker, pp. 37-48

Newell, H., Wilkinson, R. & Harrap, K.P. (1978) The comparative pharmacokinetics of prednimustine and chlorambucil (Abstract). *Br. J. Cancer, 38,* 187

Pajak, T.F., Nissen, N.I., Stutzman, L., Hoogstraten, B., Cooper, M.R., Glowienka, L.P., Glidewell, O. & Glicksman, A. (1979) Acute myeloid leukemia (AML) occurring during complete remission (CR) in Hodgkin's disease (Abstract no. C-425). *Proc. Am. Soc. clin. Oncol., 15,* 394

Poth, J.L., George, R.P., Jr, Creger, W.P. & Schrier, S.L. (1971) Acute myelogenous leukemia following localized radiotherapy. *Arch. intern. Med., 128,* 802-805

Preisler, H.D. & Lyman, G.H. (1977) Acute myelogenous leukemia subsequent to therapy for a different neoplasm: clinical features and responses to therapy. *Am. J. Hematol., 3,* 209-218

Raposa, T. (1978) Sister chromatid exchange studies for monitoring DNA damage and repair capacity after cytostatics *in vitro* and in lymphocytes of leukaemic patients under cytostatic therapy. *Mutat. Res., 57,* 241-251

Reeves, B.R. & Margoles, C. (1974) Preferential location of chlorambucil-induced breakage in the chromosomes of normal human lymphocytes. *Mutat. Res., 26,* 205-208

Reeves, B.R., Pickup, V.L. & Lawler, S.D. (1975) A chromosome study of patients with uveitis treated with chlorambucil. *Br. med. J., iv,* 22-23

Reimer, R.R., Hoover, R., Fraumeni, J.F., Jr & Young, R.C. (1977) Acute leukemia after alkylating-agent therapy of ovarian cancer. *New Engl. J. Med., 297,* 177-181

Richter, P., Calamera, J.C., Mosgenfeld, M.C., Kierszenbaum, A.L., Lavieri, J.C. & Mancini, R.E. (1970) Effect of chlorambucil on spermatogenesis in the human with malignant lymphoma. *Cancer, 25,* 1026-1030

Rose, M.S. (1975) Busulphan toxicity syndrome caused by chlorambucil. *Br. med. J., i,* 123

Rosenoer, V.M., Mitchley, B.C.V., Roe, F.J.C. & Connors, T.A. (1966) Walker carcinosarcoma 256 in study of anticancer agents. I. Method for simultaneous assessment of therapeutic value and toxicity. *Cancer Res., 26, Suppl.,* 937-949

Rosner, F. & Grünwald, H. (1974) Multiple myeloma terminating in acute leukaemia. Report of 12 cases and review of the literature. *Am. J. Med., 57,* 927-939

Rosner, F. & Grünwald, G. (1975) Hodgkin's disease and acute leukaemia. Report of eight cases and review of the literature. *Am. J. Med., 58,* 339-353

Rubio, F.A., Jr (1972) Possible pulmonary effects of alkylating agents. *New Engl. J. Med., 287,* 1150-1151

Ruhland, A., Fleer, R. & Brendel, M. (1978) Genetic activity of chemicals in yeast: DNA alterations and mutations induced by alkylating anti-cancer agents. *Mutat. Res., 58,* 241-250

Sadler, T.W. (1976) Chlorambucil-induced cell death in embryonic mouse limb buds (Abstract). *Anat. Rec., 184,* 519-520

Sadler, T.W. & Kochhar, D.M. (1975) Teratogenic effects of chlorambucil on *in vivo* and *in vitro* organogenesis in mice. *Teratology, 12,* 71-78

Sadler, T.W. & Kochhar, D.M. (1976) Chlorambucil-induced cell death in embryonic mouse limb buds. *Toxicol. appl. Pharmacol., 37,* 237-256

Salaman, M.G. & Roe, F.J.C. (1956) Further tests for tumour-initiating activity: *N,N*-di(2-chloroethyl)-*p*-aminophenylbutyric acid (CB 1348) as an initiator of skin tumour formation in the mouse. *Br. J. Cancer, 10,* 363-378

Schiffman, F.J., Uehara, Y., Fisher, J.M. & Rabinovitz, M. (1978) Potentiation of chlorambucil toxicity by phenylbutazone. *Cancer Lett., 4,* 211-216

Sheibani, K., Bukowski, R.M., Tubbs, R.R., Savage, R.A., Sebek, B.A. & Hoffman, G.C. (1980) Acute nonlymphocytic leukemia in patients receiving chemotherapy for nonmalignant diseases. *Hum. Pathol., 11,* 175-179

Shimkin, M.B., Weisburger, J.H., Weisburger, E.K., Gubareff, N. & Suntzeff, V. (1966) Bioassay of 29 alkylating chemicals by the pulmonary-tumor response in strain A mice. *J. natl Cancer Inst., 36,* 915-935

Shotton, D. & Monie, I.W. (1963) Possible teratogenic effect of chlorambucil on a human fetus. *J. Am. med. Assoc., 186,* 74-75

Sigwald, J., Mazalton, A., Raymondeaud, C., Piot, C. & Jacquillat, C. (1973) Critical study of the treatment of multiple sclerosis with chlorambucil and intraspinal corticotherapy (Fr.). *Rev. Neurol., 128,* 72-77

Smith, R.B.W., Sheehy, J.W. & Rothberg, H. (1958) Hodgkin's disease and pregnancy. *Arch. intern. Med., 102,* 777-789

Sotrel, G., Jafari, K., Lash, A.F. & Stepto, R.C. (1976) Acute leukaemia in advanced ovarian carcinoma after treatment with alkylating agents. *Obstet. Gynecol., 47,* 67S-71S

Soukup, S., Takacs, E. & Warkany, J. (1967) Chromosome changes in embryos treated with various teratogens. *J. Embryol. exp. Morphol., 18,* 215-226

Stacey, K.A., Cobb, K., Cousens, S.F. & Alexander, P. (1958) The reactions of the 'radiomimetic' alkylating agents with macromolecules *in vitro. Ann. N.Y. Acad. Sci., 68,* 682-701

Stachowiak, J., Gorin, N.-C., Najman, A. & Duhamel, G. (1976) Acute leukaemia after long-term treatment with chlorambucil: study of two cases (Fr.). *Ann. Méd. intern., 127,* 584-589

Steigbigel, R.T., Kim. H., Potolsky, A. & Schrier, S.L. (1974) Acute myeloproliferative disorder following long-term chlorambucil therapy. *Arch. intern. Med., 134,* 728-731

Steinberg, M.H., Geary, C.G. & Crosby, W.H. (1970) Acute granulocytic leukemia complicating Hodgkin's disease. *Arch. intern. Med., 125,* 496-502

Stevenson, A.C. & Patel, C. (1973) Effects of chlorambucil on human chromosomes. *Mutat. Res., 18,* 333-351

Szybalski, W. (1958) Special microbiological systems. II. Observations on chemical mutagenesis in microorganisms. *Ann. N.Y. Acad. Sci., 76,* 475-489

Tchernia, G., Mielot, F., Subtil, E. & Parmentier, C. (1976) Acute myeloblastic leukemia after immunodepressive therapy for primary nonmalignant disease. *Blood Cells, 2,* 67-80

Tew, K.D. & Taylor, D.M. (1978) Tissue distribution and nucleic acid binding of chlorambucil-^{3}H in tumor-bearing rats. *Experientia, 34,* 1215-1216

Thraves, P.J., Wilkinson, R. & Harrap. K.R. (1979) Effect of chlorambucil on nuclear protein phosphatases (Abstract). *Br. J. Cancer, 40,* 318

Tulliez, M., Ricard, M.F., Jan, F. & Sultan, C. (1974) Preleukaemic abnormal myelopoiesis induced by chlorambucil: a case study. *Scand. J. Haematol., 13,* 179-183

US International Trade Commission (1979) *Imports of Benzenoid Chemicals and Products, 1978,* USITC Publication 990, Washington DC, US Government Printing Office, p. 82

US Pharmacopeial Convention, Inc. (1980) *The US Pharmacopeia,* 20th rev., Rockville, MD, pp. 129-130

Videbaek, A. (1971) Unusual cases of myelomatosis. *Br. med. J., ii,* 326

Wade, A., ed. (1977) *Martindale, The Extra Pharmacopoeia,* 27th ed., London, The Pharmaceutical Press, pp. 131-133

Wall, R.L. & Clausen, K.P. (1975) Carcinoma of the urinary bladder in patients receiving cyclophosphamide. *New Engl. J. Med., 293,* 271-273

Weisburger, E.K. (1977) Bioassay program for carcinogenic hazards of cancer chemotherapeutic agents. *Cancer, 40,* 1935-1949

Weisburger, J.H., Griswold, D.P., Prejean, J.D., Casey, A.E., Wood, H.B. & Weisburger, E.K. (1975) The carcinogenic properties of some of the principal drugs used in clinical cancer chemotherapy. *Recent Results Cancer Res., 52,* 1-17

Westberg, N.G. & Swolin, B. (1976) Acute myeloid leukaemia appearing in two patients after prolonged continuous chlorambucil treatment for Wegener's granulomatosis. *Acta med. scand., 199,* 373

Williams, S.A., Makker, S.P. & Grupe, W.E. (1978) Seizures: a significant side effect of chlorambucil therapy in children. *J. Paediatr., 93,* 516-518

Williams, S.A., Makker, S.P., Ingelfinger, J.R. & Grupe, W.E. (1980) Long-term evaluation of chlorambucil plus prednisone in the idiopathic nephrotic syndrome in childhood. *New Engl. J. Med., 302,* 929-933

Windholz, M., ed. (1976) *The Merck Index,* 9th ed., Rahway, NJ, Merck & Co., Inc., pp. 260-261

Witz, F., Lederlin, P., Aymard, J.-P., Thibaut, G. & Guerci, O. (1978) Acute myeloblastic leukaemia after chlorambucil treatment. Two new cases (Fr.). *Nouv. Presse méd., 7,* 2392

Worlledge, S.M., Brain, M.C., Cooper, A.C., Hobbs, J.R. & Dacie, J.V. (1968) Immunosuppressive drugs in the treatment of autoimmune haemolytic anaemia. *Proc. R. Soc. Med., 61,* 1312-1315

Zarrabi, M.H., Rosner, F. & Bennett, J.M. (1979) Non-Hodgkin's lymphoma and acute myeloblastic leukemia. A report of 12 cases and review of the literature. *Cancer, 44,* 1070-1080

Zimmermann, F.K. (1971) Induction of mitotic gene conversion by mutagens. *Mutat. Res., 11,* 327-337

Zittoun, R., Debré, P., Gardais, J., Thuau, F.P., Renier, J.C. & Simon, F. (1972) Lymphosarcoma of the small intestine after treatment of rheumatoid polyarthritis with chlorambucil (Fr.). *Nouv. Presse méd., 1,* 2477-2479

1. CHEMICAL AND PHYSICAL DATA

1.1 Synonyms and trade names

Chem. Abstr. Services Reg. No.: 13010-47-4

Chem. Abstr. Name: Urea, *N*-(2-chloroethyl)-*N'*-cyclohexyl-*N*-nitroso-

IUPAC Systematic Name: 1-(2-Chloroethyl)-3-cyclohexyl-1-nitrosourea

Synonyms: CCNU; chloroethylcyclohexylnitrosourea; 1-(2-chloroethyl)-3-cyclohexylnitrosourea; lomustine

Trade names: Belustine; Cee NU; ICIG 1109; NSC 79037

1.2 Structural and molecular formulae and molecular weight

$$\text{cyclohexyl}-NH-\overset{\overset{\textstyle O}{\|}}{C}-\underset{\underset{\textstyle NO}{|}}{N}-CH_2-CH_2Cl$$

$C_9H_{16}ClN_3O_2$ Mol. wt: 233.7

1.3 Chemical and physical properties of the pure substance

From Baker (1980), unless otherwise specified

(a) *Description:* Yellow powder
(b) *Melting-point:* 90°C
(c) *Solubility:* Soluble in 10% ethanol (0.05 mg per ml) and absolute ethanol (70 mg per ml) and slightly soluble in water ($<$0.05 mg per ml)
(d) *Stability:* Sensitive to oxidation and hydrolysis; forms alkylating and carbamoylating intermediates. Its half-life at 25°C at neutral pH is 117 min (Schein *et al.*, 1978).

1.4 Technical products and impurities

CCNU is available in the US in capsules containing 10, 40 or 100 mg (Baker, 1980).

2. PRODUCTION, USE, OCCURRENCE AND ANALYSIS

2.1 Production and use

(a) Production

CCNU was first synthesized in 1966 (Johnston *et al.*, 1966). The first step was the reaction of ethyl 5-(2-chloroethyl)-5-nitrosohydantoate with cyclohexylamine (see IARC, 1980). Nitrosation of the resulting 1-(2-chloroethyl)-3-cyclohexylurea with formic acid and aqueous nitrite solution produced CCNU. It is not known whether this is the method used for commercial production.

One US company is believed to produce this chemical, but no data were available on the quantities made or sold (see preamble, p. 20-21).

Apparently, CCNU has never been produced in Europe or Japan.

(b) Use

CCNU is an antineoplastic agent, administered orally, for the treatment of Hodgkin's disease and various solid tumours, such as primary and metastatic brain tumours, where it is given alone or in combination; for colorectal tumours, where it is given in association with 5-fluorouracil; and for certain pulmonary malignancies. The recommended dose for adults and children is 130 mg/m^2 body surface, given as a single dose every 6 weeks (Wade, 1977; Baker, 1980).

2.2 Occurrence

CCNU is not known to be produced in Nature.

2.3 Analysis

No information on analytical methods for the determination of CCNU was available to the Working Group.

3. BIOLOGICAL DATA RELEVANT TO THE EVALUATION
OF CARCINOGENIC RISK TO HUMANS

3.1 Carcinogenicity studies in animals

(a) Oral administration

Rat: A group of 20 female Sprague-Dawley rats, 50 - 55 days old, were administered a single dose by gavage of 5.0 mg/rat CCNU suspended in 1 ml sesame oil. A group of 20 rats treated with 18 mg/rat 7,12-dimethylbenz[a] anthracene (DMBA) served as positive controls; 89 rats that received sesame oil alone were used as solvent controls.   The cumulative 6-month mortality was 4/20 (20%) in DMBA-treated rats, 5/89 (4%) in solvent controls and 2/20 (10%) in CCNU-treated rats. All of the tumours seen in 18 (90%) positive controls were multiple breast tumours, of which 13 (65%) were mammary carcinomas.   Among the solvent controls, 1 rat had a fibroadenomatous hyperplasia of the mammary gland; in addition, 1 kidney carcinoma, 1 lung carcinoma and 1 precancerous change in the bronchus were reported.   Of the 18 CCNU-treated rats that survived the 6-month experimental period, 1 (5%) developed diffuse fibrous hyperplasia of the breast (Griswold *et al.*, 1966). [Because of limitations in experimental design, the Working Group considered the absence of carcinogenic effect to be inconclusive.]

(b) Intraperitoneal administration

Mouse: Two groups, each of 25 male and 25 female outbred Swiss-Webster-derived mice, 6 weeks old, were given i.p. injections of CCNU 3 times weekly for 6 months. Animals that survived over 100 days were observed for 12 further months, at which time they were killed.   The males received doses of 1.25 and 2.5 mg/kg bw, and females were treated with 1.25 and 5.0 mg/kg bw. A dilution of 10 ml/kg bw in physiological saline was used.   Controls consisted of 254 untreated mice.   The survival times of the treated animals were reported as percentages of that of the controls [no precise definition of the mode of calculation was given] : the survival times of male mice were 34% and 120%, respectively, that of untreated controls, and the corresponding figures for females were 27% and 59%.   Animals that died before day 100 on test were excluded from evaluation.   The incidence of 25/38 (66%) female tumour-bearing mice was 2-3 times higher than that of controls (38/153, 25%); 11 lymphosarcomas, 5 leukaemias, 3 lung tumours and 2 skin tumours were recorded.   Of treated male mice, 14/26 (54%) developed tumours, including 3 lymphosarcomas, 3 lung tumours and 1 leukaemia; 28/101 (28%) male control animals developed tumours, including 1/101 lymphosarcoma and 10/101 lung tumours (Weisburger *et al.*, 1975; Weisburger, 1977). [The overall tumour incidence and the frequency of animals with lymphosarcomas were reported to be significantly greater than in controls. The Working Group considered that the inadequate reporting of certain items, such as survival times, the amalgamation of various experimental groups and tumour types, as well as lack of age-adjustment in the analyses precluded a complete evaluation of this study.]

Rat: Two groups, each of 25 male and 25 - 28 female Sprague-Dawley-derived Charles River (CD) rats, about 30 days old, were given i.p. injections of 3 or 6 mg/kg bw CCNU 3 times a week for 6 months. Animals that survived over 100 days were observed for up to 12 further months, at which time they were killed. Tumours were seen in 60/179 (34%) untreated males and in 105/181 (58%) untreated females. The survival times of the treated animals were reported as percentages of that of the controls [no precise definition of the mode of calculation was given] : the survival times of treated females were reported to be 44% and 96% that of controls; the corresponding figures for treated males were 37% and 82%. Animals that died before day 100 on test were excluded from evaluation. Of treated females, 16/35 (46%) developed tumours: 8 lung tumours, 6 breast tumours and 1 brain tumour were recorded. The incidence of lung tumours in treated female rats was significantly greater than that in controls (1/181; 0.5%). Of treated males, 13/28 (46%) developed tumours: 6 lung tumours, 3 leukaemias and 2 sarcomas were recorded. The incidence of lung tumours in treated males was significantly greater than that in controls (3/179; 2%) (Weisburger *et al.*, 1975; Weisburger, 1977). [The Working Group considered that the inadequate reporting of certain items, such as survival times, the amalgamation of various experimental groups and tumour types, as well as the lack of age-adjustment in the analyses precluded a complete evaluation of this study.]

(c) Intravenous administration

Rat: CCNU was included in a chronic toxicity and carcinogenicity study on cytostatic *N*-nitroso(2-chloroethyl)ureas, still in progress at the time of reporting. Groups of 30 male Wistar rats [age unspecified] received i.v. injections every 6 weeks of 19, 38, 75 or 150 mg/m^2 CCNU (1.5, 4, 8 or 20 mg/kg bw) dissolved in Cremophor EL (a surfactant based on castor oil), ethanol and water (1.5:1.5:20 vol/vol). Controls consisted of 120 rats that received the same amount of solvent. Treatment was discontinued when severe lethal toxicity became apparent, i.e., after 7 applications of the highest dose or after 10 applications of any of the other doses. All animals were observed for life. Median survival times after the start of treatment were 621 days for controls, 369 days for the group treated with 150 mg/m^2 (20 mg/kg bw), 530 days for the group treated with 75 mg/m^2 (8 mg/kg bw), 601 days for the group treated with 38 mg/m^2 (4 mg/kg bw) and 661 days for the group treated with 19 mg/m^2 (2 mg/kg bw). Malignant tumours occurred in 8% (10/120) of solvent controls, in 10% of animals treated with the highest dose of CCNU and in 7% of rats treated with 75 mg/m^2. The total incidences of premalignant changes and benign and malignant tumours were 17% in the group that received the highest dose, 30% in the group treated with 75 mg/m^2, 10% in the group treated with 38 mg/m^2, 3% in the group treated with 19 mg/m^2 and 15% in the controls. The induced tumours occurred in the lung (5 adenomas and 1 adenoacanthoma) and in the forestomach (5 papillomas or premalignant basal-cell proliferations with atypia). A lung adenoma was observed in 1 control animal, and papillomas of the forestomach were recorded in 7 controls. It was stated that histopathological examinations had not been completed and that the results were thus preliminary (Eisenbrand & Habs, 1980 ; Eisenbrand et al., 1981). In a further report on the same study, the incidence of lung tumours was confirmed as follows: 2 in the highest dose group, 4 in the group given 75 mg/m^3, 1 in each of the groups given 38 and 19 mg/m^3, and none in the lowest dose group, while 1 lung tumour occurred among 120 controls. The histological diagnoses were indicated as: adenomas, adenoacanthomas (which the author considered malignant) and 1 squamous-cell carcinoma. [However, the exact attribution of the histological types in relation to the tumours observed in the various groups was not given.] (Habs, 1980).

3.2 Other relevant biological data

(a)   Experimental systems

Toxic effects

CCNU is half as toxic as its analogue BCNU in a number of species (rat, mouse, dog, monkey) and has an LD_{50} of 71 - 73 mg/kg bw after a single oral dose in corn oil in rats of both sexes and 51 mg/kg bw in male mice and 38 mg/kg bw in females. The LD_{50} value was similar if the injections were given intraperitoneally or subcutaneously or dissolved in 95% ethanol (Thompson & Larson, 1972). The lethal dose of CCNU in dogs was about 10 mg/kg bw when given as a single dose and 1.25 mg/kg bw when given daily for 14 consecutive days. In monkeys, the lethal dose by oral intubation was 5 mg/kg bw given for 14 days (Oliverio, 1973).

A characteristic feature of the antitumour nitrosoureas is their delayed bone-marrow toxicity (Young et al., 1971). In a toxicological evaluation of a single i.v. infusion of CCNU in dogs and monkeys, both species exhibited toxic changes in bone marrow and lymphoid tissue, with neutropenia and lymphopenia. Neutropenia was particularly severe in dogs, and doses of 5 mg/kg bw or above were lethal. Monkeys survived haematopoietic toxicity, but chronic interstitial nephritis developed in several animals treated with 20 or 30 mg/kg bw, and they died 16 days or more after treatment. Monkeys treated with an i.v. dose of 10 mg/kg bw exhibited nephritis 100 days after treatment. Transient hepatotoxicity developed in dogs 20 - 30 days after administration of doses exceeding 2.5 mg/kg bw. It was concluded that the highest nontoxic dose was 0.625 mg/kg bw for dogs and 1.25 mg/kg bw for monkeys. I.v. treatment caused toxicity that was qualitatively and quantitatively similar to that with oral treatment (Schaeppi *et al.*, 1974). CCNU also has cardiopulmonary toxicity in dogs and gastro-intestinal toxicity in dogs and monkeys (Oliverio, 1973).

Effects on reproduction and prenatal toxicity

CCNU was teratogenic when given to pregnant Sprague-Dawley rats in i.p. doses of 2, 4 or 8 mg/kg bw per day during various 4-day periods of organogenesis, or 6 mg/kg bw per day throughout organogenesis (days 6 - 15 of pregnancy). The principal period of sensitivity was days 6 - 9 of pregnancy; omphalocele, ectopia cordis and aortic arch anomalies, syndactyly and anophthalmia occurred most frequently. Treatment of rabbits with i.v. or i.p. doses of 1.5 - 3 mg/kg bw once daily on days 6 - 18 caused no teratogenic effect, but a high incidence of abortion was observed with the highest dose (Thompson *et al.*, 1975,a,b).

Absorption, distribution, excretion and metabolism

CCNU undergoes spontaneous decomposition under physiological conditions to release both alkylating and carbamoylating entities (Reed & May, 1975; Reed *et al.*, 1975). It disappears from plasma within 5 minutes following its oral administration, but the antitumour effect of its metabolites may persist for up to 15 minutes (Oliverio, 1976).

Following its i.p. or i.v. injection or oral administration, C^{14}-labelled CCNU was rapidly distributed to many tissues in mice, rats, rabbits and dogs (Oliverio *et al.*, 1970; Litterst *et al.*, 1974; Levin *et al.*, 1978). About 80% of label was excreted in the urine of mice 24 hours after a single parenteral or oral dose of 50 mg/kg bw (Oliverio *et al.*, 1970).

In addition to chemical decomposition, CCNU may be converted by microsomal metabolism to 6 isomeric hydroxylated derivatives, some of which may differ in their biological properties from CCNU (May *et al.*, 1974; Wheeler *et al.*, 1977).

After administration of ^{14}C-labelled CCNU, radioactivity was found bound to proteins (Schmall *et al.*, 1973; Connors & Hare, 1974) and to nucleic acids (Cheng *et al.*, 1972; Connors & Hare, 1974). CCNU reacts with calf thymus DNA to form 7-hydroxyethyldeoxyguanosine, 3-hydroxyethyldeoxycytidine and 3,N^4-ethano-deoxycytidine. In addition, small amounts of 7-aminoethylguanine were found (Gombar *et al.*, 1980).

Mutagenicity and other short-term tests

CCNU induced mutations in *Salmonella typhimurium* tester strains *his* G46 (Zimmer & Bhuyan, 1976; Auletta *et al.*, 1978), TA1530 (Auletta *et al.*, 1978), TA1535 and TA100 (Franza *et al.*, 1980) without metabolic activation, as well as in strain *his* G46 in the mouse host-mediated assay (Auletta *et al.*, 1978).

CCNU also induced mutations at the hypoxanthine-guanine phosphoribosyl transferase locus in V79 Chinese hamster cells *in vitro* (Bradley *et al.*, 1980).

(b) Humans

Toxic effects

Toxicity of CCNU (reviewed by Katz & Glick, 1979) is largely haematological and is delayed: thrombocytopenia is maximal between 3 and 5 weeks after a single dose and leucopenia between 4 and 7 weeks. This toxicity is schedule-dependent (Israel & Chahinian, 1973). Nausea and vomiting occur during 24 hours after dosage (Katz & Glick, 1979), and nephrotoxicity has been reported (Silver & Morton, 1979). Although hepatic and pulmonary toxicity are found with other nitrosoureas (Lokich *et al.*, 1974), they have not been reported after use of CCNU.

Effects on reproduction and prenatal toxicity

No data were available to the Working Group.

Absorption, distribution, excretion and metabolism

CCNU is well absorbed from the gut. Ten patients were given ^{14}C-CCNU labelled at various sites: peak plasma levels of radioactivity occurred 1, 3 and 4 hours after administration of label in the carbonyl, cyclohexyl and chloroethyl moieties, respectively. Radioactivity associated with the carbonyl and the cyclohexyl moieties decayed biphasically, with half-lives of 5 and 27 hours in the former case and 4 and 50 hours in the latter. Radioactivity in the chloroethyl moiety decayed monophasically, with a half-life of 72 hours (Sponzo *et al.*, 1973). No intact drug was found in the plasma; 25% of the radioactivity was ether-extractable and may represent hydroxylated metabolites (Walker & Hilton, 1976). From 50-77% of the administered radioactivity was excreted in the urine between 24 and 48 hours. Radioactivity in the cerebro-spinal fluid paralleled that in plasma, but at 30% of the level (Sponzo *et al.*, 1973), and did not represent intact drug.

Mutagenicity and chromosomal effects

An increase in the frequency of sister chromatid exchanges was observed in peripheral lymphocytes from CCNU-treated melanoma patients for up to 8 weeks following treatment with a dose of 130 mg/m^2 (Lambert *et al.*, 1979).

3.3 Case reports and epidemiological studies of carcinogenicity in humans

Acute nonlymphocytic leukaemia developed in 4 patients with Hodgkin's disease (Preisler & Lyman, 1977; Foucar *et al.*, 1979), 3 patients with non-Hodgkin's lymphoma (Collins *et al.*, 1977; Foucar *et al.*, 1979; Zarrabi *et al.*, 1979), 1 patient with multiple myeloma (Preisler & Lyman, 1977) and 1 patient with a brain tumour (Cohen *et al.*, 1976), all of whom had received CCNU in combination with a number of other cytotoxic agents and/or radiation. One patient with a brain tumour treated in a similar fashion developed Hodgkin's disease (Crafts *et al.*, 1978). In the only report involving use of CCNU as a single agent, a patient with a metastatic carcinoma of unknown origin developed acute nonlymphocytic leukaemia (Foucar *et al.*, 1979).

4. SUMMARY OF DATA REPORTED AND EVALUATION

4.1 Experimental data

CCNU is carcinogenic in rats following its intraperitoneal or intravenous injection, producing lung carcinomas. It was also tested in mice by intraperitoneal injection; a slight increase in the incidence of lymphomas was observed.

CCNU can induce embryo- and fetolethality in rats and rabbits at doses nontoxic to the mother and a variety of severe teratogenic effects in rats.

It is mutagenic in *Salmonella typhimurium* and in Chinese hamster lung cells.

4.2 Human data

CCNU has had limited use since the early 1970s in the treatment of lymphomas and carcinomas, usually in conjunction with other antineoplastic drugs.

The frequency of sister chromatid exchanges is increased in the lymphocytes of patients who have been treated with CCNU. No data were available to evaluate the teratogenic or mutagenic potential of this drug in humans.

Several case reports describe the development of acute nonlymphocytic leukaemia in cancer patients who received CCNU. With one exception, all such patients had also received other cytotoxic agents and/or irradiation. No epidemiological study of CCNU as a single agent was available to the Working Group.

4.3 Evaluation

There is *sufficient evidence*[1] for the carcinogenicity of CCNU in rats. The data from studies in humans are inadequate to evaluate the carcinogenicity of CCNU in man.

This chemical should be regarded for practical purposes as if it presented a carcinogenic risk to humans.

---

[1] See preamble, p. 18.

5. REFERENCES

Auletta, A.E., Martz, A.G. & Parmar, A.S. (1978) Mutagenicity of nitrosourea compounds for *Salmonella typhimurium:* brief communication. *J. natl Cancer Inst., 60,* 1495-1497

Baker, C.E., Jr, ed. (1980) *Physicians' Desk Reference,* 34th ed., Oradell, NJ, Medical Economics Co., pp. 708-709

Bradley, M.O., Sharkey, N.A., Kohn, K.W. & Layard, M.W. (1980) Mutagenicity and cytotoxicity of various nitrosoureas in V-79 Chinese hamster cells. *Cancer Res., 40,* 2719-2725

Cheng, C.J., Fujimura, S., Grunberger, D. & Weinstein, I.B. (1972) Interaction of 1-(2-chloroethyl)-3-cyclohexyl-1-nitrosourea (NSC 79037) with nucleic acids and proteins *in vivo* and *in vitro. Cancer Res., 32,* 22-27

Cohen, R.J., Wiernik, P.H. & Walker, M.D. (1976) Acute nonlymphocytic leukemia associated with nitrosourea chemotherapy: report of two cases. *Cancer Treat. Rep., 60,* 1257-1261

Collins, A.J., Bloomfield, C.D., Peterson, B.A. & McKenna, R.W. (1977) Acute nonlymphocytic leukemia in patients with nodular lymphoma. *Cancer, 40,* 1748-1754

Connors, T.A. & Hare, J.R. (1974) The binding of ^{14}C labelled 1-(2-chloroethyl)-3-cyclohexyl-1-nitrosourea (CCNU) to macromolecules of sensitive and resistant tumours. *Br. J. Cancer, 30,* 477-480

Crafts, D.C., Townsend, J., Wilson, C.B. & Levin, V.A. (1978) Development of Hodgkin's disease in a patient receiving procarbazine, CCNU, and vincristine therapy for a gemistocytic astrocytoma. *Cancer Treat. Rep., 62,* 177-178

Eisenbrand, G. & Habs, M. (1980) *Chronic toxicity and carcinogenicity of cytostatic N-nitroso(2-chloroethyl)ureas after repeated intravenous application to rats.* In: Holmstedt, B., Lauwerys, R., Mercier, M. & Roberfroid, M., eds, *Mechanisms of Toxicity and Hazard Evaluation,* Amsterdam, Elsevier/North-Holland Biomedical Press, pp. 273-278

Eisenbrand, G., Habs, M., Zeller, W.J., Fiebig, H., Berger, M., Zelesny, O. & Schmähl, D. (1981) *New nitrosoureas - therapeutic and long-term toxic effects of selected compounds in comparison to selected drugs.* In: Imbach, J.L., Serrou, B. & Schein, P., eds, *Proceedings of an International Symposium on Nitrosoureas in Cancer Treatment, Montpellier,* Amsterdam, Elsevier (in press)

Foucar, K., McKenna, R.W., Bloomfield, C.D., Bowers, T.K. & Brunning, R.D. (1979) Therapy-related leukemia. A panmyelosis. *Cancer, 43,* 1285-1296

Franza, B.R., Jr, Oeschger, N.S., Oeschger, M.P. & Schein, P.S. (1980) Mutagenic activity of nitrosourea antitumor agents. *J. natl Cancer Inst., 65,* 149-154

Gombar, C.T., Tong, W.P. & Ludlum, D.B. (1980) Mechanism of action of the nitrosoureas. IV. Reactions of bis-chloroethyl nitrosourea and chloroethyl cyclohexyl nitrosourea with deoxyribonucleic acid. *Biochem. Pharmacol., 29,* 2639-2643

Griswold, D.P., Jr, Casey, A.E., Weisburger, E.K., Weisburger, J.H. & Schabel, F.M., Jr (1966) On the carcinogenicity of a single intragastric dose of hydrocarbons, nitrosamines, aromatic amines, dyes, coumarins, and miscellaneous chemicals in female Sprague-Dawley rats. *Cancer Res., 26,* 619-625

Habs, M. (1980) *Experimentelle Untersuchungen zur Cancerogenese Wirkung Zytostatischer Arzneimittel (Experimental Studies on the Carcinogenic Effect of Cytostatic Drugs),* Thesis, Medical Faculty of Heidelberg University

IARC (1980) *IARC Monographs on the Evaluation of the Carcinogenic Risk of Chemicals to Humans,* Vol. 22, *Some Non-nutritive Sweetening Agents,* Lyon, pp. 55-109

Israel, L. & Chahinian, P. (1973) Comparative toxicity on leukocytes and platelets of two regimes of CCNU: the relationship between maximum dose and optimum dose. *Eur. J. Cancer, 9,* 799-802

Johnston, T.P., McCaleb, G.S., Opliger, P.S. & Montgomery, J.A. (1966) The synthesis of potential anticancer agents. 36. *N*-Nitrosoureas. II. Haloalkyl derivatives. *J. med. Chem., 9,* 892-911

Katz, M.E. & Glick, J.H. (1979) Nitrosoureas: a reappraisal of clinical trials. *Cancer clin. Trials, 2,* 297-316

Lambert, B., Ringborg, U. & Lindblad, A. (1979) Prolonged increase of sister-chromatid exchanges in lymphocytes of melanoma patients after CCNU treatment. *Mutat. Res., 59,* 295-300

Levin, V.A., Kabra, P.A. & Freeman-Dove, M.A. (1978) Relationship of 1,3-bis(2-chloroethyl)-1-nitrosourea (BCNU) and 1-(2-chloroethyl)-3-cyclohexyl-1-nitrosourea (CCNU) pharmacokinetics of uptake, distribution, and tissue/plasma partitioning in rat organs and intracerebral tumors. *Cancer Chemother. Pharmacol., 1,* 233-242

Litterst, C.L., Mimnaugh, E.G., Cowles, A.C., Gram, T.E. & Guarino, A.M. (1974) Distribution of ^{14}C-lomustine (^{14}C-CCNU)-derived radioactivity following intravenous administration of three potential clinical formulations to rabbits. *J. pharm. Sci., 63,* 1718-1721

Lokich, J.J., Drum, D.E. & Kaplan, W. (1974) Hepatic toxicity of nitrosourea analogues. *Clin. Pharmacol. Ther., 16,* 363-367

May, H.E., Boose, R. & Reed, D.J. (1974) Hydroxylation of the carcinostatic 1-(2-chloroethyl)-3-cyclohexyl-1-nitrosourea (CCNU) by rat liver microsomes. *Biochem. biophys. Res. Commun., 57,* 426-433

Oliverio, V.T. (1973) Toxicology and pharmacology of the nitrosoureas. *Cancer Chemother. Rep., Part 3, 4,* 13-20

Oliverio, V.T. (1976) Pharmacology of the nitrosureas: an overview. *Cancer Treat. Rep., 60,* 703-707

Oliverio, V.T., Vietzke, W.M., Williams, M.K. & Adamson, R.H. (1970) The absorption, distribution, excretion and biotransformation of the carcinostatic 1-(2-chloroethyl)-3-cyclohexyl-1-nitrosourea in animals. *Cancer Res., 30,* 1330-1337

Preisler, H.D. & Lyman, G.H. (1977) Acute myelogenous leukemia subsequent to therapy for a different neoplasm: clinical features and responses to therapy. *Am. J. Hematol., 3,* 209-218

Reed, D.J. & May, H.E. (1975) Alkylation and carbamoylation intermediates from the carcinostatic 1-(2-chloroethyl)-3-cyclohexyl-1-nitrosourea (CCNU). *Life Sci., 16,* 1263-1270

Reed, D.J., May, H.E., Boose, R.B., Gregory, K.M. & Beilstein, M.A. (1975) 2-Chloroethanol formation as evidence for a 2-chloroethyl alkylating intermediate during chemical degradation of 1-(2-chloroethyl)-3-cyclohexyl-1-nitrosourea   and   1-(2-chloroethyl)-3-(*trans*-4-methylcyclohexyl)-1-nitrosourea. *Cancer Res., 35,* 568-576

Schaeppi, U., Fleischman, R.W., Phelan, R.S., Ethier, M.F. & Luthra, Y.K. (1974) CCNU (NSC-79037): preclinical toxicologic evaluation of a single intravenous infusion in dogs and monkeys. *Cancer Chemother. Rep., Part 3, 5,* 53-64

Schein, P.S., Heal, J., Green, D. & Woolley, P.V. (1978) Pharmacology of nitrosourea antitumor agents. *Fundam. Cancer Chemother. Antibiot. Chemother., 23,* 64-75

Schmall, B., Cheng, C.J., Fujimara, S., Gersten, N., Grunberger, D. & Weinstein, I.B. (1973) Modifications of proteins by 1-(2-chloroethyl)-3-cyclohexyl-1-nitrosourea (NSC 79037) *in vitro. Cancer Res., 33,* 1921-1924

Silver, H.K.B. & Morton, D.L. (1979) CCNU nephrotoxicity following sustained remission in oat cell carcinoma. *Cancer Treat. Rep., 63,* 226-227

Sponzo, R.W., DeVita, V.T. & Oliverio, V.T. (1973) Physiologic disposition of 1-(2-chloroethyl)-3-cyclohexyl-1-nitrosourea (CCNU) and 1-(2-chloroethyl)-3-(4-methyl-cyclohexyl)-1-nitrosourea (MeCCNU) in man. *Cancer, 31,* 1154-1159

Thompson, G.R. & Larson, R.E. (1972) A toxicological comparison of the potency and activity of 1,3-bis(2-chloroethyl)-1-nitrosurea   (BCNU)   and   1-(2-chloroethyl)-3-cyclohexyl-1-nitrosourea (CCNU) in mice and rats. *Toxicol. appl. Pharmacol., 2,* 405-413

Thompson, D.J., Molello, J.A., Strebing, R.J. & Dyke, I.L. (1975a) Reproduction and teratological studies with 1-(2-chloroethyl)-3-cyclohexyl-1-nitrosourea (CCNU) in the rat and rabbit. *Toxicol. appl. Pharmacol., 34,* 456-466

Thompson, D.J., Molello, J.A., Strebing, R.J. & Dyke, I.L. (1975b) Reproduction and teratology studies with 1-(2-chloroethyl)-3-cyclohexyl-1-nitrosourea (CCNU) in the rat (Abstract). *Teratology, 11,* 36A

Wade, A., ed. (1977) *Martindale, The Extra Pharmacopoeia,* 27th ed., London, The Pharmaceutical Press, pp. 151-152

Walker, M.D. & Hilton, J. (1976) Nitrosourea pharmacodynamics in relation to the central nervous system. *Cancer Treat. Rep., 60,* 725-728

Weisburger, E.K. (1977)   Bioassay program for carcinogenic hazards of cancer chemotherapeutic agents. *Cancer, 40,* 1935-1951

Weisburger, J.H., Griswold, D.P., Prejean, J.D., Casey, A.E., Wood, H.B. & Weisburger, E.K. (1975) The carcinogenic properties of some of the principal drugs used in clinical cancer chemotherapy. *Recent Results Cancer Res., 52,* 1-17

Wheeler, G.P., Johnston, T.P., Bowdon, B.J., McCaleb, G.S., Hill, D.L. & Montgomery, J.A. (1977) Comparison of the properties of metabolites of CCNU. *Biochem. Pharmacol., 26,* 2331-2336

Young, R.C., DeVita, V.T., Jr, Serpick, A.A. & Canellos, G.P. (1971)   Treatment of advanced Hodgkin's disease with [1,3-bis(2-chloroethyl)-1-nitrosourea] BCNU. *New Engl. J. Med., 285,* 475-479

Zarrabi, M.H., Rosner, F. & Bennett, J.M. (1979) Non-Hodgkin's lymphoma and acute myeloblastic leukemia. A report of 12 cases and review of the literature. *Cancer, 44,* 1070-1080

Zimmer, D.M. & Bhuyan, B.K. (1976) Mutagenicity of streptozotocin and several other nitrosourea compounds in *Salmonella typhimurium. Mutat. Res., 40,* 281-288

CISPLATIN

1. CHEMICAL AND PHYSICAL DATA

1.1 Synonyms and trade names

Chem. Abstr. Services Reg. No.: 15663-27-1

Chem. Abstr. Name: Platinum, diamminedichloro-, (SP-4-2)-

IUPAC Systematic Name: *cis*-Diamminedichloroplatinum

Synonyms: CDDP; DDP; *cis*-DDP; *cis*-diaminodichloroplatinum; *cis*-diamino-dichloroplatinum(II); *cis*-diamminedichloroplatinum (II); *cis*-diammineplatinum(II)-chloride; *cis*-dichlorodiaminoplatinum; *cis*-dichlorodiaminoplatinum(II); *cis*-di-chlorodiammineplatinum; *cis*-dichlorodiammineplatinum(II); PDD; *cis*-platinous diaminodichloride; *cis*-platinum; *cis*-platinum diaminodichloride; *cis*-platinum(II) diaminodichloride; *cis*-platinum diamminedichloride; *cis*-platinum(II) diammine-dichloride; platinum diamminodichloride

Trade names: Cisplatyl; NSC 119875; Platinol

1.2 Structural and molecular formulae and molecular weight

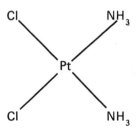

Cl$_2$H$_6$N$_2$Pt

Mol. wt: 300.1

1.3   Chemical and physical properties of the pure substance

From Kauffman & Cowan (1963)

(a) *Description:* Yellow crystals

(b) *Melting-point:* ~ 270°C (dec.)

(c) *Solubility:* Slightly soluble in cold water (1 in 400 at 25°C); insoluble in most common solvents except *N,N*-dimethylformamide

(d) *Stability:* Slowly changes to the *trans*-form in aqueous solution [reaction conditions unknown]

1.4   Technical products and impurities

Cisplatin is available in vials for injections containing 10, 25 or 50 mg of the drug. Solutions for infusion must contain 0.5% sodium chloride to enhance stability (Repta *et al.*, 1979).

2. PRODUCTION, USE, OCCURRENCE AND ANALYSIS

2.1   Production and use

(a) *Production*

Preparation of cisplatin was reported in the 1840s. A convenient synthesis method has been described (Kauffman & Cowan, 1963), in which potassium tetrachloroplatinate (II) is treated with a buffered aqueous ammonia solution to give, after recrystallization from dilute hydrochloric acid, pure cisplatin.

One US company is believed to manufacture cisplatin currently, but no data were available on the quantities made or sold (see preamble, pp. 20-21). It is not produced commercially in Europe or Japan.

(b) *Use*

Cisplatin is used in human medicine for the treatment of a variety of malignancies, usually in combination with other agents. It is used to treat testicular tumours, malignant melanoma, osteogenic sarcoma and carcinomas of the bladder, lung (non-small-cell), uterine cervix and ovary and squamous carcinoma of the head and neck region (Rozencweig *et al.*, 1977; Baker, 1980).

As a single agent, cisplatin is administered at a dose of 50 - 120 mg/m^2, intravenously once every 4 weeks. When used in combination, the dose is lowered to between 20 and 50 mg/m^2 and given every 3 weeks (usually for 3 courses). Pretreatment hydration with 1 to 2 litres of fluid infused for 8 - 12 hours is recommended. The drug is diluted in 2 litres of 5% dextrose in 0.5 or 0.3N saline containing 37.5 g mannitol, and infused over a 6 - 8-hour period. Adequate hydration should be maintained for at least 24 hours after dosing (Rozencweig et al., 1977).

2.2 Occurrence

Cisplatin is not known to be produced in Nature.

2.3 Analysis

Typical methods for the analysis of cisplatin in various matrices are summarized in Table 1.

Table 1. Methods for the analysis of cisplatin

Sample matrix	Sample preparation	Assay procedure[a]	Limit of detection	Reference
Formulations and urine	For pure samples, dissolve in sodium diethyldithiocarbamate (DDTC) and recrystallize. For urine samples, add DDTC, sodium hydroxide and sodium nitrate; seal; mix; allow to stand. Extract with chloroform; centrifuge	HPLC-UV	25 μg/l	Bannister et al. (1979)
Blood plasma	Centrifuge; filter; add ethylenediamine and let stand; filter through resin-loaded paper discs; dry discs	AAS	35 μg/l	Bannister et al. (1978)
		XF	240 μg/l	Bannister et al. (1977)
Blood plasma, tissue and urine	Freeze-dry tissues; triturate; liquify and digest with nitric and perchloric acids; dissolve residue in hydrochloric acid; evaporate; redissolve in hydrochloric acid	FAAS	∿ 30 mg/kg	LeRoy et al. (1977)

[a]Abbreviations: HPLC-UV, high-performance liquid chromatography with ultra-violet detection; AAS, atomic absorption spectrometry; XF, X-ray fluorescence; FAAS, flameless atomic absorption spectrometry

3. BIOLOGICAL DATA RELEVANT TO THE EVALUATION
OF CARCINOGENIC RISK TO HUMANS

3.1 Carcinogenicity studies in animals

Intraperitoneal administration

Mouse: Groups of 10 or 20 8-week-old female A/Jax mice were injected weekly with cisplatin in 0.85% NaCl or trioctanoin. Using NaCl solution, 1 group received 10 injections of 3.25 mg/kg bw cisplatin, for a total dose of 108 μmol/kg bw, and the second group received 19 injections of 1.62 mg/kg bw, for a total dose of 103 μmol/kg bw. The numbers of animals still alive at 8 months were 9/10 in the first group and 7/10 in the second. All of 6 control mice given 19 injections of 6.5 ml/kg bw NaCl survived for 8 months, when the experiment was terminated. Using trioctanoin, 2 groups of 20 mice were given 10 injections of 3.25 mg/kg bw cisplatin, for a total dose of 108 μmol/kg bw, and 1 group received 10 injections of 1.62 mg/kg bw and another 5 injections of 3.25 mg/kg bw, for total doses of 54 μmol/kg bw. The numbers of animals still alive at 8 months were 17 or 18 out of 20 in all groups; 19/20 control mice given 10 injections of 5 ml/kg bw trioctanoin survived to 8 months. The incidence and multiplicity of pulmonary adenomas were increased in all treated groups. With NaCl solution, 108 μmol/kg bw cisplatin produced adenomas in 100% of mice, with 14.2 adenomas/mouse; 103 μmol/kg bw produced adenomas in 100% of mice, with 15.8 adenomas/mouse; and there was an incidence of 67% in the control group, with 0.8 adenomas/mouse. In the two groups which received 108 μmol/kg bw in trioctanoin, there was also a 100% incidence of adenomas, with 10.4 or 11.4 adenomas/mouse. Administration of 54 μmol/kg bw as 10 injections produced a 94% incidence, with 5.4 adenomas/mouse, while the same total dose given as 5 injections produced a 100% incidence, with 7.2 adenomas/mouse. The control group that received only trioctanoin had a 26% incidence of adenomas, with 0.5 adenomas/mouse (Leopold *et al.*, 1979). [The Working Group noted the limited sizes of the controls groups, and especially that in the experiment with NaCl.]

Two groups of 40 8-week-old female CD-1 mice were given weekly injections of 1.62 mg cisplatin in 5 ml/kg bw 0.85% NaCl for 16 weeks. One group also received applications to shaved areas of the skin of 0.15 ml 0.6% croton oil in redistilled acetone twice weekly (1 and 4 days after the injections of cisplatin) for the entire experimental period (52 weeks), at which time all survivors were killed. Control groups of 40 mice were given either NaCl injections alone or NaCl injections plus croton oil application. The numbers of animals still alive at 41 weeks were 30/40 in the group injected with cisplatin alone, 30/40 in the group given cisplatin plus croton oil, 33/40 in the NaCl control group and 35/40 in the group given NaCl plus croton oil. At 41 weeks, 15/30 mice given cisplatin injections plus croton oil had skin papillomas, with an average of 3.2 papillomas/mouse. No skin tumour was seen in animals in other groups at that time. By 52 weeks, 3 mice in the group given injections of cisplatin plus croton oil had epidermoid carcinomas, 1 a thymic lymphoma and 1 a pulmonary adenoma; of the mice given cisplatin alone, 1 had an epidermoid carcinoma in the external ear, 2 had thymic lymphomas, 1 a pulmonary adenoma, 3 mammary adeno-carcinomas and 1 a subcutaneous fibroliposarcoma; and of the group given croton oil and NaCl, 1 mouse had a pulmonary adenoma and 1 a reticulum-cell sarcoma of the spleen. No tumour occurred in the group given the vehicle only (Leopold *et al.*, 1979). [The Working Group noted the limited reporting of the data.]

3.2 Other relevant biological data

(a) Experimental systems

Toxic effects

The LD_{50} of cisplatin after a single i.p. injection in peanut oil to female BALB/c mice was 13.0 mg/kg bw (Connors *et al.*, 1972). In Swiss mice, the LD_{50} following a single i.v. dose was 13.36 mg/kg bw in males and 12.32 mg/kg bw in females (Schaeppi *et al.*, 1973). The LD_{50} in male Sprague-Dawley rats after a single i.p. injection in saline was 12.0 mg/kg bw (Kociba & Sleight, 1971).

In Sprague-Dawley rats, a single i.p. injection of 12.2 mg/kg bw caused leucopenia, with decreased numbers of neutrophils, lymphocytes and circulating platelets. Generalized lymphoid depletion, intestinal epithelial injury and bone-marrow depression were most severe 2 - 4 days after the injection. Sloughing of the renal tubular epithelium also occurred (Kociba & Sleight, 1971). The nephrotoxicity of cisplatin may be reduced by hydration, by forced diuresis using mannitol and by use of probenecid (Krakoff, 1979; Ross & Gale, 1979).

In a preclinical evaluation of the toxicity of cisplatin in monkeys and dogs, the minimum lethal dose for dogs was a single i.v. injection of 2.5 mg/kg bw or 5 daily consecutive injections of 0.75 mg/kg bw. Five daily injections of 2.5 mg/kg bw was the minimum lethal dose for monkeys. Severe morbidity occurred within 5 - 17 days in dogs; toxic symptoms included severe haemorrhagic enterocolitis, severe damage to bone marrow and lymphoid tissue, and marked renal tubular necrosis in dogs and nephrosis in monkeys. Dogs also showed occasional pancreatitis, and monkeys myocarditis and some degeneration of spermatogenic cells. Recovery from toxicity occurred within 55 - 124 days (Schaeppi *et al.*, 1973).

Ototoxicity observed in early clinical trials of cisplatin has been studied in detail in guinea-pigs (Fleischman *et al.*, 1975).

Effects on reproduction and prenatal toxicity

An i.p. dose of 13 mg/kg bw cisplatin given to Swiss-Webster mice on day 8 of pregnancy was lethal to all fetuses of 10 dams; and a dose of 8 mg/kg bw was lethal to 98% of the fetuses of 13 dams and a dose of 3 mg/kg bw to 31% of fetuses of 12 dams. The surviving 88 and 3 fetuses of dams given 3 and 8 mg/kg bw cisplatin, respectively, showed growth retardation and had a number of apparently minor skeletal anomalies (Lazar *et al.*, 1979).

Absorption, distribution, excretion and metabolism

The distribution of cisplatin has been followed in many animal species by determining platinum by atomic absorption spectrometry (LeRoy *et al.*, 1979; Litterst *et al.*, 1979) or by the use of radioactive isotopes (Conran, 1974). After i.v. administration, many species (rat, mouse, dog) show the same general organ distribution. All tissues take up platinum, followed within the first hour by an accumulation in kidney, liver, muscle and skin. After 24 hours, tissue:plasma drug ratios are greater than 1 in other tissues; these are maintained for at least a week in dogs and in other species. Up to 4 weeks after a single dose, platinum is still detectable in kidney, liver, skin and lung (Litterst *et al.*, 1979). Cisplatin labelled with ^{193m}Pt was also distributed in most tissues 18 hours after i.v. injection into rabbits; kidney and liver showed the highest levels of radioactivity (Lange *et al.*, 1972). Although most species rapidly excrete about 80% of administered platinum in the urine within 24 hours (Litterst *et al.*, 1979), there is also a much slower clearance, possibly from a metabolite of cisplatin (LeRoy *et al.*, 1979).

Cisplatin reacts with nucleosides and nucleic acids (Robins, 1974; Thomson, 1974) and can cross-link the DNA of cells (Roberts, 1974; Bradley *et al.*, 1979; Zwelling *et al.*, 1979). Cisplatin also inhibits a number of enzymes that contain a catalytically active sulphydryl group (Aull *et al.*, 1979).

Mutagenicity and other short-term tests

Cisplatin was mutagenic in *Salmonella typhimurium* strains *his* G46/pkM101 (Monti-Bragadin *et al.*, 1975), TA100 and TA98, without metabolic activation (Benedict *et al.*, 1977; Andersen, 1979; Beck & Fisch, 1980).

In CHO or V79 Chinese hamster cells the drug induced a dose-dependent increase in 8-azaguanine-resistant mutants or thioguanine-resistant mutants (O'Neill *et al.*, 1977; Bradley *et al.*, 1979; Taylor *et al.*, 1979; Turnbull *et al.*, 1979; Zwelling *et al.*, 1979), but not ouabain-resistant mutants (Taylor *et al.*, 1979). Cisplatin also induced post-replication repair in V79 cells (van den Berg & Roberts, 1975, 1976a,b; van den Berg *et al.*, 1977) and HeLa cells (van den Berg *et al.*, 1977). Sister chromatid exchanges were also induced in V79 cells (Turnbull *et al.*, 1979).

Treatment of human lymphocyte cultures *in vitro* with cisplatin resulted in a dose-dependent induction of chromosomal damage (non-randomly distributed breakpoints) (Meyne & Lockhart, 1978) and sister chromatid exchanges (Wiencke *et al.*, 1979).

In a study in mice *in vivo*, an i.p. injection of 13.85 mg/kg bw cisplatin induced significant increases in the number of sister chromatid exchanges and chromosome aberrations in bone-marrow cells (Wiencke *et al.*, 1979).

After exposure to cisplatin, morphological transformation was observed in Syrian hamster embryo cells (Turnbull *et al.*, 1979).

(b)   Humans

Toxic effects

The toxic effects of cisplatin in humans have been reviewed (Prestayko *et al.*, 1979; Von Hoff *et al.*, 1979).

Cisplatin, like several heavy metals, causes toxicity to the kidney, bone marrow, peripheral nerves and gut. The effects on kidney take the form of reversible acute tubular necrosis, as shown by biopsy (Piel & Perlia, 1975), aminoaciduria, selective proteinuria, and magnesium loss (Fleming *et al.*, 1979; Schilsky *et al.*, 1979; Jones *et al.*, 1980). Since cisplatin is now given to patients with a concomitant fluid load (and, sometimes, mannitol), renal toxicity no longer limits the therapeutic dose which can be given (Rainey & Alberts, 1978 ; Hayes *et al.*, 1979).   Rather, acute, intractable nausea and vomiting, resistant to antiemetics, is the main toxicity effect in patients; diarrhoea is much less frequent. With high single and total doses, leucopenia and thrombocytopenia occur. Progressive anaemia has been noted in about 33% of patients (Rossof *et al.*, 1972; Piel & Perlia, 1975), and direct antiglobulin-positive haemolysis has been observed recently in the presence of the drug (Getaz *et al.*, 1980).

Loss of hearing at high frequencies (above 4000 herz) and tinnitus have been reported in about 9% of patients given cisplatin (Piel *et al.*, 1974; Von Hoff *et al.*, 1979). Oto-toxicity is rarely a clinical problem, except in young children and elderly patients. Peripheral neuropathy has been reported in 2 patients; in one it was reversible, in the other it was disabling and permanent (Hadley & Herr, 1979). In these patients and in another reported by Becher *et al.* (1980), it was manifested by distal sensory loss; in the last individual, diminished visual acuity was also noted after receiving 1 g cisplatin. Cortical blindness and epileptiform fits not related to tumour have been reported after administration of only 180 mg of the drug (Berman & Mann, 1980). Reversible jaundice has been reported with cisplatin, and the response was reproducible after a challenge dose of the drug (Cavalli *et al.*, 1978).

Other, isolated reports of toxic effects include allergic phenomena, angioneurotic oedema, rash, asthma (Von Hoff *et al.*, 1976), cardiac arrest (Vogl *et al.*, 1980), gingival discolouration (Ettinger & Freeman, 1979) and tetany due to hypocalcaemia and hypomagnesaemia (Hayes *et al.*, 1979). The mechanism of the last may be related to the renal loss of magnesium noted previously (Schilsky *et al.*, 1979), which is due to platinum-induced tubular necrosis.

Intra-arterial administration causes toxicity similar to that seen with i.v. injections (Pritchard *et al.*, 1979).

Effects on reproduction and prenatal toxicity

No data were available to the Working Group.

Absorption, distribution, excretion and metabolism

A current review of the pharmacokinetics of cisplatin is given by Prestayko *et al.* (1979). A study with ^{193}Pt (DeConti *et al.*, 1973) indicated that cisplatin has 2 half-lives after i.v. injection: 25.5 - 49 minutes and 58.5 - 73 hours. Vermorken *et al.* (1980a) found a similar result in a study utilizing atomic absorption spectrometry to measure urine and non-protein-bound plasma platinum. In a number of patients they found a consistently longer half-life (5. 7 -8.5 days). Even after meticulous urine collection for 1 month, only 50% of the injected dose of cisplatin was retrieved. Enterohepatic circulation was suggested by this study. Plasma levels of sequential courses of cisplatin increased, indicating accumulation (Vermorken *et al.*, 1980b). During the second phase, about 90% of plasma radioactivity is bound to protein (DeConti *et al.*, 1973). Cisplatin also penetrates to cerebrospinal fluids (Berman & Mann, 1980).

Mutagenicity and chromosomal effects

No data were available to the Working Group.

3.3 Case reports and epidemiological studies of carcinogenicity in humans

No data were available to the Working Group.

4. SUMMARY OF DATA REPORTED AND EVALUATION

4.1 Experimental data

Cisplatin was tested by intraperitoneal administration in mice, increasing the incidence of lung tumours. When cisplatin was administered intraperitoneally, alternately with croton oil application to the skin, papillomas and carcinomas of the skin were produced, along with small numbers of internal neoplasms.

In mice, high doses of cisplatin can induce embryolethality. The limited data available do not allow an evaluation of the teratogenic potential of the drug.

Cisplatin is a mutagen in bacterial and cultured mammalian cells. It also induces chromosomal aberrations in various cells in culture and in mice *in vivo*. Additionally, treatment of Syrian hamster embryo cells in culture with the drug resulted in the induction of morphological transformation.

4.2 Human data

Cisplatin has been used since the 1970s primarily in the treatment of testicular and ovarian cancer, often in combination with other antineoplastic drugs.

No data were available to evaluate the teratogenic potential or the mutagenicity or chromosomal effects of cisplatin in humans.

No case report or epidemiological study was available to the Working Group.

4.3 Evaluation

There is *limited evidence*[1] that cisplatin is carcinogenic in mice. No data from studies in humans were available.

The available data were insufficient for the Working Group to evaluate the carcinogenicity of cisplatin to humans.

---

[1] See preamble, p. 19.

5. REFERENCES

Andersen, K.S. (1979) Platinum(II) complexes generate frame-shift mutations in test strains of *Salmonella typhimurium*. *Mutat. Res., 67,* 209-214

Aull, J.L., Allen, R.L., Bapat, A.R., Daron, H.H., Friedman, M.E. & Wilson, J.F. (1979) The effects of platinum complexes on seven enzymes. *Biochim. biophys. Acta, 571,* 352-358

Baker, C.E., Jr, ed. (1980) *Physicians' Desk Reference,* 34th ed., Oradell, NJ, Medical Economics Co., pp. 722-723

Bannister, S.J., Sternson, L.A., Repta, A.J. & James, G.W. (1977) Measurement of free-circulating *cis*-dichlorodiammineplatinum(II) in plasma. *Clin. Chem., 23,* 2258-2262

Bannister, S.J., Chang, Y., Sternson, L.A. & Repta, A.J. (1978) Atomic absorption spectrophotometry of free circulating platinum species in plasma derived from *cis*-dichlorodiammineplatinum(II). *Clin. Chem., 24,* 877-880

Bannister, S.J., Sternson, L.A. & Repta, A.J. (1979) Urine analysis of platinum species derived from *cis*-dichlorodiammineplatinum(II) by high-performance liquid chromatography following derivatization with sodium diethyldithiocarbamate. *J. Chromatogr., 173,* 333-342

Becher, R., Schütt, P., Osieka, R. & Schmidt, C.G. (1980) Peripheral neuropathy and ophthalmologic toxicity after treatment with *cis*-dichlorodiaminoplatinum II. *J. Cancer Res. clin. Oncol., 96,* 219-221

Beck, D.J. & Fisch, J.E. (1980) Mutagenicity of platinum coordination complexes in *Salmonella typhimurium*. *Mutat. Res., 77,* 45-54

Benedict, W.F., Baker, M.S., Haroun, L., Choi, E. & Ames, B.N. (1977) Mutagenicity of cancer chemotherapeutic agents in the *Salmonella*/microsome test. *Cancer Res., 37,* 2209-2213

van den Berg, H.W. & Roberts, J.J. (1975) Post-replication repair of DNA in Chinese hamster cells treated with *cis* platinum(II) diamine dichloride. Enhancement of toxicity and chromosome damage by caffeine. *Mutat. Res., 33,* 279-284

van den Berg, H.W. & Roberts, J.H. (1976a) *Inhibition by caffeine of post-replication DNA repair in hamster cells treated with* cis *platinum(II) diamine dichloride.* In: Hellmann, K. & Connors, T.A., eds, *Chemotherapy, Proceedings of the 9th International Congress on Chemotherapy, 1975,* Vol. 8, New York, Plenum, pp. 139-144

van den Berg, H.W. & Roberts, J.H. (1976b) Inhibition by caffeine of post-replication repair in Chinese hamster cells treated with *cis* platinum (II) diamminedichloride: the extent of platinum binding to template DNA in relation to the size of low molecular weight nascent DNA. *Chem.-biol. Interactions, 12,* 375-390

van den Berg, H.W., Fraval, H.N.A. & Roberts J.J. (1977) Repair of DNA damaged by neutral platinum complexes. *J. clin. Hematol. Oncol., 7,* 349-373

Berman, I.J. & Mann, M.P. (1980) Seizures and transient cortical blindness associated with *cis*-platinum(II)-diamminedichloride (PDD) therapy in a thirty-year-old man. *Cancer, 45,* 764-766

Bradley, M.O., Hsu, I.C. & Harris, C.C. (1979) Relationships between sister chromatid exchange and mutagenicity, toxicity and DNA damage. *Nature, 282,* 318-320

Cavalli, F., Tschopp, L., Sonntag, R.W. & Zimmermann, A. (1978) A case of liver toxicity following *cis*-dichlorodiammine platinum (II) treatment. *Cancer Treat. Rep., 62,* 2125-2126

Connors, T.A., Jones, M., Ross, W.C.J., Braddock, P.D., Khokhar, A.R. & Tobe, M.L. (1972) New platinum complexes with anti-tumour activity. *Chem.-biol. Interactions, 5,* 415-424

Conran, P.B. (1974) Pharmacokinetics of platinum compounds. *Recent Results Cancer Res., 48,* 124-136

DeConti, R.C., Toftness, B.R., Lange, R.C. & Creasey, W.A. (1973) Clinical and pharmacological studies with *cis*-diamminedichloroplatinum(II). *Cancer Res., 33,* 1310-1315

Ettinger, L.J. & Freeman, A.I. (1979) The gingival platinum line. A new finding following *cis*-dichlorodiammine platinum (II) treatment. *Cancer, 44,* 1882-1884

Fleischman, R.W., Stadnicki, S.W., Ethier, M.F. & Schaeppi, U. (1975) Ototoxicity of *cis*-dichlorodiammine platinum (II) in the guinea pig. *Toxicol. appl. Pharmacol., 33,* 320-332

Fleming, J.J., Collis, C. & Peckham, M.J. (1979) Renal damage after *cis*-platinum. *Lancet, ii,* 960

Getaz, E.P., Beckley, S., Fitzpatrick, J. & Dozier, A. (1980) Cisplatin-induced hemolysis. *New Engl. J. Med., 302,* 334-335

Hadley, D. & Herr, H.W. (1979) Peripheral neuropathy associated with *cis*-dichlorodiammineplatinum (II) treatment. *Cancer, 44,* 2026-2028

Hayes, F.A., Green, A.A., Senzer, N. & Pratt, C.B. (1979) Tetany: a complication of *cis*-dichlorodiammine-platinum(II) therapy. *Cancer Treat. Rep., 63,* 547-548

Jones, B.R., Bhalla, R.B., Mladek, J., Kaleya, R.N., Gralla, R.J., Alcock, N.W., Schwartz, M.K., Young, C.W. & Reidenberg, M.M. (1980) Comparison of methods of evaluating nephrotoxicity of *cis*-platinum. *Clin. Pharmacol. Ther., 27,* 557-562

Kauffman, G.B. & Cowan, D.O. (1963) *cis- and trans- Dichlorodiammineplatinum(II).* In: Kleinberg, J., ed., *Inorganic Synthesis,* Vol. 7, New York, McGraw-Hill, pp. 239-245

Kociba, R.J. & Sleight, S.D. (1971) Acute toxicologic and pathologic effects of *cis*-diamminedichloro-platinum (NSC-119875) in the male rat. *Cancer Chemother. Rep., Part 1, 55,* 1-8

Krakoff, I.H. (1979) Nephrotoxicity of *cis*-dichlorodiammineplatinum (II). *Cancer Treat. Rep., 63,* 1523-1525

Lange, R.C., Spencer, R.P. & Harder, H.C. (1972) Synthesis and distribution of a radiolabeled antitumor agent: cis-diamminedichloroplatinum(II). J. nuclear Med., 13, 328-330

Lazar, R., Conran, P.C. & Damjanov, I. (1979) Embryotoxicity and teratogenicity of cis-diamminedichloroplatinum. Experientia, 35, 647-648

Leopold, W.R., Miller, E.C. & Miller, J.A. (1979) Carcinogenicity of antitumor cis-platinum(II) coordination complexes in the mouse and rat. Cancer Res., 39, 913-918

LeRoy, A.F., Wehling, M.L., Sponseller, H.L., Friauf, W.S., Solomon, R.E., Dedrick, R.L., Litterst, C.L., Gram, T.E., Guarino, A.M. & Becker, D.A. (1977) Analysis of platinum in biological materials by flameless atomic absorption spectrophotometry. Biochem. Med., 18, 184-191

LeRoy, A.F., Lutz, R.J., Dedrick, R.L., Litterst, C.L. & Guarino, A.M. (1979) Pharmacokinetic study of cis-dichlorodiammineplatinum(II) (DDP) in the beagle dog: thermodynamic and kinetic behavior of DDP in a biologic milieu. Cancer Treat. Rep., 63, 59-71

Litterst, C.L., LeRoy, A.F. & Guarino, A.M. (1979) Disposition and distribution of platinum following parenteral administration of cis-dichlorodiammineplatinum(II) to animals. Cancer Treat. Rep., 63, 1485-1492

Meyne, J. & Lockhart, L.H. (1978) Cytogenetic effects of cis-platinum(II)diamminedichloride on human lymphocyte cultures. Mutat. Res., 58, 87-97

Monti-Bragadin, C., Tamaro, M. & Banfi, E. (1975) Mutagenic activity of platinum and ruthenium complexes. Chem.-biol. Interactions, 11, 469-472

O'Neill, J.P., Couch, D.B., Machanoff, R., San Sebastian, J.R., Brimer, P.A. & Hsie, A.W. (1977) A quantitative assay of mutation induction at the hypoxanthine-guanine phosphoribosyl transferase locus in Chinese hamster ovary cells (CHO/HGPRT system): utilization with a variety of mutagenic agents. Mutat. Res., 45, 103-109

Piel, I.J. & Perlia, C.P. (1975) Phase II study of cis-dichlorodiammineplatinum(II) (NSC-119875) in combination with cyclophosphamide (NSC-26271) in the treatment of human malignancies. Cancer Chemother. Rep., 59, 995-999

Piel, I.J., Meyer, D., Perlia, C.P. & Wolfe, V.I. (1974) Effects of cis-diamminedichloroplatinum (NSC-119875) on hearing function in man. Cancer Chemother. Rep., 58, 871-875

Prestayko, A.W., D'Aoust, J.C., Issell, B.F. & Crooke, S.T. (1979) Cisplatin (cis-diamminedichloroplatinum II). Cancer Treat. Rev., 6, 17-39

Pritchard, J.D., Mavligit, G.M., Benjamin, R.S., Patt, Y.Z., Calvo, D.B., Hall, S.W., Bodey, G.P. & Wallace, S. (1979) Regression of regionally confined melanoma with intra-arterial cis-dichlorodiammineplatinum-(II). Cancer Chemother. Rep., 63, 555-558

Rainey, J.M. & Alberts, D.S. (1978) Safe, rapid administration schedule for cis-platinum-mannitol. Med. paediatr. Oncol., 4, 371-375

Repta, A.J., Long, D.F. & Hincal, A.A. (1979) *cis*-Dichlorodiammineplatinium (II) stability in aqueous vehicles. *Cancer Treat. Rep., 63,* 229-230

Roberts, J.J. (1974) Bacterial, viral and tissue culture studies on neutral platinum complexes. *Recent Results Cancer Res., 48,* 79-97

Robins, A.B. (1974) Interactions with biomacromolecules. *Recent Results Cancer Res., 48,* 63-78

Ross, D.A. & Gale, G.R. (1979) Reduction of the renal toxicity of *cis*-dichlorodiammineplatinum(II) by probenecid. *Cancer Treat. Rep., 63,* 781-787

Rossof, A.H., Slayton, R.E. & Perlia, C.P. (1972) Preliminary clinical experience with *cis*-diamminedi-chloroplatinum (II) (NSC 119875, CACP). *Cancer, 30,* 1451-1456

Rozencweig, M., Von Hoff, D.D., Slavik, M. & Muggia, F.M. (1977) *cis*-Diamminedichloroplatinum(II). A new anticancer drug. *Ann. intern. Med., 86,* 803-812

Schaeppi, U., Heyman, I.A., Fleischman, R.W., Rosenkrantz, H., Ilievski, V., Phelan, R., Cooney, D.A. & Davis, R.D. (1973) *cis*-Dichlorodiammineplatinum(II) (NSC-119-875): preclinical toxicologic evalua-tion of intravenous injection in dogs, monkeys and mice. *Toxicol. appl. Pharmacol., 25,* 230-241

Schilsky, R.L., Anderson, T. & Weiss, R.B. (1979) Hypomagnesemia and renal magnesium wasting in patients receiving *cis*-diamminedichloroplatinum II (DDP) (Abstract no. C-261). *Proc. Am. Soc. clin. Oncol., 20,* 354

Taylor, R.T., Carver, J.H., Hanna, M.L. & Wandres, D.L. (1979) Platinum-induced mutations to 8-aza-guanine resistance in Chinese hamster ovary cells. *Mutat. Res., 67,* 65-80

Thomson, A.J. (1974) The interactions of platinum compounds with biological molecules. *Recent Results Cancer Res., 48,* 38-62

Turnbull, D., Popescu, N.C., DiPaolo, J.A. & Myhr, B.C. (1979) *cis*-Platinum(II) diamine dichloride causes mutation, transformation, and sister-chromatid exchanges in cultured mammalian cells. *Mutat. Res., 66,* 267-275

Vermorken, J.B., van der Vijgh, W.J.F. & Pinedo, H.M. (1980a) Pharmacokinetic evidence for an entero-hepatic circulation in a patient treated with *cis*-dichlorodiammineplatinum (II). *Res. Commun. chem. Pathol. Pharmacol., 28,* 319-328

Vermoken, J.B., van der Vijgh, W.J.F., McVie, J.G. & Pinedo, H.M. (1980b) Some new pharmacokinetic aspects of *cis* diammine dichloroplatinum (DDP) (Abstract no. C-77). *Proc. Am. Soc. clin. Oncol., 21,* 338

Vogl, S.E., Zaravinos, T. & Kaplan, B.H. (1980) Toxicity of *cis*-diamminedichloroplatinum II given in a two-hour outpatient regimen of diuresis and hydration. *Cancer, 45,* 11-15

Von Hoff, D.D., Slavik, M. & Muggia, F.M. (1976) Allergic reactions to cisplatinum. *Lancet, i,* 90

Von Hoff, D.D., Schilsky, R., Reichert, C.M., Reddick, R.L., Rozencweig, M., Young, R.C. & Muggia, F.M. (1979) Toxic effects of *cis*-dichlorodiammineplatinum (II) in man. *Cancer Treat. Rep., 63,* 1527-1531

Wiencke, J.K., Cervenka, J. & Paulus, H. (1979) Mutagenic activity of anticancer agent *cis*-dichlorodiammine platinum-II. *Mutat. Res., 68,* 69-77

Zwelling, L.A., Bradley, M.O., Sharkey, N.A., Anderson, T. & Kohn, K.W. (1979) Mutagenicity, cytotoxicity and DNA crosslinking in V79 Chinese hamster cells treated with *cis*- and *trans*-Pt(II) diamminedichloride. *Mutat. Res., 67,* 271-280

This substance was considered by a previous Working Group, in April 1975 (IARC, 1975). Since that time new data have become available, and these have been incorporated into the monograph and taken into consideration in the present evaluation.

1. CHEMICAL AND PHYSICAL DATA

1.1 Synonyms and trade names

Chem. Abstr. Services Reg. No.: 6055-19-2; anhydrous form, 50-18-0

Chem. Abstr. Name: 2*H*-1,3,2-Oxazaphosphorin-2-amine, *N,N*-bis(2-chloroethyl)-tetrahydro-, 2-oxide monohydrate

IUPAC Systematic Name: 2-[Bis(2-chloroethyl)amino] tetrahydro-2*H*-1,3,2-oxazaphosphorine 2-oxide monohydrate

Synonyms: 2-[Bis(*β*-chloroethyl)amino]-1-oxa-3-aza-2-phosphacyclohexan-2-oxide monohydrate; 1-bis(2-chloroethyl)amino-1-oxo-2-aza-5-oxaphosphoridin monohydrate; *N-N*-bis(2-chloroethyl)-*N'*-(3-hydroxypropyl)phosphorodiamidic acid intramolecular ester monohydrate; bis(2-chloroethyl)phosphamide cyclic propanolamide ester monohydrate; bis(2-chloroethyl)phosphoramide cyclic propanolamide ester monohydrate; *N-N*-bis(2-chloroethyl)-*N'-O*-propylenephosphoric acid ester diamide monohydrate; *N,N*-bis(*β*-chloroethyl)-*N',O*-propylenephosphoric acid ester diamide monohydrate; *N,N*-bis(*β*-chloroethyl)-*N',O*-trimethylenephosphoric acid ester diamide monohydrate; CP monohydrate; cyclophosphamid monohydrate; 2-[di(2-chloroethyl)amino]-1-oxa-3-aza-2-phosphacyclohexane 2-oxide monohydrate

Trade names: Asta B 518; B 518; B 518-Asta; Ciclofosfamide; Clafen; Claphene; Cyclophospham; Cyclophosphan; Cyclophosphane; Cytophosphan; Cytoxan; Endoxan; Endoxana; Endoxan-ASTA; Enduxan; Genoxal; Mitoxan; NSC 26271; Procytox; Sendoxan; Syklofosfamid; Zytoxan

1.2 Structural and molecular formulae and molecular weight

*2 optical isomers

$$C_7H_{15}Cl_2N_2O_2P.H_2O$$ Mol. wt: 279.1

1.3 Chemical and physical properties of the pure substance

From Wade (1977) or Windholz (1976)

(a) *Description:*   Fine, white, odourless or almost odourless, crystalline powder with a slightly bitter tase

(b) *Melting-point:* 41-45°C (Windholz, 1976), 49.5-53°C (Wade, 1977)

(c) *Solubility:*   Soluble in water (1 in 25) and ethanol (1 in 1); slightly soluble in benzene, ethylene glycol, carbon tetrachloride and dioxane; sparingly soluble in diethyl ether and acetone

(d) *Stability:* Sensitive to oxidation, moisture and light

1.4 Technical products and impurities

Various national and international pharmacopoeias give specifications for the purity of cyclophosphamide in pharmaceutical products. For example, it is available in the US as a USP grade measured as containing 95.0 - 105.0% active ingredient calculated as the mono-hydrate, 5.7 - 6.8% max. water content, 0.002% max. heavy metals, and producing an aqueous solution (1 in 100) at pH 3.9 - 7.1. It is also available as 25 and 50 mg tablets measured as containing 90.0 - 110.0% of the stated amount of anhydrous cyclophospha-mide, and in vials for injection in amounts of 100, 200 or 500 mg measured as containing 90.0 - 110.0% of the stated amount of anhydrous cyclophosphamide (Wade, 1977; US Pharmacopeial Convention, Inc., 1980).

In Europe, cyclophosphamide is available in tablets, in crystalline powder form and in vials for injection in the same amounts as in the US (Wade, 1977).

In Japan, cyclophosphamide is available as tablets containing 50 mg.

2. PRODUCTION, USE, OCCURRENCE AND ANALYSIS

2.1 Production and use

(a) Production

Synthesis of cyclophosphamide was first reported by Arnold & Bourseaux (1958) by treating N,N-bis(β-chloroethyl)phosphamide dichloride with propanolamine in the presence of triethylamine and dioxane (see IARC, 1976). It is not known whether this is the method used for commercial production.

Cyclophosphamide is produced by one company each in the Federal Republic of Germany, the UK and Finland. It is not produced in the US, and no data were available on the quantities imported. Cyclophosphamide is not produced in Japan. It was first used there in 1962; imports in 1978 amounted to 327 kg.

(b) Use

Cyclophosphamide is used in human medicine as an antineoplastic agent in a variety of applications. It is administered by both the oral and parenteral routes in the treatment of Hodgkin's disease and non-Hodgkin's lymphoma, particularly in combination with a corticosteroid and vincristine (Anon., 1977). It is also used in the treatment of chronic lymphocytic leukaemia, chronic granulocytic leukaemia, acute myelogenous and monoblastic leukaemia and acute lymphoblastic leukaemia in children. Cyclophosphamide is also used in the treatment of the following neoplastic diseases: multiple myeloma, mycosis fungoides, neuroblastoma, adenocarcinoma of the ovary, retinoblastoma, carcinoma of the breast and certain malignant neoplasms of the lung. It is also used for conditioning patients for bone-marrow transplantation (Harvey, 1975; Wade, 1977; Baker, 1980).

Cyclophosphamide is a potent immunosuppressive agent and is used to prevent rejection episodes following renal, hepatic and cardiac homotransplantation and in non-neoplastic disorders where there is altered immune reactivity, such as Wegener's granulomatosis, rheumatoid arthritis, the nephrotic syndrome in children, autoimmune ocular diseases, etc. (Goodman & Gilman, 1975).

The usual range of intravenous doses for cancer patients with no haematological deficiency is 10 - 15 mg/kg bw repeated thrice weekly. When therapy is given orally, the dose is 1 - 5 mg/kg bw per day, depending upon the patient's tolerance. I.v. doses of 144 - 270 mg/kg bw have been given over 4 days to condition patients for bone-marrow transplantation (Wade, 1977; Mills & Roberts, 1979; Baker, 1980).

Cyclophosphamide has been used in veterinary practice for fleecing sheep (Windholz, 1976).

2.2 Occurrence

Cyclophosphamide is not known to be produced in Nature.

2.3 Analysis

Typical methods of analysis for cyclophosphamide in various matrices are summarized in Table 1.

Table 1. Methods for the analysis of cyclophosphamide

Sample matrix	Sample preparation	Assay procedure[a]	Reference
Formulations	Add sample to phosphate buffer; filter; heat; dilute with water	HPLC-UV	Kensler et al. (1979)
	Dissolve sample in water; add methyl stearate in chloroform (as an internal standard) and sodium hydroxide solution; mix	GC-FID	US Pharmacopeial Convention, Inc. (1980)
Blood and urine	Add isophosphamide in diethyl ether (as an internal standard), saturated sodium bicarbonate solution and sodium chloride; mix; extract with diethyl ether; evaporate; add ethyl acetate and trifluoroacetic anhydride	GC-NPD	Whiting et al. (1978)
	Inject labelled cyclophosphamide; extract with dichloromethane; add benzyl mercaptan and trichloroacetic acid	TLC-SS	Wagner et al. (1977)

[a]Abbreviations: HPLC-UV, high-performance liquid chromatography with ultra-violet detection; GC-FID, gas chromatography with flame ionization detection; GC-NPD, gas chromatography with nitrogen phosphorous detection; TLC-SS, thin-layer chromatography with scintillation spectrometry

3. BIOLOGICAL DATA RELEVANT TO THE EVALUATION
OF CARCINOGENIC RISK TO HUMANS

3.1 Carcinogenicity studies in animals

(a)   Oral administration

Rat: Groups of 40 female and 40 male outbred Sprague-Dawley rats, about 100 days old, received cyclophosphamide in drinking-water or were untreated.   Doses of 2.5, 1.25, 0.63 or 0.31 mg/kg bw were administered 5 times a week for life; animals were observed until death or killed when moribund.   The median survival times (MST) for untreated animals were 759 days for males and 985 days for females; in the group treated with 2.5 mg/kg bw, the MSTs were 638 and 642 days, respectively; in the group treated with 1.25 mg/kg bw, they were 646 and 720 days, respectively; in the group that received 0.63 mg/kg bw, they were 808 and 889 days, respectively; and in animals treated with 0.31 mg/kg bw, they were 906 and 934 days, respectively.   Malignant tumours occurred in 4/38 (11%) male and in 5/34 (15%) female controls; in 13/31 (42%) males and in 9/27 (33%) females that received 2.5 mg/kg bw; in 15/35 (43%) males and 11/33 (33%) females that received 1.25 mg/kg bw; in 14/36 (39%) males and 13/37 (35%) females that received 0.63 mg/kg bw; and in 11/34 (32%) males and 11/37 (30%) females given 0.31 mg/kg bw. In the groups that received the three higher doses, cyclophosphamide proved to be carcinogenic ($P < 0.05$). Using an age-standardization method, a log-linear dose-response relationship of the overall carcinogenicity was observed, after eliminating biases due to mortality.   In 97 treated rats (53 males and 44 females), a total of 115 malignant tumours were found in a wide spectrum of organs: 16 male and 1 female treated rats developed transitional-cell carcinomas of the urinary bladder; a further 18 males and 10 females had bladder papillomas.   No carcinomas of the urinary bladder were observed in controls; only 1 female showed a papilloma.   The difference in the number of urinary bladder neoplasms was sex-related, being significantly greater in males than in females ($P < 0.05$). For treated rats, an increased risk of developing tumours of the haematopoietic tissues was also calculated; thus, there were 19/270 (7%) *versus* 0/72 in controls.   Neurogenic sarcomas arising from the peripheral nerves occurred in 19/270 (7%) treated rats *versus* 1/72 (1.4%) controls (Schmähl & Habs, 1979). [The Working Group wished to draw attention to two conclusions that emerged from the experimental data: 1) doses that produced carcinogenic effects in animals were in some studies lower on a mg/kg bw basis than therapeutic doses; 2) the organ-specific effect of cyclophosphamide on the bladder is the same in animals and in humans.   These statements are not intended to provide a basis for a quantitative risk evaluation with regard to humans.]

(b)   Subcutaneous and/or intramuscular administration

Mouse: Two groups of 17 and 21 female New Zealand Black/New Zealand White (NZB/NZW) hybrid mice, mean age 7 - 9 weeks, were given daily s.c. injections of 5.7 and 16 mg/kg bw cyclophosphamide, respectively. A group of 15 females (mean age, 11 weeks) were given the solvent only (0.1 ml of isotonic saline).   NZB/NZW mice spontaneously develop antinuclear antibodies and immune complex glomerulonephritis and thus serve as models of systemic lupus erythematosus.   Animals were observed for life, or killed when moribund or when tumours developed.   Mean age at death was 46 weeks in controls, 59 weeks in mice treated with 16 mg/kg bw for 65 weeks and 80 weeks for mice treated with 5.7 mg/kg bw for 96 weeks. Total doses of cyclophosphamide in the high-dose group varied between 158 and 218 mg/kg bw. None of 13 controls developed a neoplasm, and they died of vasculitis and severe proliferative glomerulonephritis. Neoplasms occurred in 17/19 mice that could be evaluated and that received 16 mg/kg bw and in 15/15 mice that could be evaluated and that received 5.7 mg/kg/bw; 8 (42%) and 11 (73%) in the two groups, respectively, had multiple neoplasms.   The neoplasms were mostly mammary carcinomas (16 in the high-dose group and 5 in the low-dose group).   Other neoplasms specified included lymphomas, pulmonary adenomas and sarcomas.   The authors stated that early deaths in mice treated with the high dose reflected premature appearance of neoplasms and that earlier appearance of tumours in such mice, as compared with animals that received the low dose, supports the concept that cyclophosphamide has oncogenic properties and not only increases survival times (Walker & Anver, 1979).   [No age-standardized comparison of tumour incidences was carried out.   The Working Group noted that in the absence of age-adjusted comparisons, early death of NZB/NZW hybrid strain mice from autoimmune disease precluded direct comparison with treated mice.]

Two groups of 10 male and 10 female 4 - 24-week-old NZB/NZW hybrid mice were given daily s.c. injections of 1 mg/kg bw or 8 mg/kg bw cyclophosphamide in 0.1 ml saline for up to 93 weeks; 20 males and 20 females were injected with saline alone and served as controls.   Fifty percent of female controls had died by the 31st week of the study, compared with 41 and 60 weeks for those given the low and high dose levels. Fifty percent of male controls had died by 57 weeks, compared with 71 and 80 weeks for the treated animals.   Tumours were observed in treated males after 60 weeks of treatment and in females after 40 weeks.   Eight males and 9 females given the highest dose level developed neoplasms, including 3 generalized lymphoreticular neoplasms in males and 3 in females as well as a poorly differentiated sarcoma.   Three squamous-cell carcinomas occurred at the site of injection in females. Pulmonary adenomas were also observed in 3 male and 1 female mice.   Of animals given the low dose level, 3 males and 1 female developed neoplasms. Among controls 2 male and 1 female mice had reticulum-cell sarcomas (Walker & Bole, 1973a,b).   In a similar experiment, 6/10 females treated with the high dose developed neoplasms, mainly lymphoreticular, after 36 - 64 weeks of treatment, compared with 0/16 controls.   The average lifespans were 67 weeks in treated animals and 48 weeks in controls (Walker & Bole, 1971). [The Working Group noted that in the absence of age-adjusted comparisons, early death of NZB/NZW hybrid strain mice from autoimmune disease precluded direct comparison with treated animals.]

A group of 50 female NMRI mice, 65 days old, received 52 weekly s.c. injections of 26 mg/kg bw (7% of LD_{50}) cyclophosphamide (total dose, 1352 mg/kg bw); another group of 50 females served as controls. The average lifespan of treated and control animals was 630 ± 130 days. In the control group, 3/46 (6%) mice developed stem-cell leukaemia, and no other malignant tumour was observed. Of the treated mice, 28/46 (61%) developed malignant tumours: 3 leukaemias, 12 mammary carcinomas and 1 other mammary tumour, 4 ovarian carcinomas, 1 fibrosarcoma of the thorax, 1 skin carcinoma, 2 sarcomas at the injection site and 4 lung tumours (Schmähl & Osswald, 1970). [$P < 0.001$.]

(c)   Intraperitoneal administration

Mouse: Four groups of 15 male and 15 female A/J mice, 4 - 6 weeks old, were given i.p. injections of cyclophosphamide in water 3 times a week for 4 weeks (total doses, 420, 135, 34 and 8 mg/kg bw). Of 165 male and 195 female controls injected with water only, 37% of male and 27% of female survivors developed lung tumours within 39 weeks, with 0.48 and 0.29 tumours per mouse. After 39 weeks, 4/30, 27/30, 26/30 and 30/30 animals were still alive in the respective dose groups. Among surviving animals, the numbers with lung neoplasms were 2/4 (2.5 tumours/mouse), 20/27 (74%; 1.3 tumours/mouse), 11/26 (42%; 0.6 tumour/mouse) and 12/30 (40%; 0.4 tumour/mouse), respectively (Shimkin *et al.*, 1966). [The incidence of lung tumours in treated mice was significantly greater than that in controls only for those given the second highest dose level ($P < 0.001$).]

A group of 29 dd mice and a group of 25 A mice of both sexes, 4 - 5 weeks old, received i.p. injections of 5 mg/kg bw cyclophosphamide in saline twice weekly for 15 successive weeks; 20 and 16 control mice of each strain were injected with isotonic saline only. All mice were observed until death. Neoplasms developed in various organs in 12/22 dd mice that survived more than 48 weeks after the beginning of the treatment; these occurred predominantly in the lung, liver, testis and mammary gland. Three of 10 control dd mice that lived beyond the same period also had neoplasms. Neoplasms developed in 6/16 strain A mice that survived more than 42 weeks and included 6 in the lungs and 1 in the orbit. Two of 11 control A mice had neoplasms, both in the lung (Tokuoka, 1965).

Two groups, each of 25 male and 25 female outbred Swiss-Webster-derived mice, 6 weeks old, were given i.p. injections of 12 or 25 mg/kg bw cyclophosphamide 3 times a week for 6 months. Animals that survived over 100 days were observed for up to 12 further months, at which time they were killed. Lung neoplasms occurred in 7/30 males combined from both treatment groups and in 10/35 females; bladder papillomas were found in 4/30 males. The incidences of the two tumour types were reported to be statistically greater than those in pooled controls (Weisburger et al., 1975). [The Working Group considered that the inadequate reporting of certain items, such as survival times, the amalgamation of various experimental groups and tumour types, as well as the lack of age-adjustment in the analyses precluded a complete evaluation of this study.]

Groups of 20 female BALB/c mice, 8 weeks old, were injected intraperitoneally with 200 mg/kg bw cyclophosphamide once, twice or four times in saline at week 0, at weeks 0 and 20, or at weeks 0, 10, 20 and 30 or remained untreated. All animals were observed for 55 weeks and then killed for histological examination; mice that died within 40 weeks were excluded from evaluation. The results reported are restricted to the liver and urinary bladder. No alteration in the liver was described in 17 untreated controls or in 14 mice treated once, in 14 mice treated twice or in 13 mice treated four times with cyclophosphamide. No alteration in the urinary bladder was noted in controls; no vesicular calculus was observed in any of the mice. Diffuse hyperplasia was observed in 8/14 (57%) animals treated once, in 11/14 (79%) animals treated twice and in 9/13 (69%) animals treated four times. Papillary epithelial hyperplasia was described in 5 (36%), 5 (36%) and 4 (31%) animals treated once, twice and four times, respectively. Thus, no clear dose-response relationship was observed. The incidences of histological changes recorded were significantly greater in the combined groups of treated animals than in controls (P < 0.05). No carcinoma of the urinary bladder was noted (Yoshida et al., 1979). [The Working Group noted that the study was of short duration and that results on only two organs were reported.]

Rat: Two groups, each of 25 male and 25 - 28 female Charles River CD rats, 6 weeks old, were given i.p. injections of 5 or 10 mg/kg bw cyclophosphamide 3 times a week for 6 months. Animals that survived over 100 days were observed for 12 further months, at which time they were killed. Mammary carcinomas occurred in 9/53 females combined from both treatment groups and in 1/50 males, and mammary adenomas occurred in 24/53 females. The incidence of adenocarcinomas in control females was 13/181; the incidences of the two mammary tumour types were reported to be increased to a statistically significant extent over those in pooled female controls (Weisburger et al., 1975). [The Working Group considered that the inadequate reporting of certain items, such as survival times, the amalgamation of various experimental groups and tumour types, as well as the lack of age-adjustment in the analyses precluded a complete evaluation of this study.]

In a study reported as an abstract, a group of 10-week-old male Fischer rats (number not specified) were given i.p. injections of 10 mg/kg bw cyclophosphamide twice a week for an unspecified duration. Of 19 rats examined for lesions of the urinary bladder, only 2 survived more than 64 weeks of age; most died of haemorrhagic cystitis. One rat had a bladder papilloma, another 2 had carcinomas in situ, and 7 had severe epithelial dysplasia of the mucosa. Hyperplastic epithelial lesions were common, so that only 1 animal showed a normal epithelium (Cohen et al., 1979). [No information was given on median life expectancy or induction time of the observed lesions.]

(d)   Intravenous administration

Rat: An increased incidence of benign and malignant neoplasms was reported in 40 male BR 46 rats, 3 months old, given once weekly i.v. injections of 15 mg/kg bw (7% of LD_{50}) cyclophosphamide (total dose, 750 mg/kg bw). The average time for induction of tumours was 18 months. Neoplasms (9 malignant and 5 benign) occurred at various sites in 14/26 (54%)   animals still alive at the time of appearance of the first tumour and included 6 sarcomas of the peritoneal cavity. One benign thymoma was found in 1/50 (2%) control animals at 26 months [P < 0.001] (Schmähl, 1967).

In two further experiments with male BR 46 rats, 65 control animals had incidences of 3/65 (5%) benign and 4/65 (6%) malignant tumours; and of 48 rats given 52 weekly i.v. injections of 13 mg/kg bw cyclophosphamide, 36 alive at the time of appearance of the first tumour had incidences of 4/36 (11%) benign and 6/36 (17%) malignant tumours [P > 0.05]. Of 96 rats given 5 doses of 33 mg/kg bw every 2 weeks, 66 still alive at the time of appearance of the first tumour had incidences of 5/66 (8%) benign and 16/66 (24%) malignant tumours [P < 0.01]. The average observation time of treated rats was 16 - 18 months and that of controls, 23 months (Schmähl & Osswald, 1970).

A group of 32 male Sprague-Dawley rats, 3 months old, received weekly i.v. injections of 13 mg/kg bw cyclophosphamide (total dose, 670 mg/kg bw). A group of 52 untreated rats served as controls. Malignant tumours developed in 14/32 treated rats within 510 ± 90 days: there were 3 reticulum-cell sarcomas, 6 haemangioendotheliomas in various organs, 1 neurogenic sarcoma of the mediastinum, 1 sarcoma of the heart and 1 leukaemia; 2 rats had 2 malignant tumours each: one had an osteosarcoma of the paranasal sinus and a pheochromocytoma, and the other had an angiosarcoma of the abdomen and a pheochromocytoma.   Of the controls, 6/52 developed malignant tumours within 670 ± 150 days: 3 reticulum-cell sarcomas, 1 pheochromocytoma, 1 haemangiosarcoma of the lung and 1 sarcoma of the kidney [P < 0.001.] (Schmähl, 1974).

(e)   Perinatal exposure

Mouse: Groups of 30 male and 30 female Charles River CD-1 mice were given i.p. injections of 0.8, 4.0 or 20.0 mg/kg bw cyclophosphamide in isotonic saline within 24 hours of birth and again at 3 and 6 days of age. Mice which died during the study or were sacrificed at 79 weeks were examined grossly and microscopically. Cyclophosphamide was neither leukaemogenic nor hepatocarcinogenic, but a few pulmonary adenomas were observed (Kelly *et al.*, 1974). [The occurrence of pulmonary adenomas may have been increased in the group given 4 mg/kg bw, but the statistical analysis did not permit evaluation of this result.]

(f)   Other experimental systems

Pre- and post-natal exposure: A group of pregnant *mice*, comprised of animals of two inbred strains (XVII/Bln and AWD Dresden), were given i.p. doses of 25 mg/kg bw cyclophosphamide every 2 weeks for 60 weeks starting on day 14 of pregnancy; the maximum survival was 2 years (total dose, 750 mg/kg bw). Five hepatomas, 12 lung carcinomas and 1 skin carcinoma occurred among 33 mice still alive after 60 weeks, but no control was available for comparison. The offspring of the treated mice were either treated with 25 mg/kg bw cyclophosphamide every 2 weeks (total dose, 750 mg/kg bw) or left untreated. Of treated male offspring, 16 mice survived 60 weeks or more; 2 developed lung adenomas and 3, lung carcinomas. Of treated female offspring, 18 survived 60 weeks or more: 1 developed a lung adenoma; 4, lung carcinomas; 3, hepatomas; 1, a skin carcinoma; and 1, a skin sarcoma. In untreated offspring, lung adenomas occurred in 4/16 males and in 5/12 females that lived up to 18 months; 1 male and 2 females developed hepatomas; no lung carcinoma was observed. The historical incidences of lung adenomas and carcinomas in untreated female and male mice of these two strains were considered to be about 9% and 5% (Roschlau & Justus, 1971). [No statistical evaluation of these results was possible.]

Administration with known carcinogens: It was reported in an abstract that 2 groups of *rats* were fed with 0.2% *N*-[4-(5-nitro-2-furyl)-2-thiazolyl] formamide (FANFT) for 6 weeks. One group then received i.p. injections of 10 mg/kg bw cyclophosphamide twice a week [duration unspecified]; the other group subsequently received control diet for 6 weeks and then cyclophosphamide. Animals were examined only for lesions of the urinary bladder. In the first group, 3/18 rats developed papillary carcinomas; 2 rats showed a carcinoma *in situ*; and 8 rats developed epithelial dysplasia. In the second group, 1 papillary carcinoma was seen in 14 rats; 2 rats showed a carcinoma *in situ*; and 9 rats had dysplastic changes (Cohen *et al.*, 1979). [No information on survival times was given, and no information was available on the effects of FANFT alone.]

In a study in which female BALB/c *mice* were given i.p. injections of cyclophosphamide, it was also injected during feeding with 2 000 mg/kg of diet 2-naphthylamine. Neither cyclophosphamide nor 2-naphthylamine alone produced bladder cancer, but 1, 2 and 4 injections of 200 mg/kg bw cyclophosphamide produced a 27 - 35% incidence of transitional-cell carcinomas in 2-naphthylamine-fed mice (Yoshida *et al.*, 1979).

3.2 Other relevant biological data

(a) Experimental systems

Toxic effects

The single s.c. LD_{50} of cyclophosphamide was 370 mg/kg bw in mice (Schmähl & Osswald, 1970). The single i.v. LD_{50} was 160 mg/kg bw in rats, 400 mg/kg bw in guinea-pigs, 130 mg/kg bw in rabbits and 40 mg/kg bw in dogs. The single oral LD_{50} was 180 mg/kg bw in rats (Brock & Wilmanns, 1958) and about 400 mg/kg bw by a single i.p. injection in female rats bearing the Walker tumour (Connors et al., 1970). The i.p. LD_{50} in male mice was 360 mg/kg bw (Greco et al., 1979). The i.v. LD_{10} in mice was 310 mg/kg bw (Takamizawa et al., 1974).

The toxicity of cyclophosphamide may be reduced by prior treatment with other alkylating agents and vice versa (Millar et al., 1978). Agents that affect drug-metabolizing enzymes may also alter the cytotoxicity of cyclophosphamide (Hart & Adamson, 1969; Sladek, 1971; Ohira et al., 1974; Alberts et al., 1978).

In mice, rats and dogs the predominant haematologic effect was leucopenia; some depression of thrombocytes was also noted (Wheeler et al., 1962). Prolonged treatment of rodents with cyclophosphamide has produced pathological structural changes in a variety of organs, including lung, gut, pancreas and liver (Jáskiewicz, 1979; Mansi et al., 1979; Stoichkova et al., 1979), although in another experiment little damage was observed in liver even after prolonged administration (Hegewald & Bärenwald, 1972). In rats, cyclophosphamide given orally decreases mitosis in crypts, decreases the height of the villi and causes degeneration of the intestinal mucosa (Habibullah et al., 1979).

A single i.p. dose of cyclophosphamide caused marked necrosis of the bladder and of the renal tubular and renal pelvic epithelium in mice, rats and dogs (Philips et al., 1961; Koss, 1967; Campobasso & Berrino, 1972). It is likely that this bladder toxicity is due to the formation of acrolein from metabolism of cyclophosphamide (Brock et al., 1979a; Cox, 1979): it can be prevented by the use of agents that react with acrolein (e.g., 2-mercapto-ethane sodium sulphonate or N-acetyl-L-cysteine) (Brock et al., 1979a,b; Cox & Abel, 1979).

In an investigation of the effects of cyclophosphamide on regenerating liver parenchyma, it induced abnormal mitoses and atypical hepatic nuclei when administered to rats immediately after partial hepatectomy (Mietkiewski et al., 1973).

Effects on reproduction and prenatal toxicity

Cyclophosphamide is teratogenic in several species, including mice, rats, rabbits and chickens. It produces a variety of skeletal, soft tissue and other malformations and an increased number of resorptions; the type and frequency of malformations are strictly dose- and time-dependent (von Kreybig, 1965; Gibson & Becker, 1968; Singh, 1971; Kar *et al.*, 1974; Clavert *et al.*, 1978; Nawar *et al.*, 1979; Ujházy *et al.*, 1979).

More detailed studies of the teratogenic action of cyclophosphamide were made in rats with regard to eye anomalies (Singh & Sanyal, 1976) and skeletal defects (Schmitz *et al.*, 1972; Potturi *et al.*, 1975; Singh & Singh, 1975; Pabst & Wendler, 1976). It has been demonstrated that various kinds of embryo- and fetotoxic effects can also be induced at early gestational stages (Spielmann *et al.*, 1977; Spielmann & Eibs, 1978) and late in gestation (Stekar, 1973; Schmidt *et al.*, 1977).

Cyclophosphamide is also teratogenic in the rhesus monkey when given intra-muscularly for various periods between days 25 and 43 of pregnancy at doses ranging between 2.5 and 20 mg/kg bw. The induced abnormalities included cleft lip with cleft palate, exophthalmus, a marked underdevelopment of the midfacial bones and meningo-encephalocele (McClure *et al.*, 1979).

Abnormalities could be produced with 4-perhydroxycyclophosphamide and with 4-ketocyclophosphamide in differentiating embryonic tissues using organ culture tech-niques (Manson & Smith, 1976, 1977; Barrach *et al.*, 1978) or by adding cyclophosphamide together with a drug-metabolizing system to the organ culture medium (Barrach *et al.*, 1978; Fantel *et al.*, 1979; Manson *et al.*, 1980).

Placental transfer of ^{14}C-cyclophosphamide has been demonstrated in mice (Gibson & Becker, 1971); and a positive correlation between the alkylation of embryonic DNA and production of congenital abnormalities in mice has been reported by Murthy *et al.* (1973). A similar correlation has been found for nuclear-DNA-dependent RNA polymerases in rat embryos (Köhler & Merker, 1973).

Absorption, distribution, excretion and metabolism

In most species, cyclophosphamide is rapidly absorbed, metabolized and excreted. In rats, the specific activity in tissues is highest within 20 - 30 minutes following i.p. injection; up to 75% of the radioactivity is excreted within 5 - 8 hours (Mosienko & Pivnyuk, 1968; Chandramouli & Sivaramakrishnan, 1969; Talha *et al.*, 1980). Its metabolic fate has been studied in a number of species, including mice, rats, hamsters, rabbits, dogs, sheep and monkeys (Torkelson *et al.*, 1974; Schaumlöffel *et al.*, 1975; Voelcker *et al.*, 1976).

Cyclophosphamide is not cytotoxic *per se*, since it requires metabolic activation before it can act as an alkylating agent (Foley *et al.*, 1961; Brock & Hohorst, 1963; Cohen & Jao, 1970; Sladek, 1971). Activation takes place predominantly in the liver, although other tissues may be able to activate the drug (Brock & Hohorst, 1963; Kondo & Muragishi, 1970; Manson & Simons, 1979). Cyclophosphamide is a racemer, and stereoselective metabolism of the enantiomers of cyclophosphamide have been demonstrated in mice, rats and rabbits (Cox *et al.*, 1978).

The metabolic pathway of cyclophosphamide is shown in Figure 1. The 4-hydroxy derivative, which is the primary metabolite, exists in equilibrium with its ring-opened tautomer, aldophosphamide. Either metabolite can undergo further metabolism by mammalian enzymes to 4-ketocyclophosphamide, in the case of 4-hydroxycyclophosphamide, or to the propionic acid derivative, in the case of aldophosphamide. Both compounds have poor alkylating activity, are relatively nontoxic and represent major urinary metabolites of cyclophosphamide in a number of species. However, in the absence of enzymes to carry out the detoxification reaction, aldophosphamide can decompose to form phosphoramide mustard and acrolein (see IARC, 1979) (Colvin *et al.*, 1973; Connors *et al.*, 1974; Struck, 1974; Struck & Laster, 1975; Alarcon, 1976; Colvin, 1978; Domeyer & Sladek, 1980). An extensive study of cyclophosphamide analogues, some of which release acrolein but no phosphoramide mustard, and others which cannot undergo complete metabolism, has provided strong evidence that the metabolite of cyclophosphamide responsible for its antitumour activity is the phosphoramide mustard (Connors, 1978). The toxic side-effects of cyclophosphamide are probably due to phosphoramide mustard and acrolein, although it has been suggested that nor-nitrogen mustard may account for the renal damage sometimes observed (Colvin, 1978).

Reactive cyclophosphamide metabolites have been shown to cross-link nucleic acids both *in vivo* and *in vitro* (Wheeler, 1962; Roberts *et al.*, 1968).

Mutagenicity and other short-term tests

Cyclophosphamide gives positive results in several *in vitro* and *in vivo* short-term assays, as reported in a recent review (Hollstein *et al.*, 1979).

In the presence of a liver activation system, cyclophosphamide induced point mutations in the *Salmonella typhimurium* tester strains TA1535 (McCann *et al.*, 1975; Herbold & Buselmaier, 1976; Benedict *et al.*, 1977; Matheson *et al.*, 1978) and TA100 (McCann *et al.*, 1975; Seino *et al.*, 1978). The drug induced point mutations in several genes of *Escherichia coli* 343/113 after activation with mouse or rat liver fractions (Ellenberger & Mohn, 1975). In host-mediated assays, point mutations were induced in bacteria injected into mice (Propping *et al.*, 1972) and mitotic gene conversions in strain D4 of *Saccharomyces cerevisiae* in rats and mice (Fahrig, 1974).

Fig. 1. Metabolism of cyclophosphamide[a]

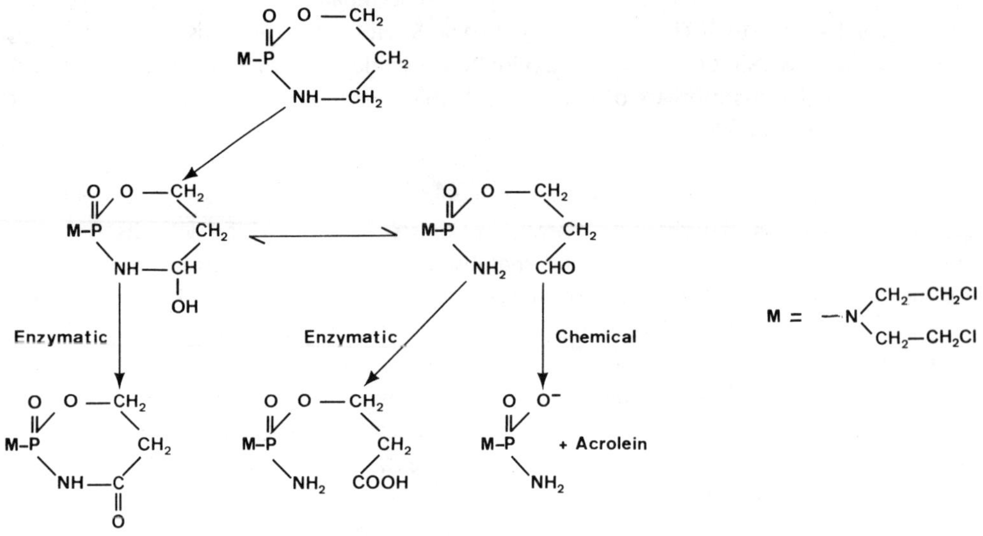

[a]From Connors (1979)

Cyclophosphamide was mutagenic in the mouse lymphoma cell line L5178Y following exogenous metabolic activation (Matheson et al., 1978; Clive et al., 1979). It induced recessive lethal mutations in the Muller-5 strain of Drosophila melanogaster (Bertram & Höhne, 1959) and produced significant dominant lethal mutations in mice and rats (Epstein et al., 1972; Machemer & Lorke, 1975a; Anderson et al., 1976, 1977a,b; Knudsen et al., 1977; Šrám & Zhurkov, 1977; Machemer & Lorke, 1978).

Cyclophosphamide also induced chromosomal aberrations in mice and hamster cells in vitro in the presence of an exogenous source of metabolic activation (Benedict et al., 1978) and in cultured human lymphocytes after exposure to the serum of C57BL/6 mice previously injected intraperitoneally with cyclophosphamide (Chebotarev et al., 1976). The drug caused a dose-dependent increase in chromatid translocations in human lymphocytes after activation by a perfusate of rat liver or by a crude homogenate of mouse liver (Madle et al., 1978). Chromosomal aberrations have also been produced in vivo in the bone marrow of mice (Röhrborn & Basler, 1977; Šrám & Zhurkov, 1977), rats (Payne et al., 1974;

Röhrborn & Basler, 1977) and Chinese hamsters (Schmid *et al.*, 1971; Röhrborn & Basler, 1977; Roszinsky-Köcher & Röhrborn, 1979). Cyclophosphamide induced chromosomal aberrations in the spermatogonia of Chinese hamsters (Machemer & Lorke, 1975b; Röhrborn & Basler, 1977) and mice (Rathenberg, 1975).

In *in vitro* assays, increases were found in the frequency of sister chromatid exchange in mouse and Syrian hamster cells (Benedict *et al.*, 1978); in Chinese hamster ovary cells (De Raat, 1977) following exposure to cyclophosphamide in the presence of an Aroclor-induced rat liver activation system; and in Chinese hamster cells cultured in diffusion chambers implanted in the peritoneal cavities of mice injected with cyclophosphamide (Sirianni & Huang, 1978). Similarly, increases in sister chromatid exchanges have been produced by cyclophosphamide *in vivo* in the bone-marrow of mice (Allen & Latt, 1976; Bauknecht *et al.*, 1977; Schreck *et al.*, 1979) and Chinese hamsters (Roszinsky-Köcher & Röhrborn, 1979), in the spermatogonia of mice (Allen & Latt, 1976) and in regenerating liver of mice (Schreck *et al.*, 1979). Increases in sister chromatid exchanges were also found in both fetal tissues and maternal bone marrow after an i.v. injection of cyclophosphamide to pregnant female mice on day 13 of gestation (Kram *et al.*, 1979). An increase in sister chromatid exchanges was induced *in vitro* in human diploid fibroblasts exposed to the urine of individuals undergoing cyclophosphamide treatment (Guerrero *et al.*, 1979).

Cyclophosphamide was positive in the micronucleus test in rats (Trzos *et al.*, 1978), Chinese hamsters (Röhrborn & Basler, 1977) and mice (Ioan *et al.*, 1977; Machemer & Lorke, 1978).

Cyclophosphamide has produced morphological transformation in C3H/10T½ clone 8 mouse cells in the presence of a supernatant fraction from Aroclor-induced rat liver (Benedict *et al.*, 1978). Morphological transformation was also observed in Syrian hamster embryo cultures following exposure to cyclophosphamide, with no exogenous source of activation (Pienta, 1980).

(b) Humans

Toxic effects

The predominant haematological effect of cyclophosphamide is leucopenia (Bergsagel *et al.*, 1968; Stott *et al.*, 1976). The reported frequency of cystitis in patients treated with cyclophosphamide ranges from 4 - 36% (Bennett, 1974); Plotz *et al.* (1979) reported haemorrhagic cystitis in 7/54 patients treated for rheumatoid arthritis or lupus erythematosus; and 25% of children treated for neoplasia with cyclophosphamide had fibrosis of the bladder wall (Johnson & Meadows, 1971). The bladder toxicity of cyclophosphamide is due to the formation of acrolein and may be prevented by the co-administration of 2-

mercaptoethane sodium sulphonate (Brock *et al.*, 1979b). Alopecia is common in patients receiving cyclophosphamide (Deshayes *et al.*, 1971). The drug has been reported to cause changes in the nucleoli of lymphocytes (Matějková, 1975); it has also been associated with water and sodium retention (Steele *et al.*, 1973), pulmonary fibrosis (reviewed by Patel *et al.*, 1976; Willson, 1978), visual blurring (Kende *et al.*, 1979) and pigmentation of the nails (Shah *et al.*, 1975). The causative role of cyclophosphamide in these effects is, however, not well established.

A fatal cardiomyopathy may result when very large doses of cyclophosphamide are given as conditioning for bone-marrow transplantation. Mills & Roberts (1979) described 2 cases and reported 9 others: doses, given over a few days, ranged from 144 - 270 mg/kg bw; deaths occurred 5 - 15 days after dosage and were associated with myocardial necrosis and haemorrhage and pericardial effusion.

Effects on reproduction and prenatal toxicity

Cyclophosphamide can cause sterility in people of either sex. It can damage the germinal cells in prepubertal, pubertal and adult males (Penso *et al.*, 1974; Gilmore *et al.*, 1979) and causes premature ovarian failure in females (Uldall *et al.*, 1972; Koyama *et al.*, 1977).

Limb reduction defects have been observed in two cases of infants exposed to cyclophosphamide *in utero*. One mother received 100 mg/day during her entire pregnancy: her infant had no big toes or their respective metatarsals and phalanges; the left fifth finger had a hypoplastic midphalange; the infant also had a prominent palatal groove (Greenberg & Tanaka, 1964). The other case was stillborn and had no toes and a single coronary artery. The mother had received 560 mg/day for 4 days followed by 100 then 150 mg/day for 2 months; she had also had multiple X-rays during the second to the fifth months of her pregnancy (Toledo *et al.*, 1971).

Absorption, distribution, excretion and metabolism

The distribution of cyclophosphamide in the body and its metabolism appear to be similar in man and animals (Brock *et al.*, 1971; Fenselau, 1976), with the formation of aldophosphamide (Fenselau *et al.*, 1977) and 4-hydroxycyclophosphamide as precursors to the reactive metabolite, phosphoramide mustard (Fenselau *et al.*, 1975). The rate of formation of aldophosphamide and 4-hydroxycyclophosphamide is, however, about 50-fold slower in man than in mouse, although their rates of elimination are similar (Wagner *et al.*, 1980).

After its i.v. injection, the drug is rapidly absorbed from the blood. In patients receiving 6.7 - 80 mg/kg bw per day of ring-labelled cyclophosphamide, radioactivity was distributed rapidly to all tissues: its half-life in the plasma was 6.5 hours. No radioactivity was found in the expired air or faeces (Bagley et al., 1973). Recovery of radioactivity in urine has been reported to be between 50 - 68%, mainly in the form of carboxyphosphamide and phosphoramide mustard (Bagley et al., 1973; Wagner et al., 1980); 10 - 40% of the drug was excreted unchanged (Cohen et al., 1971); and 56% of the reactive metabolites were bound to plasma proteins (Bagley et al., 1973).

The pharmacokinetic parameters of cyclophosphamide and its metabolites are independent of dose and do not change after 22 days' treatment (Mouridsen et al., 1976), although the half-life of the intact drug is reduced following 6 months' continuous treatment (D'Incalci et al., 1979) and increased by concurrent treatment with chloramphenicol (Faber et al., 1975). After oral administration, the first-pass hepatic metabolism extraction ratio has been estimated as 0.25 (Juma et al., 1979).

Cyclophosphamide is an asymmetrical molecule by virtue of the chiral phosphorus atom; however, there are only minor differences in the metabolism and pharmacokinetics of the (+)-enantiomer and its (-)-antipode (Jarman et al., 1979).

Cyclophosphamide and several of its metabolites have also been found in milk, sweat, saliva, cerebrospinal fluid and synovial fluid after i.v. infusion (Wiernik & Duncan, 1971; Duncan et al., 1973). The metabolism of intravenously administered ^{14}C-cyclophosphamide and the rate of excretion of its metabolites show large individual variations (Mouridsen et al., 1974).

Mutagenicity and chromosomal effects

There was an increase in the number of chromosomal aberrations in the peripheral blood lymphocytes of children treated with cyclophosphamide (3 - 5 mg daily for 6 - 8 months) for nonmalignant conditions (Dobos et al., 1974) and of patients with rheumatoid arthritis following cyclophosphamide treatment (Vormittag, 1974). Similar increases were observed in the lymphocytes of women with recurrent ovarian or uteral carcinoma 3 or 24 hours after an i.v. administration of 2.0 g (Morad & El Zawahri, 1977), and in the bone-marrow and lymph-node cells of patients with lymphogranulomatosis 24 -72 hours after a single dose of 400 mg cyclophosphamide (Neistadt et al., 1978).

Increased levels of sister chromatid exchange in peripheral blood lymphocytes have been observed in patients treated with cyclophosphamide. These have included patients with malignant lymphoma (Kurvink et al., 1978) and nephrotic syndrome (Torigoe, 1980), a patient with reticulosarcoma (Raposa, 1978), 3 patients with unspecified malignant tumours and 1 patient with acute glomerulonephritis (Musilová et al., 1979).

3.3 Case reports and epidemiological studies of carcinogenicity in humans

There have been at least 30 case reports of malignancy in patients treated with cyclo-phosphamide for nonmalignant disorders, mainly rheumatoid arthritis and chronic glomerulonephritis. These included 17 *acute nonlymphocytic leukaemias* (Cobau *et al.*, 1973; Love & Sowa, 1975; Cazalis *et al.*, 1976; Roberts & Bell, 1976; Seidenfeld *et al.*, 1976; Tchernia *et al.*, 1976; Chang & Geary, 1977; Kapadia & Kaplan, 1978; Mougeot-Martin *et al.*, 1978; Casciato & Scott, 1979; Hochberg & Shulman, 1978; Kahn *et al.*, 1979; Kapadia *et al.*, 1980; Sheibani *et al.*, 1980); 1 *chronic nonlymphocytic leukaemia* (Čáp & Mišíková, 1975); 1 *acute lymphocytic leukaemia* (Kuis *et al.*, 1976); 1 *chronic lymphocytic leukaemia* (Fosdick *et al.*, 1969); 2 *bladder cancers* (Dale & Smith, 1974; Chasko *et al.*, 1980); 1 *squamous-cell cancer of the skin* (Symington *et al.*, 1977); 3 *reticulum-cell sarcomas* (Worlledge *et al.*, 1968; Fosdick *et al.*, 1969; Tannenbaum & Schur, 1974); 1 *Hodgkin's disease* (Cameron *et al.*, 1974); 1 *melanoma* (Manny *et al.*, 1972); 2 *cerebral gliomas* (Starzl *et al.*, 1973; Cameron *et al.*, 1974); 1 *cervical cancer* (Bashour *et al.*, 1973); and 1 *pleural sarcoma* (Marks & Scholtz, 1977).

Of these, the following 10 cases involved use of other chemotherapeutic agents (other than prednisone) in addition to cyclophosphamide: 6 *acute nonlymphocytic leukaemias* (Cobau *et al.*, 1973; Cazalis *et al.*, 1976; Roberts & Bell, 1976; Seidenfeld *et al.*, 1976; Hochberg & Shulman, 1978; Sheibani *et al.*, 1980); 2 *bladder cancers* (Dale & Smith, 1974; Chasko *et al.*, 1980); 1 *reticulum-cell sarcoma* (Worlledge *et al.*, 1968); and 1 *melanoma* (Manny *et al.*, 1972).

In addition, the following 83 cases of second malignancy have been reported following cyclophosphamide therapy for malignant diseases: 17 *bladder cancers* (Worth, 1971; Rupprecht & Blessing, 1973; Dale & Smith, 1974; Ansell & Castro, 1975; Richtsmeier, 1975; Wall & Clausen, 1975; Weinstein *et al.*, 1975; West, 1976; Beyer-Boon *et al.*, 1978; Lenzin *et al.*, 1978; Pearson & Soloway, 1978); 56 *acute nonlymphocytic leuk-aemias* (Durant & Tassoni, 1967; Edwards & Zawadzki, 1967; Andersen & Videbaek, 1970; Sypkens Smit & Meyler, 1970; Osserman, 1971; Schaefer & Kanzler, 1972; Castro *et al.*, 1973; Davis *et al.*, 1973; Khaleeli *et al.*, 1973; Karchmer. *et al.*, 1974; Pariser, 1974; Rosner & Grünwald, 1975; Wall & Clausen, 1975; Baer & Wilkinson, 1976; Kapadia & Kaplan, 1976; West, 1976; Collins *et al.*, 1977; Ligorsky *et al.*, 1977; Preisler & Lyman, 1977; Rowley *et al.*, 1977; Smithson *et al.*, 1978; West, 1978; Casciato & Scott, 1979; Portugal *et al.*, 1979; Zarrabi *et al.*, 1979; Kapadia *et al.*, 1980); 1 *reti-culum-cell lymphoma* (Mundy & Baikie, 1973); 1 *squamous-cell carcinoma of the skin* (West, 1976); and 2 *plasma-cell reticulosarcomas* (Holt *et al.*, 1972; Holt & Robb-Smith, 1973).

Most of these cases involved exposure to other chemotherapeutic agents in addition to cyclophosphamide; only the following 23 cases occurred after treatment with cyclophosphamide alone: 12 *bladder cancers* (Worth, 1971; Dale & Smith, 1974; Ansell & Castro, 1975; Richtsmeier, 1975; Wall & Clausen, 1975; Weinstein *et al.*, 1975; West, 1976; Beyer-Boon *et al.*, 1978); 8 *acute nonlymphocytic leukaemias* (Andersen & Videbaek, 1970; Karchmer *et al.*, 1974; Wall & Clausen, 1975; West, 1976; Ligorsky *et al.*, 1977; Portugal *et al.*, 1979; Zarrabi *et al.*, 1979); 1 *reticulum-cell sarcoma* (Mundy & Baikie, 1973); and 2 *plasma-cell reticulosarcomas* (Holt *et al.*, 1972; Holt & Robb-Smith, 1973).

Kinlen and his colleagues (1979, 1981) investigated the incidence of cancer in 1349 non-transplant patients treated for at least 3 months with azathioprine, cyclophosphamide or chlorambucil for nonmalignant diseases, of whom 430 received cyclophosphamide. A significant excess of bladder cancer was found in association with use of cyclophosphamide (3 observed *versus* 0.29 expected), and 2 further cases occurred after the last follow-up date used in the analysis. An excess was recorded for non-Hodgkin's lymphoma (1 observed *versus* 0.10 expected), squamous-cell carcinoma of the skin (1 observed *versus* 0.11 expected) and other cancers (13 observed *versus* 5.86 expected).

Plotz *et al.* (1979) investigated the incidence of bladder cancer among 54 patients treated with cyclophosphamide for systemic lupus erythematosus or rheumatoid arthritis. Two cases (one in a patient who had haemorrhagic cystitis) were observed, compared with 0.02 expected.

Li *et al.* (1975) followed up 414 long-term survivors of childhood cancer for up to 20 years; 17 had been treated with cyclophosphamide as the only chemotherapeutic agent. Fifteen of the 414 children, all of whom had received radiation, subsequently developed new cancers, compared with 0.7 expected (P < 0.001); most appeared at irradiated sites and were attributed by the authors to radiation. One child who had received cyclophosphamide developed a rhabdomyosarcoma.

Reimer *et al.* (1977) studied 5455 women with ovarian cancer treated at centres where alkylating agents were used regularly and found 15 who later developed leukaemia (13 acute nonlymphocytic and 2 other), compared with 1.62 expected. Three of the women with acute nonlymphocytic leukaemia had received cyclophosphamide, two as the only chemotherapeutic agent. The total number of women who were at risk of developing leukaemia after receiving this drug was not stated.

Bergsagel *et al.* (1979) investigated the incidence of leukaemia in patients with myeloma treated with different combinations of melphalan, cyclophosphamide, BCNU and prednisone. An excess of acute nonlymphocytic leukaemia was found, with 14 cases observed compared with 0.07 expected; 9 cases were in patients who had received all 4 agents.

4. SUMMARY OF DATA REPORTED AND EVALUATION

4.1 Experimental data

Cyclophosphamide is carcinogenic in rats after its oral or intravenous administration, producing benign and malignant tumours at various sites, including the bladder. It is carcinogenic in mice following its subcutaneous injection, producing benign and malignant tumours at the site of injection and at distant sites. There was some evidence of its onco-genicity in mice and rats following intraperitoneal injection. The combined administration of cyclophosphamide intraperitoneally and of 2-naphthylamine orally to mice resulted in the induction of carcinomas of the bladder at doses of the compounds which, given indi-vidually, did not produce bladder cancer.

The teratogenic effects of cyclophosphamide are well established in many animal species. The drug can also be embryolethal at doses nontoxic to the mother.

Cyclophosphamide demonstrated mutagenic activity in several different assays (bacteria, yeast and mammalian cells *in vitro*, and *Drosophila* and mice *in vivo*). The agent also induced chromosomal aberrations in mammalian cells of several species *in vitro* and *in vivo*. Moreover, it induced morphological transformation of mammalian cells *in vitro*.

4.2 Human data

Cyclophosphamide has been widely used since the early 1950s in the treatment of malignant lymphoma, multiple myeloma, and cancers of the breast, ovary and lung. It has also been used in the treatment of certain chronic diseases, such as rheumatoid arthritis and chronic glomerulonephritis and other nonmalignant diseases.

Although two cases of limb reduction defects have been reported among the offspring of women treated with cyclophosphamide during pregnancy, no epidemiological data were available to the Working Group for assessing the embryotoxic risk to man. Increases in chromosomal aberrations and sister chromatid exchanges were seen in peripheral blood lymphocytes of patients treated with cyclophosphamide.

There is epidemiological evidence that cyclophosphamide increases the incidence of bladder cancer, and there is a suggestion that the incidence of other cancers may also be increased. There are also many cases reports of cancer, particularly bladder cancer and acute nonlymphocytic leukaemia, following cyclophosphamide therapy.

4.3 Evaluation

There is *sufficient evidence*[1] for the carcinogenicity of cyclophosphamide in mice and rats. There is *sufficient evidence*[2] that cyclophosphamide is carcinogenic in humans.

---

[1] See preamble, p. 18.

[2] See preamble, p. 17.

5. REFERENCES

Alarcon, R.A. (1976) Studies on the *in vivo* formation of acrolein: 3-hydroxypropylmercapturic acid as an index of cyclophosphamide (NSC-26271) activation. *Cancer Treat. Rep., 60,* 327-335

Alberts, D.S., Peng, Y.M., Chen, H.S. & Struck, R.F. (1978) Effect of phenobarbital on plasma levels of cyclophosphamide and its metabolites in the mouse. *Br. J. Cancer, 38,* 316-324

Allen, J.W. & Latt, S.A. (1976) *In vivo* BrdU-33258 Hoechst analysis of DNA replication kinetics and sister chromatid exchange formation in mouse somatic and meiotic cells. *Chromosoma, 58,* 325-340

Andersen, E. & Videbaek, A. (1970) Stem cell leukaemia in myelomatosis. *Scand. J. Haematol., 7,* 201-207

Anderson, D., McGregor, D.B. & Purchase, I.F.H. (1976) Dominant lethal studies with Paraquat and Diquat in male CD-1 mice. *Mutat. Res., 40,* 349-358

Anderson, D., Hodge, M.C.E. & Purchase, I.F.H. (1977a) Dominant lethal studies with the halogenated olefins vinyl chloride and vinylidene dichloride in male CD-1 mice. *Environ. Health Perspect., 21,* 71-78

Anderson, D., McGregor, D.B., Purchase, I.F.H., Hodge, M.C.E. & Cuthbert, J.A. (1977b) Dominant-lethal test results with known mutagens in two laboratories. *Mutat. Res., 43,* 231-246

Anon. (1977) *AMA Drug Evaluations,* 3rd ed., Littleton, MA, PSG Publishing Co., pp. 1112-1113

Ansell, I.D. & Castro, J.E. (1975) Carcinoma of the bladder complicating cyclophosphamide therapy. *Br. J. Urol., 47,* 413-418

Arnold, H. & Bourseaux, F. (1958) Synthesis and degradation of active cytostatic cyclic *N*-phosphamide esters of bis(β-chloroethyl)amine (Ger.). *Angew. Chem., 70,* 539-544

Baer, D. & Wilkinson, L.S. (1976) Daunomycin, adryamicin, and recall effect. *Ann. intern. Med., 85,* 259-260

Bagley, C.M., Jr, Bostick, F.W. & DeVita, V.T., Jr (1973) Clinical pharmacology of cyclophosphamide. *Cancer Res., 33,* 226-233

Baker, C.E., Jr, ed. (1980) *Physicians' Desk Reference,* 34th ed., Oradell, NJ, Medical Economics Co., pp. 1110-1111

Barrach, H.-J., Baumann, I. & Neubert, D. (1978) *The applicability of* in vitro *systems for the evaluation of the significance of pharmacokinetic parameters for the induction of an embryotoxic effect.* In: Neubert, D., Merker, H.-J., Nau, H. & Langman, J., eds, *Role of Pharmacokinetics in Prenatal and Perinatal Toxicology,* Stuttgart, Georg Thieme, pp. 323-336

Bashour, B.N., Mancer, K. & Rance, C.P. (1973) Malignant mixed Mullerian tumor of the cervix following cyclophosphamide therapy for nephrotic syndrome. *J. Pediatr., 82,* 292-293

Bauknecht, T., Vogel, W., Bayer, U. & Wild, D. (1977) Comparative *in vivo* mutagenicity testing by SCE and micronucleus induction in mouse bone marrow. *Hum. Genet., 35,* 299-307

Benedict, W.F., Baker, M.S., Haroun, L., Choi, E. & Ames, B.N. (1977) Mutagenicity of cancer chemo-therapeutic agents in the *Salmonella*/microsome test. *Cancer Res., 37,* 2209-2213

Benedict, W.F., Banerjee, A. & Venkatesan, N. (1978) Cyclophosphamide-induced oncogenic transforma-tion, chromosomal breakage, and sister chromatid exchange following microsomal activation. *Cancer Res., 38,* 2922-2924

Bennett, A.H. (1974) Cyclophosphamide and hemorrhagic cystitis. *J. Urol., 111,* 603-606

Bergsagel, D.E., Robertson, G.L. & Hasselback, R. (1968) Effect of cyclophosphamide on advanced lung cancer and the hematological toxicity of large, intermittent intravenous doses. *Can. med. Assoc. J., 98,* 532-538

Bergsagel, D.E., Bailey, A.J., Langley, G.R., MacDonald, R.N., White, D.F. & Miller, A.B. (1979) The chemotherapy of plasma-cell myeloma and the incidence of acute leukemia. *New Engl. J. Med., 301,* 743-748

Bertram, C. & Höhne, G. (1959) On the radiomimetic action of some cytostatic compounds in mutation studies on *Drosophila* (Ger.). *Strahlentherapie, 43,* 388-391

Beyer-Boon, M.E., de Voogt, H.J. & Schaberg, A. (1978) The effects of cyclophosphamide treatment on the epithelium and stroma of the urinary bladder. *Eur. J. Cancer, 14,* 1029-1035

Brock, N. & Hohorst, H.-J. (1963) On the activation of cyclophosphamide *in vivo* and *in vitro* (Ger.). *Arzneimittel-Forsch., 13,* 1021-1031

Brock, N. & Wilmanns, H. (1958) Action of a cyclic *N*-substituted phosphamide ester on the experimental production of tumours in rats (Ger.). *Dtsch. med. Wochenschr., 83,* 453-458

Brock, N., Gross, R., Hohorst, H.-J., Klein, H.O. & Schneider, B. (1971) Activation of cyclophosphamide in man and animals. *Cancer, 27,* 1512-1529

Brock, N., Stekar, J., Pohl, J., Niemeyer, U. & Scheffler, G. (1979a) Acrolein, the causative factor of urotoxic side-effects of cyclophosphamide, ifosfamide, trofosfamide and sufosfamide. *Arzneimittel-Forsch./Drug Res., 29,* 659-661

Brock, N., Stekar, J., Pohl, J. & Scheef, W. (1979b) Antidote against the urotoxic effects of the oxazaphos-phorine derivatives cyclophosphamide, ifosfamide and trofosfamide (Ger.). *Naturwissenschaften, 66,* 60-61

Cameron, J.S., Chantler, C., Ogg, C.S. & White, R.H.R. (1974) Long-term stability of remission in nephrotic syndrome after treatment with cyclophosphamide. *Br. med. J., iv,* 7-11

Campobasso, O. & Berrino, F. (1972) Early effects of cyclophosphamide on mouse bladder epithelium. *Pathol. Microbiol., 38,* 144-157

Čáp, J. & Mišíková, Ž. (1975) Chronic myelogenous leukaemia as a possible consequence of immunosuppressive treatment of nephrotic syndrome (Ger.). *Monatsschr. Kinderheilkd., 123,* 718-720

Casciato, D.A. & Scott, J.L. (1979) Acute leukemia following prolonged cytotoxic agent therapy. *Medicine, 58,* 32-47

Castro, G.A.M., Church, A., Pechet, L. & Synder, L.M. (1973) Leukemia after chemotherapy of Hodgkin's disease. *New Engl. J. Med., 289,* 103-104

Cazalis, P., Caroit, M., Zittoun, R., Kahn, M.-F. & de Sèze, S. (1976) A particular risk in long-term immunosuppressive treatment: a case of acute myelomonocytic leukaemia after treatment with chlorambucil for severe rheumatoid polyarthritis (Fr.). *Rev. Rhum., 43,* 431-435

Chandramouli, K. & Sivaramakrishnan, V.M. (1969) Radiation and radiomimetic agents. I. The distribution of P^{32}-labelled cyclophosphamide in albino rats and in humans. *Indian J. Cancer, 6,* 153-164

Chang, J. & Geary, C.G. (1977) Therapy-linked leukaemia. *Lancet, i,* 97

Chasko, S.B., Keuhnelian, J.G., Gutowski, W.T., III & Gray, G.F. (1980) Spindle cell cancer of bladder during cyclophosphamide therapy for Wegener's granulomatosis. *Am. J. surg. Pathol., 4,* 191-196

Chebotarev, A.N., Telegin, L.Y. & Derzhavets, E.M. (1976) Cytogenetic effects of cyclophosphamide in cultured human lymphocytes after its activation in mice (Russ.). *Genetika, 12,* 151-157

Clavert, J.M., Brun, B., Clavert, A. & Buck, P. (1978) Limb anomalies obtained with cyclophosphamide in rabbit embryos (Fr.). *Chir. Pédiatr., 19,* 205-207

Clive, D., Johnson, K.O., Spector, J.F.S., Batson, A.G. & Brown, M.M.M. (1979) Validation and characterization of the L5178Y/TK$^{+/-}$ mouse lymphoma mutagen assay system. *Mutat. Res., 59,* 61-108

Cobau, C.D., Sheon, R.P. & Kirsner, A.B. (1973) Immunosuppressive drugs and acute leukemia. *Ann. intern. Med., 79,* 131 - 132

Cohen, J.L. & Jao, J.Y. (1970) Enzymatic basis of cyclophosphamide activation by hepatic microsomes of the rat. *J. Pharmacol. exp. Ther., 174,* 206-210

Cohen, J.L., Jao, J.Y. & Jusko, W.J. (1971) Pharmacokinetics of cyclophosphamide in man. *Br. J. Pharmacol., 43,* 677-680

Cohen, S.M., Arai, M., Jacobs, J.B. & Friedell, G.H. (1979) Induction of papillary tumors and flat carcinoma-*in-situ* (CIS) of the urinary bladder by cyclophosphamide in male Fischer rats (Abstract). *Proc. Am. Assoc. Cancer Res., 20,* 231

Collins, A.J., Bloomfield, C.D., Peterson, B.A. & McKenna, R.W. (1977) Acute nonlymphocytic leukemia in patients with nodular lymphoma. *Cancer, 40,* 1748-1754

Colvin, M. (1978) *A review of the pharmacology and clinical use of cyclophosphamide.* In: Pinedo, H.M., ed., *Clinical Pharmacology of Anti-neoplastic Drugs,* Amsterdam, Elsevier/North-Holland Biomedical Press, pp. 245-261

Colvin, M., Padgett, C.A. & Fenselau, C. (1973) A biologically active metabolite of cyclophosphamide. *Cancer Res., 33,* 915-918

Connors, T.A. (1978) Antitumour drugs with latent activity. *Biochimie, 60,* 979-987

Connors, T.A. (1979) *Alkylating drugs, nitrosourea and dialkyltriazenes.* In: Pinedo, H.M., ed., *Cancer Chemotherapy 1979. The EORTC Cancer Chemotherapy Annual,* Amsterdam, Oxford, Excerpta Medica, pp. 25-55

Connors, T.A., Grover, P.L. & McLoughlin, A.M. (1970) Microsomal activation of cyclophosphamide *in vivo. Biochem. Pharmacol., 19,* 1533-1535

Connors, T.A., Cox, P.J., Farmer, P.B., Foster, A.B. & Jarman, M. (1974) Some studies of the active intermediates formed in the microsomal metabolism of cyclophosphamide and isophosphamide. *Biochem. Pharmacol., 23,* 115-129

Cox, P.J. (1979) Cyclophosphamide cystitis - identification of acrolein as the causative agent. *Biochem. Pharmacol., 28,* 2045-2049

Cox, P.J. & Abel, G. (1979) Cyclophosphamide-induced cystitis: its cause and possible clinical significance (Abstract). *Br. J. Cancer, 40,* 311

Cox, P.J., Farmer, P.B., Jarman, M., Kinas, R.W. & Stec, W.J. (1978) Stereoselectivity in the metabolism of the enantiomers of cyclophosphamide in mice, rats and rabbits. *Drug. Metab. Disposition, 6,* 617-622

Dale, G.A. & Smith, R.B. (1974) Transitional cell carcinoma of the bladder associated with cyclophosphamide. *J. Urol., 112,* 603-604

Davis, H.L., Jr, Prout, M.N., McKenna, P.J., Cole, D.R. & Korbitz, B.C. (1973) Acute leukemia complicating metastatic breast cancer. *Cancer, 31,* 543-546

De Raat, W.K. (1977) The induction of sister chromatid exchanges by cyclophosphamide in the presence of differently induced microsomal fractions of rat liver. *Chem.- biol. Interactions, 19,* 125-131

Deshayes, P., Rénier, J.-C., Bregeon, C. & Houdent, G. (1971) Incidents and accidents with immunosuppressive therapy for rheumatoid polyarthritis (Fr.). *Rev. Rhum., 38,* 797-806

D'Incalci, M., Bolis, G., Facchinetti, T., Mangioni, C., Morasca, L., Morazzoni, P. & Salmona, M. (1979) Decreased half life of cyclophosphamide in patients under continual treatment. *Eur. J. Cancer, 15,* 7-10

Dobos, M., Schuler, D. & Fekete, G. (1974) Cyclophosphamide-induced chromosomal aberrations in nontumorous patients. *Humangenetik, 22,* 221-227

Domeyer, B.E. & Sladek, N.E. (1980) Kinetics of cyclophosphamide biotransformation *in vivo. Cancer Res., 40,* 174-180

Duncan, J.H., Colvin, O.M. & Fenselau, C. (1973) Mass spectrometric study of the distribution of cyclophosphamide in humans. *Toxicol. appl. Pharmacol., 24,* 317-323

Durant, J.R. & Tassoni, E.M. (1967) Coexistent DiGuglielmo's leukemia and Hodgkin's disease. A case report with cytogenetic studies. *Am. J. med. Sci., 254,* 824-830

Edwards, G.A. & Zawadzki, Z.A. (1967) Extraosseus lesions in plasma cell myeloma. A report of six cases. *Am. J. Med., 43,* 194-205

Ellenberger, J. & Mohn, G. (1975) Mutagenic activity of cyclophosphamide, ifosfamide, and trofosfamide in different genes of *Escherichia coli* and *Salmonella typhimurium* after biotransformation through extracts of rodent liver. *Arch. Toxicol., 33,* 225-240

Epstein, S.S., Arnold, E., Andrea, J., Bass, W. & Bishop, Y. (1972) Detection of chemical mutagens by the dominant lethal assay in the mouse. *Toxicol. appl. Pharmacol., 23,* 288-325

Faber, O.K., Mouridsen, H.T. & Skovsted, L. (1975) The effect of chloramphenicol and sulphaphenazole on the biotransformation of cyclophosphamide in man. *Br. J. clin. Pharmacol., 2,* 281-285

Fahrig, R. (1974) Development of host-mediated mutagenicity tests. I. Differential response of yeast cells injected into the testes of rats and the peritoneum of mice and rats to mutagens. *Mutat. Res., 26,* 29-36

Fantel, A.G., Greenaway, J.C., Juchau, M.R. & Shepard, T.H. (1979) Teratogenic bioactivation of cyclophosphamide *in vitro. Life Sci., 25,* 67-72

Fenselau, C. (1976) Review of the metabolism and mode of action of cyclophosphamide. *J. Assoc. off. anal. Chem., 59,* 1028-1036

Fenselau, C., Kan, M.-N.N., Billets, S. & Colvin, M. (1975) Identification of phosphorodiamidic acid mustard as a human metabolite of cyclophosphamide. *Cancer Res., 35,* 1453-1457

Fenselau, C., Kan, M.-N.N., Rao, S.S., Myles, A., Friedman, O.M. & Colvin, M. (1977) Identification of aldophosphamide as a metabolite of cyclophosphamide *in vitro* and *in vivo* in humans. *Cancer Res., 37,* 2538-2543

Foley, G.E., Friedman, O.M. & Drolet, B.P. (1961) Studies on the mechanism of action of cytoxan. Evidence of activation *in vivo* and *in vitro. Cancer Res., 21,* 57-63

Fosdick, W.M., Parsons, J.L. & Hill, D.F. (1969) Long-term cyclophosphamide (CP) therapy in rheumatoid arthritis: a progress report, six years' experience. *Arthritis-Rheum., 12,* 663

Gibson, J.E. & Becker, B.A. (1968) The teratogenicity of cyclophosphamide in mice. *Cancer Res., 28,* 475-480

Gibson, J.E. & Becker, B.A. (1971) Effect of phenobarbital and SKF 525A on placental transfer of cyclophosphamide in mice. *J. Pharmacol. exp. Ther., 177,* 256-262

Gilmore, I.T., Cowan, R.E., Axon, A.T.R. & Thompson, R.P.H. (1979) Controlled trial of cyclophosphamide in active chronic hepatitis. *Br. med. J., ii,* 1120-1121

Goodman, L.S. & Gilman, A., eds (1975) *The Pharmacological Basis of Therapeutics,* 5th ed., New York, Macmillan, pp. 1262-1264

Greco, C., Corsi, A., Caputo, M., Cavallari, A. & Calabresi, F. (1979) Cyclophosphamide and iphosphamide against Lewis lung carcinoma: evaluation of toxic and therapeutic effects. *Tumori, 65,* 169-180

Greenberg, L.H. & Tanaka, K.R. (1964) Congenital anomalies probably induced by cyclophosphamide. *J. Am. med. Assoc., 188,* 423-426

Guerrero, R.R., Rounds, D.E. & Hall, T.C. (1979) Bioassay procedure for the detection of mutagenic metabolites in human urine with the use of sister chromatid exchange analysis. *J. natl Cancer Inst., 62,* 805-809

Habibullah, C.M., Chhuttani, P.N. & Sehgal, A.K. (1979) Effect of oral cyclophosphamide on the rat intestine. *Indian J. med. Sci., 33,* 180-184

Hart, L.G. & Adamson, R.H. (1969) Effect of microsomal enzyme modifiers on toxicity and therapeutic activity of cyclophosphamide in mice. *Arch. int. Pharmacodyn., 180,* 391-401

Harvey, S.C. (1975) *Antineoplastic and immunosuppressive drugs.* In: Osol, A., ed., *Remington's Pharmaceutical Sciences,* 15th ed., Easton, PA, Mack Publishing Co., p. 1077

Hegewald, G. & Bärenwald, G. (1972) Morphological changes in rat liver after long-term cyclophosphamide medication (Ger.). *Acta hepatogastroenterol., 19,* 85-90

Herbold, B. & Buselmaier, W. (1976) Comparative investigations with different bacterial strains (Abstract no. 32). *Mutat. Res., 38,* 118

Hochberg, M.C. & Shulman, L.E. (1978) Acute leukemia following cyclophosphamide therapy for Sjögren's syndrome. *Johns Hopkins med. J., 142,* 211-214

Hollstein, M., McCann, J., Angelosanto, F.A. & Nichols, W.W. (1979) Short-term tests for carcinogens and mutagens. *Mutat. Res., 65,* 133-226

Holt, J.M. & Robb-Smith, A.H.T. (1973) Multiple myeloma: development of plasma cell sarcoma during apparently successful chemotherapy. *J. clin. Pathol., 26,* 649-659

Holt, J.M., Robb-Smith, A.H.T., Callender, S.T. & Spriggs, A.I. (1972) Multiple myeloma - development of alternative malignancy following successful chemotherapy (Abstract). *Br. J. Haematol., 22,* 633

IARC (1975) *IARC Monographs on the Evaluation of Carcinogenic Risk of Chemicals to Man,* Vol. 9, *Some aziridines,* N-, S- & O-*mustards and selenium,* Lyon, pp. 135-156

IARC (1976) *IARC Monographs on the Evaluation of Carcinogenic Risk of Chemicals to Man,* Vol. 11, *Cadmium, nickel, some epoxides, miscellaneous industrial chemicals and general considerations on volatile anaesthetics,* Lyon, pp. 247-256

IARC (1979) *IARC Monographs on the Evaluation of the Carcinogenic Risk of Chemicals to Humans,* Vol. 19, *Some Monomers, Plastics and Synthetic Elastomers, and Acrolein,* Lyon, pp. 479-494

Ioan, D., Petrescu, M. & Maximilian, C. (1977) The mutagenic effect of ^{131}I and of two cytostatistics revealed by the micronucleus test (MT). *Rev. Roum. Med. -Endocrinol., 15,* 119-122

Jarman, M., Milsted, R.A.V., Smyth, J.F., Kinas, R.W., Pankiewicz, K. & Stec, W.J. (1979) Comparative metabolism of 2-[bis(2-chloroethyl)amino] tetrahydro-2H-1,3,2-oxazaphosphorine-2-oxide (cyclophosphamide) and its enantiomers in humans. *Cancer Res., 39,* 2762-2767

Jaśkiewicz, K. (1979) Cyclophosphamide induced lesions of tissues of the lung in mice (Pol.). *Ann. Acad. Med. Gedanenses, 9,* 71-77

Johnson, W.W. & Meadows, D.C. (1971) Urinary-bladder fibrosis and telangiectasia associated with long-term cyclophosphamide therapy. *New Engl. J. Med., 284,* 290-294

Juma, F.D. Rogers, H.J. & Trounce, J.R. (1979) First pass hepatic metabolism of cyclophosphamide. *Br. J. clin. Pharmacol., 7,* 422P

Kahn, M.F., Arlet, J., Bloch-Michel, H., Caroit, M., Chaouat, Y. & Renier, J.C. (1979) Acute leukaemias after treatment with cytotoxic agents in rheumatology: 19 observations among 2006 patients (Fr.). *Nouv. Presse méd., 8,* 1393-1397

Kapadia, S.B. & Kaplan, S.S. (1976) Simultaneous occurrence of non-Hodgkin's lymphoma and acute myelomonocytic leukemia. *Cancer, 38,* 2557-2560

Kapadia, S.B. & Kaplan, S.S. (1978) Acute myelogenous leukemia following immunosuppressive therapy for rheumatoid arthritis. *Am. J. clin. Pathol., 70,* 301-302

Kapadia, S.B., Krause, J.R., Ellis, L.D., Pan, S.F. & Wald, N. (1980) Induced acute non-lymphocytic leukemia following long-term chemotherapy. A study of 20 cases. *Cancer, 45,* 1315-1321

Kar, A.K., Singh, S. & Sanyal, A.K. (1974) Cyclophosphamide induced hydrocephalus in chick embryos. *Indian J. med. Res., 62,* 905-908

Karchmer, R.K., Amare, M., Larsen, W.E., Mallouk, A.G. & Caldwell, G.G. (1974) Alkylating agents as leukemogens in multiple myeloma. *Cancer, 33,* 1103-1107

Kelly, W.A., Nelson, L.W., Hawkins, H.C. & Weikel, J.H., Jr (1974) An evaluation of the tumorigenicity of cyclophosphamide and urethan in newborn mice. *Toxicol. appl. Pharmacol., 27,* 629-640

Kende, G., Sirkin, S.R., Thomas, P.R.M. & Freeman, A.I. (1979) Blurring of vision. A previously undescribed complication of cyclophosphamide therapy. *Cancer, 44,* 69-71

Kensler, T.T., Behme, R.J. & Brooke, D. (1979) High-performance liquid chromatographic analysis of cyclophosphamide. *J. pharm. Sci., 68,* 172-174

Khaleeli, M., Keane, W.M. & Lee, G.R. (1973) Sideroblastic anemia in multiple myeloma: a preleukemic change. *Blood, 41,* 17-25

Kinlen, L.J., Sheil, A.G.R., Peto, J. & Doll, R. (1979) Collaborative United Kingdom - Australasian study of cancer in patients treated with immunosuppressive drugs. *Br. med. J., iv,* 1461-1466

Kinlen, L.J., Peto, J., Doll, R. & Sheil, A.G.R. (1981) Cancer in patients treated with immunosuppressive drugs. *Br. med. J., i,* 474

Knudsen, I., Hansen, E.V., Meyer, O.A. & Poulsen, E. (1977) A proposed method for the simultaneous detection of germ-cell mutations leading to fetal death (dominant lethality) and of malformations (male teratogenicity) in mammals. *Mutat. Res., 48,* 267-270

Köhler, E. & Merker, H.-J. (1973) Effect of cyclophosphamide pretreatment of pregnant animals on the activity of nuclear DNA-dependent RNA-polymerases in different parts of rat embryos. *Naunyn-Schmiedeberg's Arch. Pharmacol., 277,* 71-88

Kondo, T. & Muragishi, H. (1970) Mechanisms of cyclophosphamide activation. *Gann, 61,* 145-151

Koss, L.G. (1967) A light and electron microscopic study of the effects of a single dose of cyclophosphamide on various organs in the rat. I. The urinary bladder. *Lab. Invest., 16,* 44-65

Koyama, H., Wada, T., Nishizawa, Y., Iwanaga, T., Aoki, Y., Terasawa, T., Kosaki, G., Yamamoto, T. & Wada, A. (1977) Cyclophosphamide-induced ovarian failure and its therapeutic significance in patients with breast cancer. *Cancer, 39,* 1403-1409

Kram, D., Bynum, G.D., Senula, G.C. & Schneider, E.L. (1979) *In utero* sister chromatid exchange analysis for detection of transplacental mutagens. *Nature, 279,* 531

von Kreybig, T. (1965) Teratogenic effect of cyclophosphamide during the embryonal development phase in rats (Ger.). *Naunyn-Schmiedeberg's Arch. exp. Pathol. Pharmakol., 252,* 173-195

Kuis, W., de Kraker, J., Kuijten, R.H., Doncker-Wolcke, R.A.M.G. & Voûte, P.A. (1976) Acute lymphoblastic leukaemia after treatment of nephrotic syndrome with immunosuppressive drugs. *Helv. paediatr. Acta, 31,* 91-95

Kurvink, K., Bloomfield, C.D., Keenan, K.M., Levitt, S. & Cervenka, J. (1978) Sister chromatid exchanges in lymphocytes from patients with malignant lymphoma. *Hum. Genet., 44,* 137-144

Lenzin, A., Cavalli, F., Sonntag, R. & Zimmermann, A. (1978) Bladder carcinoma associated with long-term treatment with cyclophosphamide for multiple myeloma (Ger.). *Urologe, A17,* 105-108

Li, F.P., Cassady, J.R. & Jaffe, N. (1975) Risk of second tumors in survivors of childhood cancer. *Cancer,* *35,* 1230-1235

Ligorsky, R.D., Axelrod, A.R., Mandell, R.H., Palutke, M. & Prasad, A.S. (1977) Acute myelomonocytic leukemia in a patient with macroglobulinemia and malignant lymphoma. *Cancer, 39,* 1156-1162

Love, R.R. & Sowa, J.M. (1975) Myelomonocytic leukaemia following cyclophosphamide therapy of rheumatoid disease. *Ann. rheum. Dis., 34,* 534-535

Machemer, L. & Lorke, D. (1975a) Experiences with the dominant lethal test in female mice: effects of alkylating agents and artificial sweeteners on pre-ovulatory oocyte stages. *Mutat. Res., 29,* 209-214

Machemer, L. & Lorke, D. (1975b) Method for testing mutagenic effects of chemicals on spermatogonia of the Chinese hamster. Results obtained with cyclophosphamide, saccharin and cyclamate. *Arznei-mittel-Forsch./Drug Res., 25,* 1889-1896

Machemer, L. & Lorke, D. (1978) Mutagenicity studies with Praziquantel, a new anthelmintic drug, in mammalian systems. *Arch. Toxicol., 39,* 187-197

Madle, S., Westphal, D., Hilbig, V. & Obe, G. (1978) Testing *in vitro* of an indirect mutagen (cyclophosphamide) with human leukocyte cultures. Activation by liver perfusion and by incubation with crude liver homogenate. *Mutat. Res., 54,* 95-99

Manny, N., Rosenman, E. & Benbassat, J. (1972) Hazard of immunosuppressive therapy. *Br. med. J., ii,* 291

Mansi, C., Dodero, M., Savarino, V., Picciotto, A., Ciravegna, G., Testa, R. & Celle, G. (1979) Toxic effects on mucosa of the oesophagus, stomach and colon and on the pancreas after chronic administration of azathioprine and cyclophosphamide to rats (Ital.). *Pathologica, 71,* 235-241

Manson, J.M. & Simons, R. (1979) *In vitro* metabolism of cyclophosphamide in limb bud culture. *Teratology, 19,* 149-157

Manson, J.M. & Smith, C.C. (1976) Teratogenic studies utilizing cultured embryonic mouse limb buds (Abstract). *Toxicol. appl. Pharmacol., 37,* 151

Manson, J.M. & Smith, C.C. (1977) Influence of cyclophosphamide and 4-ketocyclophosphamide on mouse limb development. *Teratology, 15,* 291-299

Manson, J.M., Simons, R. & Boyd, C. (1980) *Mechanism of cyclophosphamide-induced teratogenesis* (Abstract no. 265). In: *Abstracts of Papers. Society of Toxicology Incorporated, Nineteenth Annual Meeting, Washington DC,* Washington DC, Society of Toxicology Inc.

Marks, J.S. & Scholtz, C.L. (1977) Sarcoma complicating therapy with cyclophosphamide. *Postgrad. med. J., 53,* 48-49

Matějková, E. (1975) The effects of combined administration of cytembena and cyclophosphamide on the blood count and morphology of nucleoli in peripheral-blood lymphocytes in patients with malignant tumors. *Neoplasma, 22,* 45-54

Matheson, D., Brusick, D. & Carrano, R. (1978) Comparison of the relative mutagenic activity for eight antineoplastic drugs in the Ames *Salmonella*/microsome and TK$^{+/-}$ mouse lymphoma assays. *Drug chem. Toxicol., 1,* 277-304

McCann, J., Simmon, V., Streitwieser, D. & Ames, B.N. (1975) Mutagenicity of chloroacetaldehyde, a possible metabolic product of 1,2-dichloroethane (ethylene dichloride), chloroethanol (ethylene chlorohydrin), vinyl chloride, and cyclophosphamide. *Proc. natl Acad. Sci. USA, 72,* 3190-3193

McClure, H.M., Wilk, A.L., Horigan, E.A. & Pratt, R.M. (1979) Induction of craniofacial malformations in rhesus monkeys *(Macaca mulatta)* with cyclophosphamide. *Cleft Palate J., 16,* 248-256

Mietkiewski, K., Karoń, H. & Warchol, J.B. (1973) The effect of cyclophosphamide (Endoxan) on histo-enzymatic reactions in the liver. II. Studies on liver regeneration during cyclophosphamide administration. *Acta histochem., 45,* 185-198

Millar, J.L., Hudspith, B.N., McElwain, T.J. & Phelps, T.A. (1978) Effect of high-dose melphalan in marrow and intestinal epithelium in mice pretreated with cyclophosphamide. *Br. J. Cancer, 38,* 137-142

Mills, B.A. & Roberts, R.W. (1979) Cyclophosphamide-induced cardiomyopathy. A report of two cases and review of the English literature. *Cancer, 43,* 2223-2226

Morad, M. & El Zawahri, M. (1977) Non-random distribution of cyclophosphamide-induced chromosome breaks. *Mutat. Res., 42,* 125-130

Mosienko, V.S. & Pivnyuk, V.M. (1968) Distribution of thio-TEPA and cyclophosphamide in rats and their renal excretion (Russ.). *Vrach. Delo, 8,* 52-54 [*Chem. Abstr., 70,* 2014b]

Mougeot-Martin, M., Krulik, M., Harousseau, J.-L., Audebert, A.-A., Chaouat, Y. & Debray, J. (1978) Acute leukaemias arising in a case of Behçet's disease and a case of multiple sclerosis treated with immunosuppressors (Fr.). *Ann. Méd. intern. (Paris), 129,* 175-180

Mouridsen, H.T., Faber, O. & Skovsted, L. (1974) The biotransformation of cyclophosphamide in man: analysis of the variation in normal subjects. *Acta pharmacol., 35,* 98-106

Mouridsen, H.T., Faber, O. & Skovsted, L. (1976) The metabolism of cyclophosphamide. Dose dependency and the effect of long-term treatment with cyclophosphamide. *Cancer, 37,* 665-670

Mundy, G.R. & Baikie, A.G. (1973) Myeloma treated with cyclophosphamide and terminating in reticulum cell sarcoma. *Med. J. Aust., 1,* 1240-1241

Murthy, V.V., Becker, B.A. & Steele, W.J. (1973) Effects of dosage, phenobarbital, and 2-diethylamino-ethyl-2,2-diphenylvalerate on the binding of cyclophosphamide and/or its metabolites to the DNA, RNA, and protein of the embryo and liver in pregnant mice. *Cancer Res., 33,* 664-670

Musilová, J., Michalová, K. & Urban, J. (1979) Sister-chromatid exchanges and chromosomal breakage in patients treated with cytostatics. *Mutat. Res., 67,* 289-294

Nawar, N.N.Y., Sakla, F.B. & Mahran, Z.Y. (1979) Effects of maternal administration of Endoxan, vitamin A and vitamin B$_{12}$ on the development of the fetal spinal cord of the albino mouse. *Appl. Neurophysiol., 42,* 203-211

Neistadt, E.L., Gershanovich. M.L., Kolygin, B.A., Ogorodnikova, B.N., Fedoreev, G.A., Chekharina, E.A. & Filov, V.A. (1978) Effect of chemotherapy on the lymph node and bone marrow cell chromosomes in patients with Hodgkin's disease. *Neoplasma, 25,* 91-94

Ohira, S., Maezawa, S., Irinoda, Y., Watanabe, K., Kitada, K. & Saito, T. (1974) Increased antitumor activity of cyclophosphamide (Endoxan) following pretreatment with inducer of drug-metabolizing enzymes (cytochrome P-450). *Tohoku J. exp. Med., 114,* 55-60

Osserman, E.F. (1971) Monocytic and monomyelocytic leukaemia with increased serum and urine lysozyme as a late complication in plasma cell myeloma. *Br. med. J., ii,* 327

Pabst, R. & Wendler, D. (1976) Evaluation of chronic administration of drugs in teratology (Ger.). *Anat. Anz., 140,* 413-422

Pariser, S. (1974) Myeloblastic leukemia following cyclophosphamide therapy of plasma cell dyscrasia. *New York State J. Med., 74,* 2016-2020

Patel, A.R., Shah, P.C., Rhee, H.L., Sassoon, H. & Rao, K.P. (1976) Cyclophosphamide therapy and interstitial pulmonary fibrosis. *Cancer, 38,* 1542-1549

Payne, H.G., Nelson, L.W. & Weikel, J.H., Jr (1974) Effect of cyclophosphamide on somatic cell chromosomes in rats. *Toxicol. appl. Pharmacol., 30,* 360-368

Pearson, R.M. & Soloway, M.S. (1978) Does cyclophosphamide induce bladder cancer? *Urology, 11,* 437-447

Penso, J., Lippe, B., Ehrlich, R. & Smith, F.G., Jr (1974) Testicular function in prepubertal and pubertal male patients treated with cyclophosphamide for nephrotic syndrome. *J. Pediatr., 84,* 831-836

Philips, F.S., Sternberg, S.S., Cronin, A.P. & Vidal, P.M. (1961) Cyclophosphamide and urinary bladder toxicity. *Cancer Res., 21,* 1577-1589

Pienta, R.J. (1980) *A transformation bioassay employing cryopreserved hamster embryo cells.* In: Mishra, N., Dunkel, V.C. & Mehlman, M., eds, *Mammalian Cell Transformation by Chemical Carcinogens,* Princeton Junction, NJ, Senate Press, pp. 47-83

Plotz, P.H., Klippel, J.H., Decker, J.L., Grauman, D., Wolff, B., Brown, B.C. & Rutt, G. (1979) Bladder complications in patients receiving cyclophosphamide for systemic lupus erythematosus or rheumatoid arthritis. *Ann. intern. Med., 91,* 221-223

Portugal, M.A., Falkson, H.C., Stevens, K. & Falkson, G. (1979) Acute leukemia as a complication of long-term treatment of advanced breast cancer. *Cancer Treat. Rep., 63,* 177-181

Potturi, B.R., Singh, S. & Sanyal, A.K. (1975) Ossification patterns of sternum in rat fetuses after maternal administration of cyclophosphamide. *Congenital Anomalies, 15,* 99-106

Preisler, H.D. & Lyman, G.H. (1977) Acute myelogenous leukemia subsequent to therapy for a different neoplasm: clinical features and responses to therapy. *Am. J. Hematol., 3,* 209-218

Propping, P., Röhrborn, G. & Buselmaier, W. (1972) Comparative investigations on the chemical induction of point mutations and dominant lethal mutations in mice. *Mol. gen. Genet., 117,* 197-209

Raposa, T. (1978) Sister chromatid exchange studies for monitoring DNA damage and repair capacity after cytostatics *in vitro* and in lymphocytes of leukaemic patients under cytostatic therapy. *Mutat. Res., 57,* 241-251

Rathenberg, R. (1975) Cytogenetic effects of cyclophosphamide on mouse spermatogonia. *Humangenetik, 29,* 135-140

Reimer, R.R., Hoover, R., Fraumeni, J.F., Jr & Young, R.C. (1977) Acute leukemia after alkylating-agent therapy of ovarian cancer *New Engl. J. Med., 297,* 177-181

Richtsmeier, A.J. (1975) Urinary-bladder tumors after cyclophosphamide. *New Engl. J. Med., 293,* 1045-1046

Roberts, J.J., Brent, T.P. & Crathorn, A.R. (1968) *The mechanism of the cytotoxic action of alkylating agents on mammalian cells.* In: Campbell, P.N., ed., *The Interaction of Drugs and Subcellular Components in Animal Cells,* London, Churchill, pp. 5-27

Roberts, M.M. & Bell, R. (1976) Acute leukaemia after immunosuppressive therapy. *Lancet, ii,* 768-770

Röhrborn, G. & Basler, A. (1977) Cytogenetic investigations of mammals. Comparison of the genetic activity of cytostatics in mammals. *Arch. Toxicol., 38,* 35-43

Roschlau, G. & Justus, J. (1971) Carcinogenic action of methotrexate and cyclophosphamide in animal experiments (Ger.). *Dtsch. Gesundheitswes., 26,* 219-222

Rosner, F. & Grünwald, H. (1975) Hodgkin's disease and acute leukemia. Report of eight cases and review of the literature. *Am. J. Med., 58,* 339-353

Roszinsky-Köcher, G. & Röhrborn, G. (1979) Effects of various cyclophosphamide concentrations *in vivo* on sister chromatid exchanges (SCE) and chromosome aberrations of Chinese hamster bone marrow cells. Comparison of two methods measuring the mutagenicity of a test compound. *Hum. Genet., 46,* 51-55

Rowley, J.D., Golomb, H.M. & Vardiman, J. (1977) Nonrandom chromosomal abnormalities in acute nonlymphocytic leukemia in patients treated for Hodgkin disease and non-Hodgkin lymphomas. *Blood, 50,* 759-770

Rupprecht, L. & Blessing, M.H. (1973) Fibrosarcoma of the bladder after seven-year chemotherapy of Hodgkin's disease in childhood. *Dtsch. med. Wochenschr., 98,* 1663-1665

Schaefer, U.W. & Kanzler, G. (1972) Leukaemia along with Hodgkin's disease. A result of carcinogenic therapy (Ger.). *Med. Klin., 67,* 1024-1028

Schaumlöffel, E., Clausnitzer, M. & Kreyling, H. (1975) Radiochromatographic investigation on the metabolism of ^{3}H-cyclophosphamide in sheep (Ger.). *Arzneimittel-Forsch./Drug Res., 25,* 1385-1392

Schmähl, D. (1967) Carcinogenic action of cyclophosphamide and triaziquone in rats (Ger.). *Dtsch. med. Wochenschr., 92,* 1150-1152

Schmähl, D. (1974) Investigation on the influence of immunodepressive means on the chemical carcino-genesis in rats. *Z. Krebsforsch., 81,* 211-215

Schmähl, D. & Habs, M. (1979) Carcinogenic action of low-dose cyclophosphamide given orally to Sprague-Dawley rats in a lifetime experiment. *Int. J. Cancer, 23,* 706-712

Schmahl, D. & Osswald, H. (1970) Experimental studies on carcinogenic effects of anticancer chemo-therapeutics and immunosuppressives (Ger.). *Arzneimittel-Forsch./Drug Res., 20,* 1461-1467

Schmidt,W., Arakaki, D.T., Breslau, N.A. & Culbertson, J.C. (1971) Chemical mutagenesis. The Chinese hamster bone marrow as an *in vivo* system. I. Cytogenetic results on basic aspects of the method-ology, obtained with alkylating agents. *Humangenetik, 11,* 103-118

Schmidt, W., Kreutz, R., Wendler, D. & Gabler, W. (1977) Production of skeletal defects after admin-istration of aminoacetonitrile and cyclophosphamide during fetogenesis in rats (Ger.). *Verh. Anat. Ges., 71,* 635-638

Schmitz, R., Busch, W. & von Kreybig, T. (1972) Chemically produced malformations of the jaws in animal experiments. I. Action of cyclophosphamide and 6-mercaptopurine on embryonal and fetal development of rats. *Dtsch. Zahnheilkd. Mundheilkd. Kieferheilkd., 59,* 385-398

Schreck, R.R., Paika, I.J. & Latt, S.A. (1979) *In vivo* induction of sister-chromatid exchanges in liver and marrow cells by drugs requiring metabolic activation. *Mutat. Res., 64,* 315-328

Seidenfeld, A.M., Smythe, H.A., Ogryzlo, M.A., Urowitz, M.B. & Dotten, D.A. (1976) Acute leukemia in rheumatoid arthritis treated with cytotoxic agents. *J. Rheumatol., 3,* 295-304

Seino, Y., Nagao, M., Yahagi, T., Hoshi, A., Kawachi, T. & Sugimura, T. (1978) Mutagenicity of several classes of antitumor agents to *Salmonella typhimurium* TA98, TA100, and TA92. *Cancer Res., 38,* 2148-2156

Shah, P.C., Rao, K.R.P. & Patel, A.R. (1975) Cyclophosphamide-induced nail pigmentation. *Lancet, ii,* 548-549

Sheibani, K., Bukowski, R.M., Tubbs, R.R., Savage, R.A., Sebek, B.A. & Hoffman, G.C. (1980) Acute nonlymphocytic leukemia in patients receiving chemotherapy for nonmalignant diseases. *Hum. Pa-thol., 11,* 175-179

Shimkin, M.B., Weisburger, J.H., Weisburger, E.K., Gubareff, N. & Suntzeff, V. (1966) Bioassay of 29 alkylating chemicals by the pulmonary-tumor response in strain A mice. *J. natl Cancer Inst., 36,* 915-935

Singh, S. (1971) The teratogenicity of cyclophosphamide (Endoxan-asta) in rats. *Indian J. med. Res., 59,* 1128-1135

Singh, S. & Sanyal, A.K. (1976) Eye anomalies induced by cyclophosphamide in rat fetuses. *Acta anat., 94,* 490-496

Singh, S. & Singh, M. (1975) Histochemical changes in the malformed forelimbs of rat fetuses induced by cyclophosphamide. *J. anat. Soc. India, 24,* 53-59

Sirianni, S.R. & Huang, C.C. (1978) Sister chromatid exchange induced by promutagens/carcinogens in Chinese hamster cells cultured in diffusion chambers in mice. *Proc. Soc. exp. Biol. Med., 158,* 269-274

Sladek, N.E. (1971) Metabolism of cyclophosphamide by rat hepatic microsomes. *Cancer Res., 31,* 901 908

Smithson, W.A., Burgert, E.O., Jr, Childs, D.S. & Hoagland, H.C. (1978) Acute myelomonocytic leukemia after irradiation and chemotherapy for Ewing's sarcoma. *Mayo Clin. Proc., 53,* 757-759

Spielmann, H. & Eibs, H.-G. (1978) Recent progress in teratology. A survey of methods for the study of drug actions during the preimplantation period. *Arzneimittel-Forsch./Drug Res., 28,* 1733-1742

Spielmann, H., Eibs, H.-G. & Merker, H.-J. (1977) Effects of cyclophosphamide treatment before implantation on the development of rat embryos after implantation. *J. Embryol. exp. Morphol., 41,* 65-78

Šrám, R.J. & Zhurkov, V.S. (1977) *The significance of long-term exposures to chemical mutagens in mice.* In: Böhme, H. & Schöneich, J., eds, *Environmental Mutagens,* Berlin, Akademie-Verlag, pp. 119-132

Starzl, T.E., Groth, C.G., Putnam, C.W., Corman, J., Halgrimson, C.G., Penn, I., Husberg, B., Gustafsson, A., Cascardo, S., Geis, P. & Iwatsuki, S. (1973) Cyclophosphamide for clinical renal and hepatic transplantation. *Transplant. Proc., 5,* 511-516

Steele, T.H., Serpick, A.A. & Block, J.B. (1973) Antidiuretic response to cyclophosphamide in man. *J. Pharmacol. exp. Ther., 185,* 245-253

Stekar, J., (1973) Teratogenicity of cyclophosphamide in newborn rats. *Arzneimittel-Forsch./Drug Res., 23,* 922-923

Stoichkova, N., Damyanov, B. & Astardzhieva, Z. (1979) Ultrastructural changes in the liver of Yoshida tumour rats exposed to cyclophosphamide (Russ.). *Vop. Onkol., 25,* 88-92

Stott, H., Stephens, R.J., Fox, W. & Roy, D.C. (1976) 5-Year follow-up of cytotoxic chemotherapy as an adjuvant to surgery in carcinoma of the bronchus. *Br. J. Cancer, 34,* 167-173

Struck, R.F. (1974) Isolation and identification of a stabilized derivative of aldophosphamide, a major metabolite of cyclophosphamide. *Cancer Res., 34,* 2933-2935

Struck, R.F. & Laster, W.R., Jr (1975) Cyclophosphamide (CPA) metabolites in mouse blood (Abstract no. 70). *Proc. Am. Assoc. Cancer Res., 16,* 18

Symington, G.R., Mackay, I.R. & Lambert, R.P. (1977) Cancer and teratogenesis: infrequent occurrence after medical use of immunosuppressive drugs. *Aust. N.Z. J. Med., 7,* 368-372

Sypkens Smit, C.G. & Meyler, L. (1970) Acute myeloid leukaemia after treatment with cytostatic agents. *Lancet, ii,* 671-672

Takamizawa, A., Matsumoto, S., Iwata, T., Tochino, Y., Katagiri, K., Yamaguchi, K. & Shiratori, O. (1974) Synthesis and metabolic behavior of the suggested active species of isophosphamide having cytostatic activity. *J. med. Chem., 17,* 1237-1239

Talha, M.R.Z., Rogers, H.J. & Trounce, J.R. (1980) Distribution and pharmacokinetics of cyclophosphamide in the rat. *Br. J. Cancer, 41,* 140-143

Tannenbaum, H. & Schur, P.H. (1974) Development of reticulum cell sarcoma during cyclophosphamide therapy. *Arthritis Rheum., 17,* 15-18

Tchernia, G., Mielot, F., Subtil, E. & Parmentier, C. (1976) Acute myeloblastic leukemia after immunodepressive therapy for primary nonmalignant disease. *Blood Cells, 2,* 67-80

Tokuoka, S. (1965) Induction of tumor in mice with *N,N*-bis(2-chloroethyl)-*N',O*-propylenephosphoric acid ester diamide (cyclophosphamide). *Gann, 56,* 537-541

Toledo, T.M., Harper, R.C. & Moser, R.H. (1971) Fetal effects during cyclophosphamide and irradiation therapy. *Ann. intern. Med., 74,* 87-91

Torigoe, K. (1980) Sister chromatid exchanges in children treated with azathioprine and cyclophosphamide, and effect of protein-bound polysaccharide (PS-K). *Jpn. J. Hum. Genet., 25,* 15-21

Torkelson, A.R., LaBudde, J.A. & Weikel, J.H., Jr (1974) The metabolic fate of cyclophosphamide. *Drug Metab. Rev., 3,* 131-165

Trzos, R.J., Petzold, G.L., Brunden, M.N. & Swenberg, J.A. (1978) The evaluation of sixteen carcinogens in the rat using the micronucleus test. *Mutat. Res., 58,* 79-86

Ujházy, E., Preinerová, M. & Jozefík, M. (1979) Effects of cyclophosphamide on the prenatal development of the Swiss strain mice. *Neoplasma, 26,* 529-537

Uldall, P.R., Kerr, D.N.S. & Tacchi, D. (1972) Sterility and cyclophosphamide. *Lancet, i,* 693-694

US Pharmacopeial Convention, Inc. (1980) *The US Pharmacopeia,* 15th ed., Rockville, MD, pp. 189-190

Voelcker, G., Wagner, T. & Hohorst, H.-J. (1976) Identification and pharmacokinetics of cyclophosphamide (NSC-26271) metabolites *in vivo. Cancer Treat. Rep., 60,* 415-422

Vormittag, W. (1974) Cytostatic immunosuppressive therapy, chromosomal aberrations and carcinogenic effect (Ger.). *Wiener Klin. Wochenschr., 86,* 69-75

Wade, A., ed. (1977) *Martindale, The Extra Pharmacopoeia,* 27th ed., London, The Pharmaceutical Press, pp. 134-141

Wagner, T., Peter, G., Voelcker, G. & Hohorst, H.-J. (1977) Characterization and quantitative estimation of activated cyclophosphamide in blood and urine. *Cancer Res., 37,* 2592-2596

Wagner, T., Heydrich, D., Voelcker, G. & Hohorst, H.-J. (1980) Blood level and urinary excretion of activated cyclophosphamide and its deactivation products in man (Ger.). *J. Cancer Res. clin. Oncol., 96,* 79-92

Walker, S.E. & Anver, M.R. (1979) Accelerated appearance of neoplasms in female NZB/NZW mice treated with high-dose cyclophosphamide. *Arthritis Rheum., 22,* 1338-1343

Walker, S.E. & Bole, G.G. (1971) Augmented incidence of neoplasia in female New Zealand black/New Zealand white (NZB/NZW) mice treated with long-term cyclophosphamide. *J. Lab. clin. Med., 78,* 978-979

Walker, S.E. & Bole, G.G., Jr (1973a) Augmented incidence of neoplasia in NZB/NZW mice with long-term cyclophosphamide. *J. Lab. clin. Med., 82,* 619-633

Walker, S.E. & Bole, G.G., Jr (1973b) Suppressed auto-antibody response and development of lymphomas in NZB/NZW mice treated with long-term cyclophosphamide (Abstract). *Arthritis Rheum., 16,* 137

Wall, R.L. & Clausen, K.P. (1975) Carcinoma of the urinary bladder in patients receiving cyclophosphamide. *New Engl. J. Med., 293,* 271-273

Weinstein, S.H., Milleman, L.A. & Schmidt, J.D. (1975) Cyclophosphamide. *J. Urol., 114,* 157

Weisburger, J.H., Griswold, D.P., Prejean, J.D., Casey, A.E., Wood, H.B. & Weisburger, E.K. (1975) The carcinogenic properties of some of the principal drugs used in clinical cancer chemotherapy. *Recent Results Cancer Res., 52,* 1-17

West, W.O. (1976) Acute erythroid leukemia after cyclophosphamide therapy for multiple myeloma: report of two cases. *South. med. J., 69,* 1331-1332

West, W.O. (1978) Acute monocytic leukemia on stage IV neuroblastoma following radiation and cyclophosphamide therapy. *West Virginia med. J., 74,* 35-38

Wheeler A.G., Dansby, D., Hawkins, H.C., Payne, H.G. & Weikel, J.H., Jr (1962) A toxcologic and hematologic evaluation of cyclophosphamide (Cytoxan[®]) in experimental animals. *Toxicol. appl. Pharmacol., 4,* 324-343

Wheeler, G.P. (1962) Studies related to the mechanisms of action of cytotoxic alkylating agents: a review. *Cancer Res., 22,* 651-688

Whiting, B., Miller, S.H.K. & Caddy, B. (1978) A procedure for monitoring cyclophosphamide and iso-phosphamide in biological samples. *Br. J. clin. Pharmacol., 6,* 373-376

Wiernik, P.H. & Duncan, J.H. (1971) Cyclophosphamide in human milk. *Lancet, i,* 912

Willson, J.K.V. (1978) Pulmonary toxicity of antineoplastic drugs. *Cancer Treat. Rep., 62,* 2003-2008

Windholz, M., ed. (1976) *The Merck Index,* 9th ed., Rahway, NJ, Merck & Co., Inc., p. 359

Worlledge, S.M., Brain, M.C., Cooper, A.C., Hobbs, J.R. & Dacie, J.V. (1968) Immunosuppressive drugs in the treatment of autoimmune haemolytic anaemia. *Proc. R. Soc. Med., 61,* 1312-1315

Worth, P.H.L. (1971) Cyclophosphamide and the bladder. *Br. med. J., iii,* 182

Yoshida, M., Numoto, S. & Otsuka, H. (1979) Histopathological changes induced in the urinary bladder and liver of female BALB/c mice treated simultaneously with 2-naphthylamine and cyclophosphamide. *Gann, 70,* 645-652

Zarrabi, M.H., Rosner, F. & Bennett, J.M. (1979) Non-Hodgkin's lymphoma and acute myeloblastic leukemia. A report of 12 cases and review of the literature. *Cancer, 44,* 1070-1080

DACARBAZINE

1. CHEMICAL AND PHYSICAL DATA

1.1 Synonyms and trade names

Chem. Abstr. Services Reg. No.: 4342-03-4

Chem. Abstr. Name: 1H-Imidazole-4-carboxamide, 5-(3,3-dimethyl-1-triazenyl)-

IUPAC Systematic Name: 5-(3,3-Dimethyl-1-triazeno)imidazole-4-carboxamide

Synonyms: 5-(3,3-Dimethyltriazeno)imidazole-4-carboxamide; 4-(dimethyltriazeno)-imidazole-5-carboxamide; 5-(dimethyltriazeno)imidazole-4-carboxamide; dimethyl-(triazeno)imidazolecarboxamide; 5-(3,3-dimethyl-1-triazenyl)-1H-imidazole-4-car-boxamide

Trade names: Deticene; DIC; DTIC; DTIC-Dome; NSC 45388

1.2 Structural and molecular formulae and molecular weight

$C_6H_{10}N_6O$ Mol. wt: 182.2

1.3 Chemical and physical properties of the pure substance

From Wade (1977) or Windholz (1976), unless otherwise specified

(a) *Description:* White to ivory-coloured microcrystals

(b) *Melting-point:* 250-255°C (explosive dec.)

(c) *Spectroscopy data:* λ_{max} 223 nm, A_1^1 = 412 (in 0.1N HCl); 237 nm, A_1^1 = 614 (at pH 7)

(d) *Solubility:* Soluble in water (1 mg/ml at room temperature) (Goldsmith *et al.*, 1972)

(e) *Stability:* Sensitive to oxidation; stable in neutral solutions in absence of light. Extremely light-sensitive: rapidly undergoes chemical decomposition to form 4-diazoimidazole-5-carboxamide (Loo *et al.*, 1976; Karrer, 1978).

1.4 Technical products and impurities

Dacarbazine is available as powder for preparing injections in vials containing 100 and 200 mg with mannitol and citric acid (Wade, 1977).

2. PRODUCTION, USE, OCCURRENCE AND ANALYSIS

2.1 Production and use

(a) Production

Synthesis of dacarbazine was first reported (Shealy *et al.*, 1962) by the following method: 5-aminoimidazole-4-carboxamide was treated with a 20% excess of sodium nitrite to give 5-diazoimidazole-4-carboxamide, which was treated with anhydrous dimethylamine in methanol to give dacarbazine. It is not known whether this is the process used for its commercial production.

Dacarbazine is believed to be supplied by only one company in the US. However, the country in which it is manufactured and the quantities produced are not known.

(b) Use

Dacarbazine is used in human medicine as an antineoplastic agent in the treatment of diseases such as malignant melanomas, Hodgkin's disease, soft-tissue sarcomas, osteogenic sarcomas and neuroblastomas. The usual initial dose is 2-4.5 mg/kg bw intravenously or intra-arterially daily for 10 days and repeated after intervals of 4 weeks, or 100 to 250 mg/m^2 of body surface for 5 days and repeated after intervals of 3 weeks (Goodman & Gilman, 1975; Anon., 1977; Wade, 1977).

2.2 Occurrence

Dacarbazine is not known to be produced in Nature.

2.3 Analysis

Dacarbazine can be analysed colorimetrically by coupling with *N*-(1-naphthyl)ethyl-enediamine. The limits of detection in blood plasma and urine are 2 and 250 μg/ml, respectively (Loo & Stasswender, 1967).

3. BIOLOGICAL DATA RELEVANT TO THE EVALUATION
OF CARCINOGENIC RISK TO HUMANS

3.1 Carcinogenicity studies in animals

(a) Oral administration

Rat: Male and female weanling Sprague-Dawley rats [females stated to be 4 weeks old in a preliminary report (Skibba *et al.*, 1970a] were fed various dosages of dacarbazine in the diet. The group that received the high dose consisted of 16 males and 24 females that initially received 1000 mg/kg of diet for 1.5 weeks, reduced to 500 mg/kg because of toxicity and administered for 12.5 weeks. Animals were then maintained for an additional 4 weeks on control diet, at which time (18 weeks) they were killed and autopsied. Food consumption was determined for the first, second and fourth week and then monthly thereafter: from these measurements, the cumulative dose was calculated to be 974 mg/male rat and 740 mg/female rat. Groups that received lower doses consisted of 12 females given 500 mg/kg of diet for 14 weeks and then maintained for 10 weeks, 16 females given 500 mg/kg for 10 weeks and then kept for 5 weeks and 16 females given 100 mg/kg for 46 weeks and then kept for 14 weeks. The cumulative doses for these groups were 608 mg/rat, 346 mg/rat and 570 mg/rat, respectively. Control groups consisted of 8 males maintained for 18 weeks, 24 females maintained for 66 weeks, 12 females maintained for 36 weeks, 28 females maintained for 66 weeks, 8 females maintained for 34 weeks, and 48 females maintained for 66 weeks. Of the males treated with the high dose, 8/16 developed mammary adenocarcinomas, 15/16 thymic lymphosarcomas and 5/16 splenic lymphosarcomas by 18 weeks; 1 haemangioma also occurred. No neoplasm was found in the male controls at that time. Of the females that received the high dose, 24/24 had mammary adenocarcinomas, 24/24 had thymic lymphosarcomas, 21/24 had splenic lymphosarcomas, 10/24 had cerebral ependymomas and 4/24 had pulmonary alveolar carcinomas by 18 weeks. In the group given 608 mg/rat, 6/12 had mammary carcinomas, 5/12 thymic lymphosarcomas and 3/12 splenic lymphosarcomas by 24 weeks. With 346 mg/rat, 10/16 had mammary adenocarcinomas and 1/16 had a thymic lymphosarcoma by 15 weeks. With 570 mg/rat, 1/16 had a mammary adenocarcinoma, 12/16 had mammary adenofibromas, 3/16 had thymic lymphosarcomas, 2/16 had splenic lymphosarcomas, 2/16 had uterine leiomyosarcomas and 2/16 had leiomyosarcomas elsewhere. Among the 120 control females held for 34 to 66 weeks, a total of 4 mammary adenocarcinomas and 10 mammary adenofibromas occurred (Beal *et al.*, 1975).

A group of 16 female weanling Buffalo rats were fed 500 mg/kg of diet dacarbazine for 11 weeks and then control diet for 9 weeks. Food consumption was determined for the first, second and fourth weeks and then monthly thereafter: from these measurements, the cumulative dose was calculated to be 354 mg/rat. A control group of 16 females was maintained for 20 weeks. In the treated group 15/16 animals developed mammary adenocarcinomas and 5/16 thymic lymphosarcomas. No neoplasm was found in the control group (Beal *et al.*, 1975).

(b) Intraperitoneal administration

Mouse: Two groups, each of 25 male and 25 female outbred Swiss-Webster-derived mice, 6 weeks old, were given i.p. injections of 25 or 50 mg/kg bw dacarbazine dissolved in physiological saline 3 times a week for 6 months. Animals that survived over 100 days were observed for up to 12 further months, at which time they were killed. A control group of 101 male mice had a median survival time of 9.8 months, while that of 153 female control mice was 18 months. With the low dose, the median survival time was 331 days for males and 306 for females; with the high dose, the median survival time was 177 days for males and 128 for females. Animals that died before day 100 on test were excluded from evaluation. The combined tumour incidences with the two doses were 21/41 lung tumours, 15/41 lymphomas and 10/41 splenic haemangiomas in male mice, and 16/19 lung tumours and 5/19 uterine tumours in female mice. The tumour incidence in male and female controls combined was 31%, with 10 lung tumours, 3 lymphomas and no haemangiomas in 101 males, and 21 lung tumours and 3 uterine tumours in 153 females (Weisburger *et al.*, 1975; Weisburger, 1977). [The incidence of tumours at each site in treated mice was reported to be significantly greater than that in controls ($P < 0.001$). The Working Group considered that the inadequate reporting of certain items, such as survival times, the amalgation of various experimental groups and tumour types, as well as the lack of age-adjustment in the analyses precluded a complete evaluation of this study.]

Rat: Groups of 16 female Sprague-Dawley rats were given single i.p. injections of 100, 250 or 400 mg per rat dacarbazine dissolved in 1.0 ml citrate-mannitol solution. Another group was injected with 2.5 mg 3 times per week for 12 weeks (total, 76.5 mg). Control groups of 16 rats received single or multiple injections of a volume of the vehicle identical to that used in the experimental groups. All animals were observed for 66 weeks. The treated rats displayed a dose-dependent increase in mammary adenocarcinoma incidence, with 0/20 in the group that received multiple injections, 1/16 in those given 100 mg, 5/16 in those given 250 mg and 11/16 in those given 400 mg. Other tumours that occurred with increased frequency included mammary adenofibromas, thymic and splenic lymphosarcomas, leiomyosarcomas of the uterus, cerebral ependymomas, ependymoblastoma, embryonal adenosarcomas, adrenal cortical adenoma, bronchogenic adenocarcinomas and renal cortical adenocarcinoma. No tumour was observed in the control groups (Beal *et al.*, 1975).

Two groups, each of 25 male and 25 female Sprague-Dawley-derived Charles River CD rats, about 30 days old, were given i.p. injections of 50 or 100 mg/kg bw dacarbazine 3 times a week for 6 months. Animals that survived over 100 days were observed for up to 12 further months, at which time they were killed. A control group of 179 male and 181 female rats were kept untreated. The median survival times were 202 days in males and 195 days in females given the low dose and 141 days in males and 126 days in females given the high dose, compared with about 500 days in male and female controls. Animals that died before day 100 on test were excluded from evaluation. The combined tumour incidences with the two doses were 18/34 lymphomas in males and 12/22 in females; 8/34 heart tumours (type not specified) in males and 2/22 in females; 8/34 renal tumours in males; and 16/22 breast carcinomas in females. The incidences were statistically significantly increased in comparison with controls ($P = 0.01$ for heart tumours; $P = 0.001$ for breast carcinomas; and $P < 0.001$ for lymphomas and renal tumours) (Weisburger *et al.*, 1975). [The Working Group considered that the inadequate reporting of certain items, such as survival times, the amalgamation of various experimental groups and tumour types, as well as the lack of age-adjustment in the analyses precluded a complete evaluation of this study.]

3.2 Other relevant biological data

(a) Experimental systems

Toxic effects

[In view of the extreme light sensitivity of dacarbazine, the data below should be interpreted with caution, since most reports do not describe if steps were taken to protect the compound from light.]

The LD_{50} of dacarbazine was reported in one experiment to be about 350 mg/kg bw when given as a single i.p. injection; but in another experiment, tumour-bearing mice tolerated a single i.p. dose of 1200 mg/kg bw. With oral administration, no toxicity was observed in mice with dose levels up to 1000 mg/kg bw. Rats given a single i.p. dose of 500 mg/kg bw showed weight loss, pallor and bloody nares, and those given 1000 mg/kg bw orally also had a stilted gait, pulmonary congestion, pleural fluid, anaemia and leucopenia. In dogs, the maximum tolerated dose over 28 days was reported to be 2.5 mg/kg bw per day when given intraperitoneally and 5 mg/kg per day orally; in monkeys, the respective doses were 15 - 30 and 10 mg/kg bw. In all animals studied (rats, monkeys and dogs), the major toxicity involved damage to the gut, bone marrow and lymphoid tissue. Recovery from toxic effects may be complete within 6 weeks of finishing treatment (Goldsmith *et al.*, 1972).

Effects on reproduction and prenatal toxicity

When Wistar rats were injected on the 12th day of pregnancy with a single i.p. dose of 200 - 1000 mg/kg bw dacarbazine, urogenital anomalies, such as hydronephrosis, hydro-ureter and hypoplastic, ectopic testes, were observed in the fetuses. Embryolethality did not exceed that in controls (0 - 10%) with doses of 100 - 900 mg/kg bw, but 1000 mg/kg bw induced 15% embryolethality. Dose-dependent fetal growth retardation was observed with all doses (Chaube & Swinyard, 1975, 1976).

Sprague-Dawley rats (25 per group) were given i.p. injections of 30, 50 or 70 mg/kg bw dacarbazine on days 6 - 15 of pregnancy. Teratogenic effects, including anomalies of the skeletal system, eyes, cardiovascular system and abdominal wall, were seen with the two higher doses. The mean fetal weight was reduced with all three doses, and the rate of resorptions increased. Offspring of rats treated from day 15 of pregnancy through day 21 *post partum* with 7.5, 15 or 30 mg/kg bw showed a dose-dependent increase in postnatal mortality (Thompson *et al.*, 1975).

Fetuses of rabbits given i.p. injections of 10 mg/kg bw dacarbazine on days 6 - 18 of pregnancy showed skeletal abnormalities; doses of 2.5 or 5 mg/kg bw were ineffective. The rates of resorption and fetal weights did not differ from those of controls with all the doses used (Thompson *et al.*, 1975).

Absorption, distribution, excretion and metabolism

In mice, [^{14}C-2]-labelled dacarbazine (50 mg/kg bw) is rapidly absorbed from the site of its i.p. injection and distributed to tissues; and more than 90% of the dose is eliminated in the urine within 24 hours. The plasma half-life was 20 min. Studies with dacarbazine labelled at the methyl group gave similar results, except that 9% of the radioactivity was recovered in the expired air within 24 hours, and only 44% was found in the urine (Housholder & Loo, 1971).

In rats, i.p. administration of 160 mg/kg bw dacarbazine labelled at the methyl group led to recovery of 4.0% of the dose as $^{14}CO_2$ in the expired air within 6 hours. When the rats were pretreated with phenobarbital, increased amounts (10.5%) of dacarbazine were N-demethylated to $^{14}CO_2$ within 6 hours (Skibba *et al.*, 1970b).

In dogs, the cumulative urinary excretion after i.v. injection of 20 mg/kg bw [^{14}C-2]-dacarbazine was 40 - 66% over 5 hours; 36 - 84% of this was unchanged dacarbazine. The remaining part was represented mainly by the metabolite 5-aminoimidazole-4-carboxamide (Housholder & Loo, 1971). In dogs, the initial plasma half-life is 6 min, and the terminal half-life 86 min (Loo et al., 1976).

Ten min after i.v. administration of dacarbazine to dogs, it was found in the cerebrospinal fluid. At steady state, an average cerebrospinal fluid:plasma ratio of 1:7 was attained (Loo et al., 1968). Administration of [^{14}C-methyl]-dacarbazine to rats resulted in the urinary excretion of 7-methylguanine. DNA and RNA from several tissues of rats treated with methyl-labelled dacarbazine contained 7-methylguanine 4 hours after injection (Skibba & Bryan, 1971).

Although the mechanism of action of dacarbazine is not known in detail, it is demethylated by liver microsomal enzymes to form an unstable monoalkyl derivative which can decompose spontaneously into alkylating moieties. In light, dacarbazine can also rapidly undergo chemical decomposition to form 4-diazoimidazole-5-carboxamide, which is highly toxic but which has no antitumour activity in vivo (Skibba et al., 1970a,b; Bono, 1976; Karrer, 1978).

Mutagenicity and other short-term tests

Dacarbazine was not mutagenic in Salmonella typhimurium strains TA1535, TA1537, TA1538 or TA98 when tested in the presence or absence of a microsomal preparation of mouse liver. In the TK$^{+/-}$ assay with mouse lymphoma cells, dacarbazine was dose-dependently mutagenic after activation with a microsomal preparation of mouse liver (Matheson et al., 1978). [No information was given as to whether the assays were carried out in the dark.]

(b) Humans

Toxic effects

[In view of the extreme light sensitivity of dacarbazine, the data below should be interpreted with caution, since most reports do not describe if steps were taken to protect the compound from light.]

In common with most other cytotoxic drugs, the toxic effects of dacarbazine are mainly myelosuppression and gastrointestinal upset. Leucopenia and thrombocytopenia occurred from 5 to 21 days after a dose of 4.5 mg/kg bw per day for up to 10 days; blood counts recovered only after 2-3 weeks. Nausea and vomiting limit the therapeutic dose which can be given either intravenously or orally (Skibba et al., 1969). High doses of dacarbazine also cause gastrointestinal bleeding (Goldman et al., 1977), possibly due to a combination of low platelet counts and abnormal platelet function as suggested by coagulation studies in vitro (Klener & Kubisz, 1978).

Three cases of hepatic vein thrombosis leading to fatal hepatic necrosis have been reported (Frosch et al., 1979; Asbury et al., 1980; Balda & Bassermann, 1980). In each, the patient was treated for melanoma with 200-260 mg/m^2 daily intravenously for one cycle of 5 days. All patients experienced moderately severe gastrointestinal and bone-marrow toxicity and also developed symptoms of liver failure half-way through the second course of therapy, which followed about one month after the first course. Death was rapid, and autopsies confirmed recent hepatic vein thrombosis and massive hepatic necrosis.

Effects on reproduction and prenatal toxicity

No data were available to the Working Group.

Absorption, distribution, excretion and metabolism

Loo et al. (1968, 1976) reviewed the pharmacokinetics of dacarbazine. It can be absorbed orally, but this is variable; physiological availability is about 25%, increasing to 50% on a multiple, divided-dose schedule. Plasma half-life was 111 min after doses ranging from 30 to 260 mg/m^2. Only 19% of the dose was excreted in the urine in 6 hours. In contrast, after a large single i.v. injection, plasma disappearance is biphasic, with half-lives of 19 min and 5 hours; kinetics of the drug given to a patient with hepatorenal impairment were delayed to 55 min and 7.2 hours. The volume of distribution exceeds that of total body water, and some penetration into cerebrospinal fluid occurs.

Less than 5% of the drug is bound to protein (Loo et al., 1968), and half of an injected dose is excreted in the urine as 5-aminoimidazole-4-carboxamide or unchanged (Loo et al., 1968, 1976). The remainder is metabolized to alkylating components or degraded by light during preparation and delivery of the drug (Baird & Willoughby, 1978).

7-Methylguanine was detected in the urine of 2 patients following oral administration of dacarbazine, indicating DNA alkylation (Skibba & Bryan, 1971).

Mutagenicity and chromosomal effects

No sister chromatid exchange was observed in the peripheral lymphocytes of 6 melanoma patients given i.v. injections of 250 mg/m^2 dacarbazine daily for 5 days (Lambert et al., 1979). [No mention was made as to whether the compound was administered in the dark.]

3.3 Case reports and epidemiological studies of carcinogenicity in humans

One case of acute nonlymphocytic leukaemia was reported in a woman with breast cancer treated with dacarbazine and other cytotoxic agents (Portugal *et al.*, 1979).

A retrospective cohort study of 764 patients with Hodgkin's disease given several different combinations of chemotherapy and radiation was reported (Valagussa *et al.*, 1980). Fifty-five of these patients were followed for a median of 45 months after receiving a regimen consisting of dacarbazine, adriamycin, bleomycin and vinblastine sulphate. No second malignancies were observed in the subgroup.

4. SUMMARY OF DATA REPORTED AND EVALUATION

4.1 Experimental data

Dacarbazine is carcinogenic in mice and rats. Following its oral or intraperitoneal administration to rats, dacarbazine produced tumours at various sites, including breast, thymus, spleen and brain, in as little as 18 weeks after initial exposure. After its intraperitoneal administration to mice, dacarbazine produced tumours at various sites, including lung, haematopoietic tissue and uterus.

Dacarbazine can induce teratogenic effects in several species. It is mutagenic in mammalian cells in culture.

4.2 Human data

Dacarbazine has been used since the early 1970s in the treatment of malignant melanoma and is occasionally used in the therapy of other neoplastic diseases which have become resistant to alternative treatment.

The available data are insufficient to evaluate the teratogenicity, mutagenicity or chromosomal effects of dacarbazine in humans.

A single case of acute leukaemia following treatment with dacarbazine in combination with other cytotoxic agents has been reported. The only epidemiological study was small and of short duration and showed no excess of subsequent neoplasms in patients treated with a regimen consisting of dacarbazine, adriamycin, bleomycin and vinblastine.

4.3 Evaluation

There is *sufficient evidence*[1] for the carcinogenicity of dacarbazine in mice and rats. The data from studies in humans are inadequate to evaluate the carcinogenicity of dacarbazine.

This chemical should be regarded for practical purposes as if it presented a carcinogenic risk to humans.

---

[1] See preamble, p. 18.

5. REFERENCES

Anon. (1977) *AMA Drug Evaluations,* 3rd ed., Littleton, MA, PSG Publishing Co., Inc., pp. 1108, 1124

Asbury, R.F., Rosenthal, S.N., Descalzi, M.E., Ratcliffe, R.L. & Arseneau, J.C. (1980) Hepatic veno-occlusive disease due to DTIC. *Cancer, 45,* 2670-2674

Baird, G.M. & Willoughby, M.L.N. (1978) Photodegradation of dacarbazine. *Lancet, ii,* 681

Balda, B.-R. & Bassermann, R. (1980) Dacarbazine (DTIC) therapy and the Budd-Chiari syndrome (Ger.). *Münch. med. Wochenschr., 122,* 792-794

Beal, D.D., Skibba, J.L., Croft, W.A., Cohen, S.M. & Bryan, G.T. (1975) Carcinogenicity of the antineoplastic agent, 5-(3,3-dimethyl-1-triazeno)imidazole-4-carboxamide, and its metabolites in rats. *J. natl Cancer Inst., 54,* 951-957

Bono, V.H., Jr (1976) Studies on the mechanism of action of DTIC (NSC-45388). *Cancer Treat. Rep., 60,* 141-148

Chaube, S. & Swinyard, C.A. (1975) Cellular and biochemical aspects of growth retardation in rat fetuses induced by maternal administration of selected anticancer agents. *Teratology, 12,* 259-270

Chaube, S. & Swinyard, C.A. (1976) Urogenital anomalies in fetal rats produced by the anticancer agent 4(5)-(3,3-dimethyl-1-triazeno)imidazole-4-carboxamide. *Anat. Rec., 186,* 461-469

Frosch, P.J., Czarnetzki, B.M., Macher, R., Grundmann, E. & Gottschalk, I. (1979) Hepatic failure in a patient treated with dacarbazine (DTIC) for malignant melanoma. *J. Cancer Res. clin. Oncol., 95,* 281-286

Goldman, S.L., Pollak, E.W. & Wolfman, E.F., Jr (1977) Massive upper gastrointestinal bleeding during chemotherapy for malignant melanoma. *Am. Surg., 43,* 768-770

Goldsmith, M.A., Friedman, M.A. & Carter, S.K. (1972) *5-(3,3-Dimethyl-1-triazeno)imidazole-4-carboxamide (DTIC, DIC) NSC-45388, Clinical Brochure,* Bethesda, MD, Division of Cancer Treatment, National Cancer Institute

Goodman, L.S. & Gilman, A., eds (1975) *The Pharmacological Basis of Therapeutics,* 5th ed., New York, Macmillan, pp. 1250, 1257, 1268

Housholder, G.E. & Loo, T.L. (1971) Disposition of 5-(3,3-dimethyl-1-triazeno)imidazole-4-carboxamide, a new anti-tumor agent. *J. Pharmacol. exp. Ther., 179,* 386-395

Karrer, K. (1978) Pharmacology of DTIC (Ger.). *Wien. klin. Wochenschr., 90,* 858-861

Klener, P. & Kubisz, P. (1978) Influence of imidazole carboxamide on platelet functions and coagulation *in vitro. Am. J. med. Sci., 275,* 181-186

Lambert, B., Ringborg, U. & Lindblad, A. (1979) Prolonged increase of sister-chromatid exchanges in lymphocytes of melanoma patients after CCNU treatment. *Mutat. Res., 59,* 295-300

Loo, T.L. & Stasswender, E.A. (1967) Colorimetric determination of dialkyltriazenoimidazoles. *J. pharm. Sci., 56,* 1016-1018

Loo, T.L., Luce, J.K., Jardine, J.H. & Frei, E., III (1968) Pharmacologic studies of the antitumor agent 5-(dimethyltriazeno)imidazole-4-carboxamide. *Cancer Res., 28,* 2448-2453

Loo, T.L., Housholder, G.E., Gerulath, A.H., Saunders, P.H. & Farquhar, D. (1976) Mechanism of action and pharmacology studies with DTIC (NSC-45388). *Cancer Treat. Rep., 60,* 149-152

Matheson, D., Brusick, D. & Carrano, R. (1978) Comparison of the relative mutagenic activity for eight antineoplastic drugs in the Ames *Salmonella*/microsome and TK+/- mouse lymphoma assays. *Drug chem. Toxicol., 1,* 277-304

Portugal, M.A., Falkson, H.C., Stevens, K. & Falkson, G. (1979) Acute leukemia as a complication of long-term treatment of advanced breast cancer. *Cancer Treat. Rep., 63,* 177-181

Shealy, Y.F., Krauth, C.A. & Montgomery, J.A. (1962) Imidazoles. I. Coupling reactions of 5-diazo-imidazole-4-carboxamide. *J. org. Chem., 27,* 2150-2154

Skibba, J.L. & Bryan, G.T. (1971) Methylation of nucleic acids and urinary excretion of ^{14}C-labeled 7-methylguanine by rats and man after administration of 4(5)-(3,3-dimethyl-1-triazeno)imidazole 5(4)-carboxamide. *Toxicol. appl. Pharmacol., 18,* 707-719

Skibba, J.L., Ramirez, G., Beal, D.D. & Bryan, G.T. (1969) Preliminary clinical trial and the physiologic disposition of 4(5)-(3,3-dimethyl-1-triazeno)imidazole-5(4)-carboxamide in man. *Cancer Res., 29,* 1944-1951

Skibba, J.L., Ertück, E. & Bryan, G.T. (1970a) Induction of thymic lymphosarcoma and mammary adeno-carcinomas in rats by oral administration of the antitumor agent, 4(5)-(3,3-dimethyl-1-triazeno)-imidazole-5(4)-carboxamide. *Cancer, 26,* 1000-1005

Skibba, J.L., Beal, D.D., Raminez, G. & Bryan, G.T. (1970b) *N*-Demethylation of the antineoplastic agent 4(5)-(3,3-dimethyl-1-triazeno)imidazole-5(4)-carboxamide by rats and man. *Cancer Res., 30,* 147-150

Thompson, D.J., Molello, J.A., Strebing, R.J. & Dyke, I.L. (1975) Reproduction and teratology studies with oncolytic agents in the rat and rabbit. II. 5-(3,3-Dimethyl-1-triazeno)imidazole-4-carboxamide (DTIC). *Toxicol. appl. Pharmacol., 33,* 281-290

Valagussa, P., Santoro, A., Kenda, R., Fossati Bellani, F., Franchi, F., Banfi, A., Rilke, F. & Bonadonna, G. (1980) Second malignancies in Hodgkin's disease: a complication of certain forms of treatment. *Br. med. J., i,* 216-219

Wade, A., ed. (1977) *Martindale, The Extra Pharmacopoeia,* 27th ed., London, The Pharmaceutical Press, p. 143

Weisburger, E.K. (1977) Bioassay program for carcinogenic hazards of cancer chemotherapeutic agents. *Cancer, 40,* 1935-1951

Weisburger, J.H., Griswold, D.P., Prejean, J.D., Casey, A.E., Wood, H.B. & Weisburger, E.K. (1975) The carcinogenic properties of some of the principal drugs used in clinical cancer chemotherapy. *Recent Results Cancer Res., 52,* 1-17

Windholz, M., ed. (1976) *The Merck Index,* 9th ed., Rahway, NJ, Merck & Co., p. 368

5-FLUOROURACIL

1. CHEMICAL AND PHYSICAL DATA

1.1 Synonyms and trade names

Chem. Abstr. Services Reg. No.: 51-21-8

Chem. Abstr. Name: 2,4(1*H*,3*H*)-Pyrimidinedione, 5-fluoro-

IUPAC Systematic Name: 5-Fluorouracil

Synonyms: 2,4-Dioxo-5-fluoropyrimidine; 5-fluoropyrimidin-2,4-diol; 5-fluoro-2,4-(1*H*,3*H*)-pyrimidinedione; 5-fluoro-2,4-pyrimidinedione; 5-fluoropyrimidine-2,4-(1*H*,3*H*)-dione; 5-fluoropyrimidine-2,4-dione; fluorouracil; 5-fluracil; fluracilum; FU; 5-FU

Trade names: Adrucil; Efudex; Efudix; Fluoroplex; Fluoro Uracil; Fluoro-uracile; Fluracil; Fluril; NSC 19893; Phthoruracil; Ro-2-9757

1.2 Structural and molecular formulae and molecular weight

$C_4H_3FN_2O_2$ Mol. wt: 130.1

1.3 Chemical and physical properties of the pure substance

From Wade (1977) or Windholz (1976), unless otherwise specified

(a) *Description:* White to almost white, odourless, crystalline powder
(b) *Melting-point:* 282-283°C (dec.)
(c) *Spectroscopy data:* λ_{max} 265-266 nm, A_1^1 = 543 (in 0.1N HCl). Infra-red, mass and nuclear magnetic resonance spectra have been tabulated (Rudy & Senkowski, 1973).

(d) *Solubility:* Sparingly soluble in water (12 mg/ml at 25°C) (Rudy & Senkowski, 1973); slightly soluble in ethanol; practically insoluble in chloroform, benzene and diethyl ether

(e) *Stability:* Hydrolysed under strongly basic conditions

1.4 Technical products and impurities

Various national and international pharmacopoeias give specifications for the purity of 5-fluorouracil in pharmaceutical products. For example, 5-fluorouracil is available in the US as a USP grade measured as containing 98.5 - 101.0% active ingredient on a dried basis, 0.5% max. water content, 0.1% max. residue on ignition and 0.002% max. heavy metals. It is also available as 1% and 5% creams measured as containing 90.0 - 110.0% of the stated amount of 5-fluorouracil; injections containing 45 - 55 mg/ml; and topical solutions (1, 2 and 5%) measured as containing 90.0 - 110.0% of the stated amount of 5-fluorouracil (US Pharmacopeial Convention, Inc., 1980).

In most countries of western Europe, 5-fluorouracil is available as creams (1 and 5%), injections (50 mg/ml) and topical solutions (1, 2 and 5%) (Wade, 1977).

5-Fluorouracil is available in Japan in vials for injection (250 - 500 mg per vial).

2. PRODUCTION, USE, OCCURRENCE AND ANALYSIS

2.1 Production and use

(a) *Production*

Synthesis of 5-fluorouracil was first reported (Duschinsky & Pleven, 1957) by the following route: ethyl-sodio-fluoromalonaldehyde was condensed with 2-ethyl-2-thiopseudourea hydrobromide, and the product was converted by acid hydrolysis to 5-fluorouracil. It is not known whether this is the method used for its commercial production.

Two US companies are believed to produce 5-fluorouracil in undisclosed quantities (see preamble, pp. 20-21). No data were available on the amounts imported or exported.

It is believed to be produced by two companies in the Federal Republic of Germany, one in Switzerland and one in the UK. About 300 kg are used annually in western Europe.

5-Fluorouracil is not produced commercially in Japan. About 2000 kg per year have been imported for the last 3 years.

(b)   Use

5-Fluorouracil is used in human medicine as an antineoplastic agent in the management of carcinomas of the alimentary tract, breast, bladder, lung (non-small-cell), cervix, liver and pancreas (Wade, 1977; Baker, 1980) and of malignant insulinoma and cancers of the endometrium, ovary and prostate. It is also used topically in the treatment of precancerous keratoses of the skin and superficial basal-cell and squamous-cell carcinomas (Goodman & Gilman, 1975).

5-Fluorouracil has also been used as a 5% ointment for the treatment of psoriasis and plantar warts by application for 7 - 9 days (Wade, 1977; Lee *et al.*, 1980).

5-Fluorouracil is given intravenously, intramuscularly, orally or topically at a wide variety of dose levels. For instance, it is given in combination with cyclophosphamide and methotrexate (CMF) for breast cancer at a dose of 600 mg/m^2 of body surface area, intravenously, on day 1 and day 8 of the 4-week regimen. In gastrointestinal malignancy, it is often given as 500 mg/m^2 of body surface area per day for 5 days of a 4-6-week therapeutic cycle. In topical use, a 5% ointment is applied to the lesion 2 to 3 times a day.

2.2 Occurrence

5-Fluorouracil is not known to be produced in Nature.

2.3 Analysis

Analytical methods for the determination of 5-fluorouracil in bulk products, pharmaceutical preparations and biological fluids, based on elemental analysis, phase solubility analysis, thin-layer and gas-liquid chromatography, spectrophotometry and volumetric analysis, have been reviewed (Rudy & Senkowski, 1973).

Typical methods for the analysis of 5-fluorouracil in various matrices are summarized in Table 1.

Table 1. Methods for the analysis of 5-fluorouracil

Sample matrix	Sample preparation	Assay procedure[a]	Limit of detection	Reference
Formulations	Add dimethyl formamide and thymol blue solution; dilute with acetate buffer	T	not given	US Pharmacopeial Convention, Inc. (1980)
	Dissolve in water and methanol	TLC	not given	Hawrylyshyn et al. (1964)
	Dilute with acetate buffer	S	not given	US Pharmacopeial Convention, Inc. (1980)
Blood, bile and urine	Dilute with distilled water; apply sample to agar medium inoculated with Streptococcus faecalis; incubate	MA	10 ng/ml	Brandberg et al. (1977)
Blood plasma	Mix with ammonium sulphate; extract with isopropanol and chloroform; evaporate; re-dissolve in the same solvents	HPLC	100 ng/ml	Sitar et al. (1977)
	Add 5-chlorouracil and saturated ammonium sulphate; extract with diethyl ether and propanol; evaporate; add potassium phosphate	HPLC-UV	100 ng/ml	Cohen & Brown (1978)
	Add 5-chlorouracil; extract with ethyl acetate; evaporate; dissolve in hexane; add water; evaporate aqueous layer; re-dissolve in water	GC-NPD	50 ng/ml	Driessen et al. (1979)
	Add ^{15}N-5-fluorouracil; add saturated ammonium sulphate solution; wash with benzene; extract with propanol in diethyl ether; evaporate; methylate with ethereal diazomethane	GC-CIMS	2 ng/ml	Min & Garland (1978)

Table 1 (contd)

Sample matrix	Sample preparation	Assay procedure[a]	Limit of detection	Reference
Blood serum	Filter and centrifuge sample; purify on ion-exchange column; convert to trimethyl-silyl derivative	GC-MS	$<$1 ng	Lakings & Adamson (1978)
	Extract with ethyl acetate; convert to chloromethyldi-methylsilyl derivative	GC-ECD	0.05 ng	Pantarotto et al. (1979)
	Dilute with picric acid; centrifuge; add potassium hydroxide; elute with formic acid on an ion-exchange column; evaporate; dissolve in water	I	6.5 ng	Gustavvson et al. (1979)
Urine	Apply sample to polyacryl-amide gel column	CC	not given	Sitar et al. (1977)

[a]Abbreviations: T, titration; TLC, thin-layer chromatography; S, spectrophotometry; MA, microbiological assay; HPLC-UV, high-performance liquid chromatography with ultra-violet detection; GC-NPD, gas chromatography with nitrogen-phosphate detection; GC-CIMS, gas chromatography with chemical ionization mass spectrometry; GC-MS, gas chromatography with mass spectrometry; GC-ECD, gas chromatography with electron capture detection; I, isotachophoresis; CC, column chromatography

3. BIOLOGICAL DATA RELEVANT TO THE EVALUATION OF CARCINOGENIC RISK TO HUMANS

3.1 Carcinogenicity studies in animals

(a) Oral administration

Rat: Groups of Fischer rats were administered 5-fluorouracil by gastric intubation 5 times per week for 52 weeks, followed by a 6-month observation period. Four dose levels were used: 3 male and 3 female rats were given 3 mg/animal per day; 15 males and 15 females received 1 mg/rat per day, 12 males were given 0.01 mg/rat per day, and 12 female rats were given 0.3 mg per day. Surviving animals were killed after 18 months. In comparison with vehicle and untreated control rats, there was no evidence of carcinogenicity (Hadidian et al., 1968). [The experiment was limited by small group sizes, low doses, incomplete histopathological studies, and short duration.]

(b)   Intravenous administration

Mouse: A group of 50 7-week-old female A/Jax mice received i.v. injections of 1 mg 5-fluorouracil weekly for 16 weeks, at which time they were killed and their lungs examined.   No effect on the incidence of lung adenomas was observed (Homburger *et al.*, 1971). [The Working Group noted the short duration of this experiment.]

Rat: A group of 52 male BR 46 rats received a weekly i.v. injection of 33 mg/kg bw 5-fluorouracil (7% of the LD_{50}) for one year and were observed for lifetime.   One malignant tumour occurred late in the experiment, when 22 dosed animals were still alive.   In the control group (initially of 89 animals), 65 animals were still alive when the malignant tumour was found in the treated group.   Among the control rats, 4 malignant tumours were found (Schmähl & Osswald, 1970).

(c)   Other experimental systems

Administration with known carcinogens: A 1% solution of 5-fluorouracil in propylene glycol was painted daily on the cheek pouch mucosa of 5 Syrian *hamsters*.   No significant lesions were found at the application sites when the animals were killed after 1, 3, 6 or 9 days or 15 weeks.   Three groups of 5 hamsters each were also painted with a 5% solution of 7,12-dimethylbenz[a]anthracene (DMBA) in heavy mineral oil on the cheek pouch 3 times weekly for 3 weeks. 5-Fluorouracil was applied topically (i) immediately after DMBA treatment was completed;   (ii) 3 weeks after completion of DMBA treatment;   or (iii) on alternate days with DMBA treatment.   A fifth group of 5 hamsters received DMBA only. The combined treatment was reported to produce a more severe hyperplastic response, except in the group in which there was a 3-week period between the two treatments. At 15 weeks [one hamster per group], *in situ* or invasive carcinomas were reported in the group given DMBA alone and in the two groups in which the combination treatments alternated or were immediately successive (Weathers & Halstead, 1969). [This study is limited by the small group sizes.]

3.2   Other relevant biological data

(a)   Experimental systems

Toxic effects

The LD_{50} of 5-fluorouracil in CBA/J male mice after a single i.p. injection was 260 mg/kg bw (Houghton *et al.*, 1979).   Diurnal variations in toxicity were reported following single i.p. injections of doses near the LD_{50} (Lesnaya, 1972).   The LD_{10} for BDF_1 male mice given 1, 2, 3 and 4 sequential daily i.p. doses was about 200, 162, 61 and 39 mg/kg bw, respectively (Harrison et al., 1978). When administered subcutaneously to $B_6D_2F_1$ male mice, the LD_{90} of 5-fluorouracil in daily treatments of from 1 to 32 days ranged from 458 to 20.6 mg/kg bw; the slopes of the dose-mortality curves were steep. The LD_{50} with 2 treatments at various intervals was from 115 to 370 mg/kg bw. The greatest toxicity was observed when two doses were administered at a 4-day interval (Johnson et al., 1976).

The LD_{50} of 5-fluorouracil given intravenously by infusion for 72 hours to female CDF rats was 320 mg/kg bw. No rats survived doses above 450 mg/kg bw per 72 hours; 150 mg/kg bw produced no toxicity other than a 10% weight loss. I.v. infusion for 36 hours produced an LD_{50} and an LD_{95} of 520 mg/kg bw and 700 mg/kg bw, respectively (Danhauser & Rustum, 1979).

Mice administered lethal doses of 5-fluorouracil generally died within 2 weeks of the first treatment, after signs of weight loss, diarrhoea, rectal bleeding, lethargy and ataxia (Johnson et al., 1976; Houghton et al., 1979). Survivors recovered their lost weight by 21 days if administration of 5-fluorouracil was discontinued (Harrison et al., 1978).

In mice, lesions in the intestine, characterized by epithelial and villous atrophy, increased in severity and in incidence with increasing doses. Bone-marrow erythropenia and granulocytopenia were also observed (Harrison et al., 1978). Bone-marrow damage was also seen after s.c. administration of the LD_{10} (50 mg/kg bw) daily for 5 days (Johnson et al., 1976). Lymphoid atrophy in spleen and lymph nodes and lymphopenia also occurred (Harrison et al., 1978). In mice, cellular and humoral immunity were depressed following administration of 5-fluorouracil (Hršak & Pavičič, 1974; Scherf & Schmähl, 1975; Johnson et al., 1976; Berenbaum, 1979). The drug was highly immunosuppressive at doses well below the LD_{50} (Berenbaum, 1979). In rats, lethal doses produced degeneration of the kidney, necrosis of liver and spleen and haemorrhage of adrenals and lymph nodes (Danhauser & Rustum, 1979). Myocarditis with swelling of cardiac fibres has been reported in rats (Levillain, 1972; Levillain et al., 1974).

Other than lethargy and ataxia, no sign referable to the nervous system has been described in rodents. In dogs and cats, however, neurotoxicity has been associated with veterinary use of 5-fluorouracil in a small proportion of tumour-bearing animals. The signs in 5/13 dogs included hyperexcitability, nervousness, muscle tremors and ataxia shortly after treatment; multiple chemotherapeutic agents had been used, but 1 had received only 5-fluorouracil. One cat developed blindness, ataxia, apprehension and hyperexcitability. Focal malacia and necrosis were found in the brain (Harvey et al., 1977). Similar results were obtained by Henness et al. (1977): In 3 experimental cats, hyperesthesia, tremors and seizures occurred 3 hours after a third daily i.v. injection of 100 mg/m^2 5-fluorouracil. All 3 survived with no apparent ill effects except transient thrombocytopenia.

Topical application of 0.5 mg 5-fluorouracil daily for 14 days to the skin of Syrian hamsters had no apparent effect. Similar topical application to the cheek pouch, however, produced erythema, necrosis and ulceration of the mucosa with subsequent re-epithelization in those hamsters allowed to recover (Cherrick & Weissman, 1974).

Effects on reproduction and prenatal toxicity

Syrian golden hamsters were given i.m. injections of 3-9 mg/animal 5-fluorouracil on one of days 8 - 11 of pregnancy; the fetuses were evaluated on day 15 of gestation. Malformations were observed when the drug was given on day 9, 10 or 11 of pregnancy; these included defects of the tail and limbs and cleft palate. A dose of 4.5 mg/animal given on day 8 or 9 of pregnancy was lethal to all embryos; 8 mg/animal were required to obtain the same effect when given on day 10 of pregnancy. With the higher doses (and especially when applied on day 9 or 10 of pregnancy), the growth of the fetuses of treated mothers was retarded when compared with controls (Shah & MacKay, 1978).

It was reported in an abstract that 5-fluorouracil induced limb abnormalities in the fetuses of ICR-JCL mice injected with a single dose of 20 or 30 mg/kg bw on day 11 of pregnancy (Imagawa *et al.*, 1979).

Mice with and without genes that modify the limb skeleton (SL and SH mice) received i.p. injections of 20 mg/kg bw ^{14}C-labelled 5-fluorouracil on the first day of pregnancy. Incorporation of the label into DNA, RNA and protein of the embryos was studied 1, 2 and 4 hours after the injection. It was shown to be incorporated into the RNA and, to a much lesser degree, into the DNA of embryos of both strains, with little change in specific activity occurring between 1 and 4 hours after the injection. Saturation of the 5-fluorouracil-degrading enzymes by simultaneous application of uracil increased placental transfer of the label and incorporation of 5-fluorouracil into the nucleic acids (Forsthoefel *et al.*, 1978).

The fetuses of two rhesus monkeys treated with 20 and 40 mg/kg bw 5-fluorouracil on day 20 of pregnancy showed no embryotoxic effect when evaluated on day 100 of gestation by hysterotomy. When two monkeys were treated on two consecutive days (days 20 and 21, or 23 and 24) of pregnancy with 20 mg/kg bw, one produced a very small fetus (94 g *versus* 183 ± 3 g in controls), and the other showed resorption only. With doses exceeding 40 mg/kg bw given on various days between days 17 to 27, all of 8 treated monkeys aborted 5 - 39 days after treatment. The author concluded from his studies that the embryotoxic sensitivity of rats and rhesus monkeys may be about 1:2 (Wilson, 1971).

Absorption, distribution, excretion, and metabolism

5-Fluorouracil administered intravenously or intraperitoneally to mice or rats or orally to rats rapidly enters all body compartments. As much as 80% of the administered compound is eliminated through metabolic degradation and the remainder by urinary excretion during the first few hours. The plasma half-life has been reported to be of the order of 10-20 min in a number of species. No binding to plasma proteins has been reported in rabbits or rats (Gilev *et al.*, 1974; Giller *et al.*, 1975). Parent compound is distributed, apparently, to all tissues, with larger amounts generally reported in bone marrow, small intestine (non-villous mucosa), splenic red pulp, liver and kidney. Radiolabelled 5-fluorouracil has also been found to be localized in the hearts of rats and mice (Liss & Chadwick, 1974). Oral absorption of 5-fluorouracil is variable; percutaneous absorption has been reported. Selective uptake by tumour tissue has often been reported but varies considerably from tumour to tumour (Chaudhuri *et al.*, 1958; Oishi *et al.*, 1973; Anada *et al.*, 1974; Liss & Chadwick, 1974; Shani *et al.*, 1978a,b).

5-Fluorouracil requires metabolic activation (Figure 1). In mice, intracellular levels of active nucleotides reach a maximum within 24 hours of drug administration and decline slowly thereafter at a rate characteristic for each tissue. The half-time for disappearance of 5-fluorodeoxyuridylate is about 9 days in bone marrow and about 3 days in intestinal mucosa (Myers *et al.*, 1974; Chabner *et al.*, 1975). Following i.v. injection of 5-fluorouracil into rhesus monkeys (*Macaca mulatta*), 91% of the injected dose was cleared from the vascular compartment within 5 min and 98% by 1 hour. Approximately 0.126% of the total administered dose was found in the cerebrospinal fluid and 0.172% in the brain during the experimental hour (Bourke *et al.*, 1973).

The catabolic and anabolic pathways of 5-fluorouracil are shown in Figure 1. Catabolism, analogous to that of uracil, proceeds largely in the liver to α-fluoro-β-alanine, urea, carbon dioxide and ammonia. Anabolism can be channeled in the direction of either DNA or RNA synthesis, depending on the relative significance of deoxyuridine (thymidine) or uridine phosphorylase. The deoxyuridine pathway leads to the formation of 5-fluorodeoxyuridine monophosphate, which is a potent inhibitor of thymidylate synthetase, an essential enzyme in the *de novo* synthesis of DNA. A covalent complex is formed between 5-fluorodeoxyuridine monophosphate, methylenetetrahydrofolate and thymidylate synthetase which, although reversible, has a sufficiently long half-life to prevent thymidylic acid synthesis. Incorporation of fluorinated uridine into RNA has also been demonstrated. Both mechanisms may contribute to the toxicity of 5-fluorouracil (Chaudhuri *et al.*, 1958; Mukherjee & Heidelberger, 1960; Reichard, 1962; Miller, 1971; Chabner *et al.*, 1975; Rustum *et al.*, 1979; Washtien & Santi, 1979).

Fig. 1. Metabolic pathways of 5-fluorouracil[a]

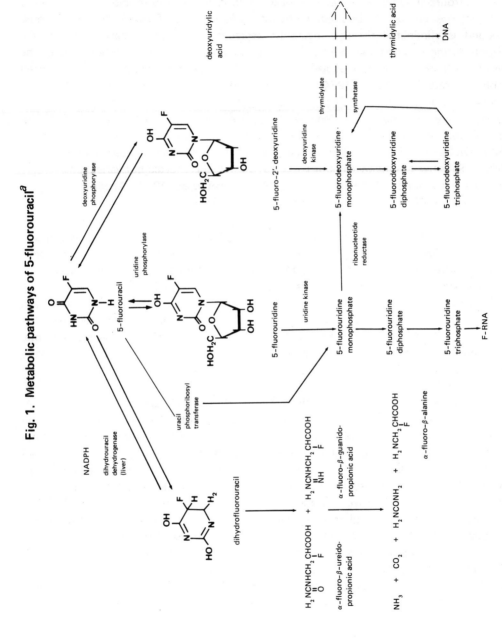

[a] Adapted from Mukherjee & Heidelberger (1960), Miller (1971) and Rustum et al. (1979)

Mutagenicity and other short-term tests

5-Fluorouracil was not mutagenic in the tester strains TA92, TA98 and TA100 of *Salmonella typhimurium* with or without addition of rat liver microsomal supernatant (Seino *et al.*, 1978). It is reported to induce 'petite mutation' in *Saccharomyces cerevisiae* (Moustacchi & Marcovich, 1963).

5-Fluorouracil produced chromosomal breakage in CHO cells but only at the high concentration of 100 μg/ml. It also produced increases in micronuclei formation in the bone marrow of outbred ICR mice (Maier & Schmid, 1976).

5-Fluorouracil produced morphological transformation of C3H/10T½ clone 8 mouse embryo cells at cytotoxic concentrations. Morphological transformation was also produced by 5-fluoro-2'-deoxyuridine, a metabolite of 5-fluorouracil, and such transformed cells produced malignant tumours when injected into immunosuppressed syngeneic mice (Jones *et al.*, 1976).

(b) Humans

Toxic effects

5-Fluorouracil has a narrow therapeutic range, and because of considerable individual variation in response, severe toxicity is occasionally associated with the commonly used dosage schedules. Jacobs *et al.* (1971) reported 8 drug-related deaths in 430 cancer patients.

The most frequently reported toxic signs reflect the effects of 5-fluorouracil on rapidly proliferating cells in the gastrointestinal mucosa, bone marrow, hair follicles and nail beds. The first signs of toxicity in treated patients are leucopenia and stomatitis. Other side effects are diarrhoea, nausea, vomiting, thrombocytopenia and a decrease in erythrocyte precursors in the marrow. These effects are reversed after cessation of therapy, when the mucosa returns to normal (Miller, 1971). In man, 5-fluorouracil is immunosuppressive in regimens of 5 - 10 mg/kg bw daily for 5 - 7 days intravenously, but not at 2.5 mg/kg bw (Berenbaum, 1979). Alopecia and dermatitis have been reported in 5 - 20% of patients. Hyperpigmentation and photosensitivity have also been reported (Miller, 1971).

Less frequent, but important, toxic effects have been reported in the nervous and cardiovascular systems. Neurotoxicity has been observed in 0.6 - 7% of small groups of patients: the clinical signs, which are those of an acute cerebellar syndrome, usually abate 1-6 weeks after discontinuing therapy. The cause of the neurotoxicity is unknown, although it is speculated that a major catabolite, α-fluoro-β-alanine may be further degraded in the nervous system to form fluoroacetate and fluorocitrate, the latter being an inhibitor of the Krebs cycle (Weiss *et al.*, 1974). Cardiotoxicity is a rare complication with signs ranging from mild stenocardia to severe myocardial infarction shortly after 5-fluorouracil administration (Stevenson *et al.*, 1977; Mikhailidis *et al.*, 1978; Pottage *et al.*, 1978; Soukop *et al.*, 1978; Villani *et al.*, 1979). Many, but not all, of the patients had also received irradiation to the chest area. Thiamine deficiency in patients has been attributed to treatment with 5-fluorouracil (Aksoy *et al.*, 1980).

Effects on reproduction and prenatal toxicity

Transient toxicity, characterized by mild respiratory distress and petechiae, was observed in a newborn whose mother had received a total dose of 7.5 g 5-fluorouracil during the second and third trimesters of pregnancy (Stadler & Knowles, 1971).

Absorption, distribution, excretion and metabolism

The distribution and metabolism of 5-fluorouracil in humans are similar to those in animals (*vide supra*) (Mukherjee *et al.*, 1963; Clarkson *et al.*, 1964; Cohen *et al.*, 1974; Chabner *et al.*, 1975; Finch *et al.*, 1979). Cancer patients exibit greater variability, however, than experimental animals in rates of absorption and degradation of 5-fluorouracil (Sitar *et al.*, 1977; MacMillan *et al.*, 1978). The early appearance and sustained presence of 5-fluorouracil in portal plasma, along with its excretion in the bile, suggest an entero-hepatic circulation after oral or i.v. administration (Douglass & Mittelman, 1974).

Mutagenicity and chromosomal effects

In 3 out of 4 patients with solid tumours who received 5-fluorouracil only, at cumulative doses of 0.24 - 1.0 g, there was a slight increase in numerical and structural chromosome aberrations in peripheral blood lymphocytes (Bridge & Melamed, 1972). No increase in sister chromatid exchanges was found in peripheral blood lymphocytes of two patients with solid tumours treated with single i.v. doses of 5 g 5-fluorouracil (Musilová *et al.*, 1979).

3.3 Case reports and epidemiological studies of carcinogenicity in humans

Acute nonlymphocytic leukaemia has been described in 5 women who received 5-fluorouracil in combination with other chemotherapy for solid tumours: 3 ovarian cancers (Kaslow *et al.*, 1972; Reimer *et al.*, 1977) and 2 breast cancers (Davis *et al.*, 1973). All 5 had received alkylating agents, and 4 had also received radiation.

In 2 case reports, a squamous-cell carcinoma of the skin occurred after local application of 5-fluorouracil to a basal-cell carcinoma (Hill, 1970; Kurtis & Rosen, 1979).

An astrocytoma appeared in a child treated with 5-fluorouracil and methotrexate for colon cancer (Regelson *et al.*, 1965).

No epidemiological study was available.

4. SUMMARY OF DATA REPORTED AND EVALUATION

4.1 Experimental data

5-Fluorouracil was tested by intravenous administration in mice and rats and by oral administration in rats. No evidence of carcinogenicity was found, but the studies suffered from limitations with regard to duration or dose.

5-Fluorouracil can induce embryotoxic and teratogenic effects in several animal species and may be embryolethal in monkeys at doses nontoxic to the mother. The available experimental data on the mutagenicity of 5-fluorouracil are inconclusive; the agent did induce transformation in a mouse cell line.

4.2 Human data

5-Fluorouracil has been used since the late 1950s as the main antineoplastic agent in the treatment of gastrointestinal tumours; it is used frequently in combination with other agents for the treatment of a variety of solid tumours.

Data available to the Working Group were insufficient to evaluate the teratogenic potential of this drug in humans. Data on chromosomal aberrations produced by 5-fluorouracil, though limited, suggest that the drug has clastogenic potential.

5-Fluorouracil has been associated in a few case reports with a variety of subsequent neoplasms. In almost all of these cases, the drug was given together with other agents known or suspected of being carcinogens. No epidemiological study was available to the Working Group.

4.3 Evaluation

There was no evidence for the carcinogenicity of 5-fluorouracil in the limited studies in experimental animals. The data from case reports in humans were insufficient to arrive at a conclusion.

On the basis of the available data, no evaluation could be made of the carcinogenic risk of 5-fluorouracil to humans.

5. REFERENCES

Aksoy, M., Basu, T.K., Brient, J. & Dickerson, J.W.T. (1980) Thiamin status of patients treated with drug combinations containing 5-fluorouracil. *Eur. J. Cancer, 16,* 1041-1045

Anada, H., Nakamura, N. & Marumo, H. (1974) Studies on the metabolic fate of 5-fluorouracil in the oral administration (Jpn.). *J. pharm. Soc. Jpn., 94,* 1131-1138

Baker, C.E., Jr, ed. (1980) *Physicians' Desk Reference,* 34th ed., Oradell, NJ, Medical Economics Co., pp. 561-562, 924, 1425-1454

Berenbaum, M.C. (1979) The immunosuppressive effects of 5-fluorocytosine and 5-fluorouracil. *Chemotherapy, 25,* 54-59

Bourke, R.S., West, C.R., Chheda, G. & Tower, D.B. (1973) Kinetics of entry and distribution of 5-fluorouracil in cerebrospinal fluid and brain following intravenous injection in a primate. *Cancer Res., 33,* 1735-1746

Brandberg, A., Almersjö, O., Falsen, E., Gustavsson, B., Hafström, L. & Lindblom, G.-B. (1977) Methodological aspects of an agar plate technique for determination of biologically active 5-fluorouracil in blood, urine and bile. *Acta pathol. microbiol. scand., Sect. B, 85,* 227-234

Bridge, M.F. & Melamed, M.R. (1972) Leukocyte chromosome abnormalities in advanced nonhematopoietic cancer. *Cancer Res., 32,* 2212-2220

Chabner, B.A., Myers, C.E., Coleman, C.N. & Johns, D.G. (1975) The clinical pharmacology of antineoplastic agents (first of two parts) *New Engl. J. Med., 292,* 1107-1113

Chaudhuri, N.K., Mukherjee, K.L. & Heidelberger, C. (1958) Studies on fluorinated pyrimidines. VII. The degradative pathway. *Biochem. Pharmacol., 1,* 328-341

Cherrick, H.M. & Weissman, D. (1974) Effects of topically applied 5-fluorouracil in the Syrian hamster. *J. invest. Dermatol., 63,* 284-286

Clarkson, B., O'Connor, A., Winston, L. & Hutchinson, D. (1964) The physiologic disposition of 5-fluorouracil and 5-fluoro-2'-deoxyuridine in man. *Clin. Pharmacol. Ther., 5,* 581-610

Cohen, J.L. & Brown, R.E. (1978) High-performance liquid chromatographic analysis of 5-fluorouracil in plasma. *J. Chromatogr., 151,* 237-240

Cohen, J.L., Irwin, L.E., Marshall, G.J., Darvey, H. & Bateman, J.R. (1974) Clinical pharmacology of oral and intravenous 5-fluorouracil (NSC-19893). *Cancer Chemother. Rep., 58,* 723-731

Danhauser, L.L. & Rustum, Y.M. (1979) A method for continuous drug infusion in unrestrained rats: its application in evaluating the toxicity of 5-fluorouracil/thymidine combinations. *J. Lab. clin. Med., 93,* 1047-1053

Davis, H.L., Jr, Prout, M.N., McKenna, P.J., Cole, D.R. & Korbitz, B.C. (1973) Acute leukemia complicating metastatic breast cancer. *Cancer, 31,* 543-546

Douglass, H.O., Jr & Mittelman, A. (1974) Metabolic studies of 5-fluorouracil. II. Influence of the route
of administration on the dynamics of distribution in man. *Cancer, 34,* 1878-1881

Driessen, O., De Vos, D. & Timmermans, P.J.A. (1979) Sensitive gas-liquid chromatographic assay of
underivatized 5-fluorouracil in plasma. *J. Chromatogr., 162,* 451-456

Duschinsky, R. & Pleven, E. (1957) The synthesis of 5-fluoropyrimidines. *J. Am. chem. Soc., 79,* 4559-
4560

Finch, R.E., Bending, M.R. & Lant, A.F. (1979) Plasma levels of 5-fluorouracil after oral and intravenous
administration in cancer patients. *Br. J. clin. Pharmacol., 7,* 613-617

Forsthoefel, P.F., Blend, M.J. & Snow, J.W. (1978) Biochemical aspects of the interactions of the teratogens 5-fluorouracil and 5-fluorodeoxyuridine with normal nucleic acid precursors in mice selected for
low and high expression of Strong's luxoid gene. *Teratology, 18,* 269-276

Gilev, A.P., Meirena, D.V., Khagi, K.B., Koptelova, M.N. & Shafro, E.A. (1974) Studies on the pharmacokinetics of fluorouracil-2-C^{14} (Russ.). *Bjull. eksp. Biol. Med., 78,* 39-41

Giller, S.A., Meiren, D.V., Khagi, K.B., Koptelova, M.N., Shafro, E.A., Zhuk, R.A. & Gilev, A.P. (1975)
A comparative study of the fate of fluorofur and 5-fluorouracil in the organism (Russ.). *Vop. Onkol.,
21,* 84-86

Goodman, L.S. & Gilman, A., eds (1975) *The Pharmacological Basis of Therapeutics,* 5th ed., New York,
Macmillan, pp. 1364-1369

Gustavsson, B., Baldesten, A., Hasselgren, P. & Almersjö, O. (1979) New assay of 5-fluorouracil in serum
by isotachophoresis. *J. Chromatogr., 179,* 151-159

Hadidian, Z., Fredrickson, T.N., Weisburger, E.K., Weisburger, J.H., Glass, R.M. & Mantel, N. (1968) Tests
for chemical carcinogens. Report on the activity of derivatives of aromatic amines, nitrosamines,
quinolines, nitroalkanes, amides, epoxides, aziridines, and purine antimetabolites. *J. natl Cancer
Inst., 41,* 985-1036

Harrison, S.D., Jr, Denine, E.P. & Peckham, J.C. (1978) Qualitative and quantitative toxicity of single and
sequential sublethal doses of 5-fluorouracil in BDF$_1$ mice. *Cancer Treat. Rep., 62,* 533-545

Harvey, H.J., MacEwen, E.G. & Hayes, A.A. (1977) Neurotoxicosis associated with use of 5-fluorouracil
in five dogs and one cat. *J. Am. vet. med. Assoc., 171,* 277-278

Hawrylyshyn, M., Senkowski, B.Z. & Wollish, E.G. (1964) Thin-layer chromatography of fluoropyrimi-
dines. *Microchem. J., 8,* 15-22

Henness, A.M., Theilen, G.H., Madewell, B.R. & Crow, S.E. (1977) Neurotoxicosis associated with use of
5-fluorouracil. *J. Am. vet. med. Assoc., 171,* 692

Hill, B.H.R. (1970)   Occurrence of squamous carcinoma in hyperkeratosis and Bowenoid lesions treated with 5-fluorouracil. *Aust. J. Dermatol., 11,* 107

Homburger, F., Treger, A. & Boger, E. (1971)   Inhibition of murine subcutaneous and intravenous benzo-(*rst*)pentaphene carcinogenesis by sweet orange oils and *d*-limonene. *Oncology, 25,* 1-10

Houghton, J.A., Houghton, P.J. & Wooten, R.S. (1979)   Mechanism of induction of gastrointestinal toxicity in the mouse by 5-fluorouracil, 5-fluorouridine, and 5-fluoro-2'-deoxyuridine. *Cancer Res., 39,* 2406-2413

Hršak, I. & Pavičič, S. (1974)   Comparison of the effects of 5-fluorouracil and ftorafur on the haematopoiesis in mice. *Biomedicine, 21,* 164-167

Imagawa, S., Tsuge, K. & Watari, S. (1979)   Morphogenesis of 5-fluorouracil induced symbrachydactyly in mice (Abstract). *Teratology, 20,* 155

Jacobs, E.M., Reeves, W.J., Jr, Wood, D.A., Pugh, R., Braunwald, J. & Bateman, J.R. (1971)   Treatment of cancer with weekly intravenous 5-fluorouracil. Study by the Western Cooperative Cancer Chemotherapy Group (WCCCG). *Cancer, 27,* 1302-1305

Johnson, R.K., Garibjanian, B.T., Houchens, D.P., Kline, I., Gaston, M.R., Syrkin, A.B. & Goldin, A. (1976)   Comparison of 5-fluorouracil and ftorafur. I. Quantitative and qualitative differences in toxicity to mice. *Cancer Treat. Rep., 60,* 1335-1345

Jones, P.A., Benedict, W.F., Baker, M.S., Mondal, S., Rapp, U. & Heidelberger, C. (1976)   Oncogenic transformation of C3H/10T½ clone 8 mouse embryo cells by halogenated pyrimidine nucleosides. *Cancer Res., 36,* 101-107

Kaslow, R.A., Wisch, N. & Glass, J.L. (1972)   Acute leukemia following cytotoxic therapy. *J. Am. med. Assoc., 219,* 75-76

Kurtis, B. & Rosen, T. (1979)   Squamous-cell carcinoma arising in a basal-cell epithelioma treated with 5-fluorouracil. *J. Dermatol. surg. Oncol., 5,* 394-396

Lakings, D.B. & Adamson, R.H. (1978)   Quantitative analysis of 5-fluorouracil in human serum by selected ion monitoring gas chromatography-mass spectrometry. *J. Chromatogr., 146,* 512-517

Lee, S., Kim, J.-G. & Chun, S.I. (1980)   Treatment of verruca plana with 5% 5-fluorouracil ointment. *Dermatologica, 160,* 383-389

Lesnaya, N.A. (1972)   Diurnal variations of the 5-fluorouracil and olivomycin toxicity (Russ.). *Farmakol. Toksikol., 35,* 218-219

Levillain, R. (1972)   Cardiac lesions observed by optic microscopy in Wistar rats after ingestion of 5-fluorouracil (Fr.). *J. Méd. Besançon, 8,* 37-44

Levillain, R., Ramona, F. & Cluzan, R. (1974)   Possible usefulness of repeated cardiac examinations in cancer patients undergoing intensive, long-term chemotherapy. (Remarks suggested by experimental results in the rat.) (Fr.). *Thérapie, 29,* 101-108

Liss, R.H. & Chadwick, M. (1974) Correlation of 5-fluorouracil (NSC-19893) distribution in rodents with toxicity and chemotherapy in man. *Cancer Chemother. Rep., 58,* 777-786

MacMillan, W.E., Wolberg, W.H. & Welling, P.G. (1978) Pharmacokinetics of fluorouracil in humans. *Cancer Res., 38,* 3479-3482

Maier, P. & Schmid, W. (1976) Ten model mutagens evaluated by the micronucleus test. *Mutat. Res., 40,* 325-338

Mikhailidis, D.P., Gillett, D.S. & Lang-Stevenson, D. (1978) Fluorouracil cardiotoxicity. *Br. med. J., ii,* 1138

Miller, E. (1971) The metabolism and pharmacology of 5-fluorouracil. *J. surg. Oncol., 3,* 309-315

Min, B.H. & Garland, W.A. (1978) Rapid assay of 5-fluorouracil (5FU) in plasma by GC-CIMS and stable isotope dilution. *Res. Commun. chem. Pathol. Pharmacol., 22,* 145-154

Moustacchi, E. & Marcovich, H. (1963) Induction of 'petite' colony mutations in yeast by 5-fluorouracil (Fr.). *C.R. Acad. Sci. Paris, 256,* 5646-5648

Mukherjee, K.L. & Heidelberger, C. (1960) Studies on fluorinated pyrimidines. IX. The degradation of 5-fluorouracil-6-C^{14}. *J. biol. Chem., 235,* 433-437

Mukherjee, K.L., Boohar, J., Wentland, D., Ansfield, F.J. & Heidelberger, C. (1963) Studies on fluorinated pyrimidines. XVI. Metabolism of 5-fluorouracil-2-C^{14} and 5-fluoro-2'-deoxyuridine-2-C^{14} in cancer patients. *Cancer Res., 23,* 49-66

Musilová, J., Michalová, K. & Urban, J. (1979) Sister-chromatid exchanges and chromosomal breakage in patients treated with cytostatics. *Mutat. Res., 67,* 289-294

Myers, C.E., Young, R.C., Johns, D.G. & Chabner, B.A. (1974) Assay of 5-fluorodeoxyuridine 5'-monophosphate and deoxyuridine 5'-monophosphate pools following 5-fluorouracil. *Cancer Res., 34,* 2682-2688

Oishi, T., Shiraki, H., Mineura, K. & Takahira, H. (1973) The study on metabolic fate of 5-fluorouracil-6-^{14}C after percutaneous administration (Jpn.). *J. pharm. Soc. Jpn., 93,* 749-755

Pantarotto, C., Fanelli, R., Filippeschi, S., Facchinetti, T., Spreafico, F. & Salmona, M. (1979) Quantitative gas-liquid chromatographic determination of ftorafur and 5-fluorouracil in biological specimens. *Analyt. Biochem., 97,* 232-238

Pottage, A., Holt, S., Ludgate, S. & Langlands, A.O. (1978) Fluorouracil cardiotoxicity. *Br. med. J., i,* 547

Regelson, W., Bross, I.D., Hananian, J. & Nigogoygan, G. (1965) Incidence of second primary tumors in children with cancer and leukemia: a seven-year survey of 150 consecutive autopsied cases. *Cancer, 18,* 58-72

Reichard, P. (1962) Biochemical changes during treatment with 5-fluorouracil. *Cancer Chemother. Rep.,*
16, 347-352

Reimer, R.R., Hoover, R., Fraumeni, J.F., Jr & Young, R.C. (1977) Acute leukemia after alkylating-agent
therapy of ovarian cancer. *New Engl. J. Med., 297,* 177-181

Rudy, B.C. & Senkowski, B.Z. (1973) *Fluorouracil.* In: Florey, K., ed., *Analytical Profiles of Drug*
Substances, Vol. 2, New York, Academic Press, pp. 222-244

Rustum, Y.M., Danhauser, L. & Wang, G. (1979) Selectivity of action of 5-FU: biochemical basis. *Bull.*
Cancer, 66, 44-47

Scherf, H.R. & Schmähl, D. (1975) Experimental investigations on immunodepressive properties of
carcinogenic substances in male Sprague-Dawley rats. *Recent Results Cancer Res., 52,* 76-87

Schmähl, D. & Osswald, H. (1970) Experimental studies on the carcinogenic effects of anticancer chemo-
therapeutics and immunosuppressives (Ger.). *Arzneimittel-Forsch./Drug Res., 20,* 1461-1467

Seino, Y., Nagao, M., Yahagi, T., Hoshi, A., Kawachi, T. & Sugimura, T. (1978) Mutagenicity of several
classes of antitumor agents to *Salmonella typhimurium* TA98, TA100, and TA92. *Cancer Res., 38,*
2148-2156

Shah, R.M. & MacKay, R.A. (1978) Teratological evaluation of 5-fluorouracil and 5-bromo-2-deoxyuridine
on hamster fetuses. *J. Embryol. exp. Morphol., 43,* 47-54

Shani, J., Berman, J.A. & Wolf, W. (1978a) Autoradiographic distribution studies of 2-^{14}C-fluorouracil
following oral or intravenous administration in mice bearing solid sarcoma-180. *J. pharm. Sci., 67,*
344-347

Shani, J., Wolf, W., Schlesinger, T., Atkins, H.L., Bradley-Moore, P.R., Casella, V., Fowler, J.S., Greenberg,
D., Ido, T., Lambrecht, R.M., MacGregor, R., Mantescu, C., Neirinckx, R., Som, P. & Wolf, A.P.
(1978b) Distribution of ^{18}F-5-fluorouracil in tumor-bearing mice and rats. *Int. J. nucl. Med. Biol.,*
5, 19-28

Sitar, D.S., Shaw, D.H., Jr, Thirlwell, M.P. & Ruedy, J.R. (1977) Disposition of 5-fluorouracil after intravenous bolus doses of a commercial formulation to cancer patients. *Cancer Res., 37,* 3981-3984

Soukop, M., McVie, J.G. & Calman, K.C. (1978) Fluorouracil cardiotoxicity. *Br. med. J., ii,* 1422

Stadler, H.E. & Knowles, J. (1971) Fluorouracil in pregnancy: effect on the neonate. *J. Am. med. Assoc.,*
217, 214-215

Stevenson, D.L., Mikhailidis, D.P. & Gillett, D.S. (1977) Cardiotoxicity of 5-fluorouracil. *Lancet, ii,*
406-407

US Pharmacopeial Convention, Inc. (1980) *The US Pharmacopeia,* 20th rev., Rockville, MD, pp. 332-334

Villani, F., Guindani, A. & Pagnoni, A. (1979) 5-Fluorouracil cardiotoxicity. *Tumori, 65,* 487-495

Wade, H., ed. (1977) *Martindale, The Extra Pharmacopoeia,* 27th ed., London, The Pharmaceutical Press, pp. 148-150

Washtien, W.L. & Santi, D.V. (1979) Assay of intracellular free and macromolecular-bound metabolites of 5-fluorodeoxyuridine and 5-fluorouracil. *Cancer Res., 39,* 3397-3404

Weathers, D.R. & Halstead, C.L. (1969) Histologic study of the effect of 5-fluorouracil on chemically induced early dysplasia of the hamster cheek pouch. *J. dent. Res., 48,* 157

Weiss, H.D., Walker, M.D. & Wiernik, P.H. (1974) Neurotoxicity of commonly used antineoplastic agents (first of two parts). *New Engl. J. Med., 291,* 75-81

Wilson, J.G. (1971) Use of rhesus monkeys in teratological studies. *Fed. Proc., 30,* 104-109

Windholz, M., ed. (1976) *The Merck Index,* 9th ed., Rahway, NJ, Merck & Co., p. 541

1. CHEMICAL AND PHYSICAL DATA

1.1 Synonyms and trade names

Chem. Abstr. Services Reg. No.: 3778-73-2

Chem. Abstr. Name: 2*H*-1,3,2-Oxazaphosphorin-2-amine, *N*,3-bis(2-chloroethyl)-tetrahydro-, 2-oxide

IUPAC Systematic Name: 3-(2-Chloroethyl)-2-[(2-chloroethyl)amino] tetrahydro-2*H*-1,3,2-oxazaphosphorine 2-oxide

Synonyms: 3-(2-Chloroethyl)-2-[(2-chloroethyl)amino] perhydro-2*H*-1,3,2-oxaza-phosphorine 2-oxide; ifosfamid; ifosfamide; iphosphamid; iphosphamide; isofosfamide; isofosfamidum

Trade names: A 4942; Asta Z 4942; Holoxan 1000; Isoendoxan; NSC 109724; Z 4942

1.2 Structural and molecular formulae and molecular weight

*2 optical isomers

$C_7H_{15}Cl_2N_2O_2P$ Mol. wt: 261.1

1.3 Chemical and physical properties of the pure substance

From Handelsman *et al.* (1974)

(a) *Description:* White crystals

(b) *Melting-point:* 48-50°C

(c) *Spectroscopy data*: Infra-red and nuclear magnetic resonance spectra have been tabulated.

(d) *Solubility:* Soluble in water (1 in 10) and carbon disulphide (1.5 in 100); very soluble in dichloromethane

(e) *Stability:* Sensitive to hydrolysis, oxidation and heat

1.4 Technical products and impurities

Isophosphamide is available in vials containing 300 mg, 1 g or 3 g of the compound, to be made up with sterile water for injection to 3, 50 or 100 mg/ml isophosphamide (Handelsman *et al.*, 1974).

2. PRODUCTION, USE, OCCURRENCE AND ANALYSIS

2.1 Production and use

(a) *Production*

A method for the synthesis of isophosphamide, first patented in 1968 (Asta-Werke AG, 1968) described the cleavage of the aziridine (ethyleneimine) ring of 3-(2-chloroethyl)-2-[1-aziridinyl] perhydro-2*H*-1,3,2-oxazaphosphorine 2-oxide with hydrogen chloride in diethyl ether to form isophosphamide.

A company in the Federal Republic of Germany is believed to be the only manu-facturer of this chemical; however, no data were available on the quantities produced.

(b) *Use*

Isophosphamide is used to a limited but increasing extent as an antineoplastic and immunosuppressive drug. Its pharmacological activity is similar to that of cyclophos-phamide. Given intravenously or orally, it is used in the treatment of oat-cell tumours of the lung, ovarian cancer, breast cancer and non-Hodgkin's lymphomas (Carter & Slavik, 1977).

2.2 Occurrence

Isophosphamide is not known to be produced in Nature.

2.3 Analysis

Analysis of isophosphamide in blood plasma of patients receiving the drug can be performed by a gas chromatography/flame ionization detection method with a detection limit of 1 μg/ml (Allen & Creaven, 1972a).

3. BIOLOGICAL DATA RELEVANT TO THE EVALUATION OF CARCINOGENIC RISK TO HUMANS

3.1 Carcinogenicity studies in animals

(a) Subcutaneous and/or intramuscular administration

Mouse: Four groups of female New Zealand Black/New Zealand White (NZB/NZW) hybrid mice, which develop antinuclear antibodies and immune complex glomerulonephritis and thus serve as models of systemic lupus erythematosus, were given s.c. injections 5 times per week of isophosphamide dissolved in normal saline. Thirty-four mice, 120 days old, and 27 mice, 180 days old, were treated with 0.2 mg/mouse; 29 mice, 120 days old, and 23 mice, 180 days old, were treated with 0.4 mg/mouse. An additional 15 mice, 120 days old, and 20 mice, 180 days old, received 2.0 mg/mouse every 7 days. Controls were 96 untreated or solvent-treated mice [proportion and age at start of experiment unspecifed]. The study was terminated at the beginning of the 21st month of age for each group. In the control group, the median survival time after the start of administration was 292 days: 3/96 (3%) mice had malignant lymphomas, and uraemia was thought to be the cause of death in 94 animals. The median survival time in the experimental groups was essentially independent of the age at the beginning of administration: for animals treated with 0.2 mg the median survival was 425 days and that of animals receiving 0.4 mg was 600 days. Animals that received weekly doses of 2 mg had a median survival of 600 days. Total tumour incidences are summarized in Table 1:

Table 1. Tumour incidence in female NZB/NZW mice treated with isophosphamide

Treatment	Tumour incidence (%)		
	All mice	According to age at start of treatment	
		120 days	180 days
Isophosphamide 0.2 mg 5 days/week	13.0	12.0	15.0
Isophosphamide 0.4 mg 5 days/week	34.5	38.0	26.0
Isophosphamide 2 mg/week	25.5	26.5	13.5
Controls	3.0	-	-

According to the authors, isophosphamide treatment resulted in a significant increase in the number of animals with neoplasms in all groups. Daily high doses of isophosphamide led to a greater tumour frequency than did low doses. Weekly isophosphamide treatment proved to be comparable in oncogenicity to daily treatment with high doses. Most tumours appeared after long-term treatment. The authors state that the age at onset of therapy did not influence the appearance of tumours [age-standardized statistical evaluation was not carried out] (Mitrou et al., 1979a). The detailed histology of the types of tumours observed in treated animals was reported later; these consisted of 23 lymphomas, 7 undifferentiated sarcomas, 1 fibrosarcoma, 6 adenocarcinomas of the lung and 1 granulocytic leukaemia (Mitrou et al., 1979b). [The Working Group noted that in the absence of age-adjusted comparisons, early death in NZB hybrid mice from autoimmune disease precluded direct comparison with treated mice.]

A similar study was carried out with younger female mice of the same strain. Four groups of 9 - 10 mice, 6, 7, 8 or 12 weeks of age, were given s.c. injections of 0.2 mg isophosphamide 5 times per week. The experiment was terminated 7 or 8 months later. The same control group as described in the previous study (Mitrou et al., 1979a) was used. Only 1 treated animal died from a lymphoma; no additional tumour was detected at autopsy. This tumour incidence was not significantly different from that of the control mice (Mitrou et al., 1979b).

(b)   Intraperitoneal administration

Mouse: Groups of 35 B6C3F$_1$ mice of each sex, 42 days old, were given i.p. injections of either 10 or 20 mg/kg bw isophosphamide in buffered saline 3 times a week for 52 weeks. Controls were 15 males and 15 females injected with vehicle alone and 15 males and 15 females that were untreated. Surviving mice were killed at 79 - 81 weeks. Of the male mice, over 90% of the untreated controls, 7% of the vehicle controls and 31% of the treated animals lived to the end of the study. The median survival times of the males in the groups receiving the high dose, the low dose and the vehicle were 53, 44 and 29 weeks, respectively. By 44 weeks of treatment, only 3 male mice in the vehicle control group, 18/35 males in the low-dose group and 22/35 males in the high-dose group were still alive. Of the female mice, 90% of the vehicle controls, 77% of the low-dose group and 66% of the high-dose group lived to the end of the study. Of untreated males, 2/14 mice had hepatocellular adenomas; no tumour was observed in the 14 male vehicle controls. Of 29 males treated with the low dose, 6 animals developed 7 tumours: 4 hepatocellular adenomas, 1 hepato-cellular carcinoma, 1 pheochromocytoma and 1 adenocarcinoma of the lung. Of 27 males treated with the high dose, 2 developed hepatocellular adenomas, 1 a carcinoma of the lung and 1 an adenoma of the Harderian gland. Tumour incidences in males were analysed only for animals surviving to week 44, when the first tumour was detected: the age-adjusted incidences of hepatic tumours were not significantly different between vehicle controls and each of the treated groups of males [however, the small size of the control group sample, 3 animals, should be noted]; when a pooled control group was used for comparison, P = 0.043. No tumour was observed in 15 untreated and 14 vehicle female controls. In the low-dose group of 32 female mice, 2 skin carcinomas, 1 subcutaneous sarcoma, 3 malignant lymphomas, 1 hepatocellular carcinoma and 1 leiomyosarcoma of the uterus occurred in a total of 7 animals. In the high-dose group, 13 malignant lymphomas, 1 leiomyosarcoma of the stomach, 1 leiomyosarcoma of the uterus and 1 ovarian haemangioma were found in a total of 15 females. The incidence of malignant lymphomas in females was significantly dose-related, by comparison with either matched vehicle controls (P = 0.001) or pooled vehicle controls (controls, 1/29; P < 0.001). The incidence of lymphomas in the high-dose group was significantly higher than that in matched vehicle controls (P = 0.005) or in pooled vehicle controls (P = 0.001) (National Cancer Institute, 1977). [The Working Group considered that insufficient matched control animals were available for evaluation. Com-parison with pooled control animals provides suggestive but inconclusive evidence for carcinogenicity.]

Groups of 10 male and 10 female A/He mice, 6 - 8 weeks old (18 - 20 g), were given 18.8 or 47 mg/kg bw isophosphamide in water 3 times per week for 8 weeks for a total of 24 applications. An additional group received 260 mg/kg bw 5 times. Controls were 30 males and 30 females which received 24 injections of 0.1 ml water. Survivors were killed after 24 weeks. Among controls, 8/30 males and 11/30 females developed lung tumours. In the group given 5 x 260 mg/kg bw, 12/20 mice survived until the end of the study, and 10 had lung tumours. In the group that received 24 x 47 mg/kg bw, 17/20 survived until the end of the study, and 13 mice developed lung tumours. In the group that received 24 x 18.8 mg/kg bw, 20/20 mice survived until the end of treatment and 12 had lung tumours. A significant increase in lung tumour incidence was observed in all treated groups (Stoner *et al.*, 1973).

Rat: Groups of 35 male (35 days old) and 35 female (42 days old) Sprague-Dawley rats were given i.p. injections of 6 or 12 mg/kg bw isophosphamide in buffered saline 3 times a week for 52 weeks. Controls consisted of 10 males and 10 females injected with the vehicle alone and 10 males and 10 females that were untreated. Surviving rats were killed at 79 - 84 weeks. Of the males, 70% of the untreated controls, 80% of the vehicle controls, 55% of the low-dose group, and 6% of the high-dose group lived to the end of the study. The median survival times of the males in the groups receiving the high and low doses were 35 and 83 weeks, respectively. Of the females, 100% of the untreated controls, 70% of the vehicle controls, 42% of the low-dose group and 3% of the high-dose group lived to the end of the study. The median survival times of the females in the high-dose and low-dose groups were 34 and 74 weeks, respectively. Of the untreated males, 4/8 animals developed 7 tumours, 2 of which were malignant. Of male vehicle controls, 5/9 animals had 7 tumours, 2 of which were malignant. Of 32 males treated with the low dose, 17 animals developed 21 tumours, 9 (26%) of which were malignant. Of 34 males in the high-dose group, 12 animals had 12 tumours, 8 (23%) of which were malignant. The 8 malignancies of the haematopoietic system observed in treated male rats were dose-related when a pooled vehicle control group was used for comparison (controls, 0/29; low dose, 3/32; high dose, 5/34; P = 0.040); and in males of the high-dose group the incidence was higher than in the pooled vehicle controls. The incidence of haematopoietic tumours was not significant when compared with that of matched vehicle controls using time-adjusted analyses; however, it should be noted that 5 of these tumours were observed in the high-dose group whose median survival was only 35 weeks. Of untreated females, 7/10 animals developed 15 tumours, 2 of which were malignant. Of female vehicle controls, 9/10 animals had 17 tumours; 7 tumours in 6 animals were malignant. All 32 females given the low dose developed a total of 84 tumours; 23 of the animals (66%) had 32 malignant tumours. Of females of the high-dose group, 15 tumours arose in 9 animals; 6 animals (17%) had 7 malignant neoplasms. The incidences of uterine leiomyosarcomas and mammary fibro-adenomas in female rats in the low-dose group were significantly higher than in pooled vehicle controls (uterus: control, 0/27, low dose, 15/32; mammary gland: control, 8/28, low dose, 28/33). The incidence of each tumour type was also significantly higher when compared with that of matched vehicle controls using time-adjusted analyses (National Cancer Institute, 1977). [The Working Group considered that insufficient matched control animals were available for evaluation. Comparison with pooled control animals provides suggestive but inconclusive evidence for carcinogenicity.]

3.2 Other relevant biological data

(a) Experimental systems

Toxic effects

In male mice the i.p. LD_{50} of isophosphamide was 540 mg/kg bw (Greco *et al.*, 1979). The i.v. LD_{10} in mice was 470 mg/kg bw (Takamizawa *et al.*, 1974).

Although its metabolic activation is very similar to that of cyclophosphamide, it is less toxic. In experiments in Sprague-Dawley rats, for example, an i.p. dose of 100 mg/kg bw of either drug caused severe leucopenia, but the effect was less in the isophosphamide-treated animals and recovery was much earlier (Marcy *et al.*, 1977).

Effects on reproduction and prenatal toxicity

When Swiss-Webster mice were given i.p. injections of 5, 10 or 20 mg/kg bw isophosphamide on day 11 of pregnancy, an increased rate of resorptions (up to 81%) was found with 20 mg/kg bw and growth retardation with 10 and 20 mg/kg bw. With the highest dose, the incidence of hydrocephalus, micromelia, adactyly, syndactyly, kidney ectopia, and missing or non-ossified skull bones, sternebrae, vertebrae and long bones was increased over that in controls. The levels of plasma-alkylating metabolites in adult mice were considerably lower than with the corresponding dose of cyclophosphamide. The authors concluded that the teratogenic response to isophosphamide, although qualitatively similar to that to cyclophosphamide, was quantitatively different (Bus & Gibson, 1973).

Absorption, distribution, excretion and metabolism

Like cyclophosphamide, isophosphamide requires metabolism by microsomal enzymes to act as a cytotoxic agent (Allen & Creaven, 1972b). It is rapidly metabolized in many species, including rodents and dogs; the urinary metabolites indicate that a series of reactions take place analogous to those in the metabolism of cyclophosphamide (Alarcon *et al.*, 1972; Allen & Creaven, 1972b; Hill *et al.*, 1973). Acrolein (see IARC, 1979) is produced during its oxidative degradation (Alarcon *et al.*, 1972), and one product of the reaction is the ring-opened carboxy derivative. Dogs also rapidly metabolize isophosphamide, and the carboxy derivative and 4-keto isophosphamide have been identified in the urine (Hill *et al.*, 1973).

Mutagenicity and other short-term tests

Isophosphamide was mutagenic in *Salmonella typhimurium* strain TA1535 when tested in the presence of an Aroclor-induced rat liver microsome preparation (Benedict *et al.*,

1977). Isophosphamide also produced a dose-dependent increase in chromosomal aberrations in Chinese hamster bone-marrow cells following its i.p. administration (Röhrborn & Basler, 1977).

(b) Humans

Toxic effects

The toxicity of isophosphamide to the urinary tract in the majority of patients limits the therapeutic dose that can be given to about 2 g/m^2 (50 mg/kg bw). This toxicity is characterized by the signs of cystitis, including frequency of micturition, haematuria and, in severe cases, a reduction in renal function. Less important side effects of isophosphamide are myelosuppression, nausea and vomiting, alopecia, lethargy, confusion and reversible glycosuria (van Dyk et al., 1972; Bremner et al., 1974; Creaven et al., 1976; Falkson & Falkson, 1976). As with cyclophosphamide, the renal toxicity may be reversed by coadministration of sodium 2-mercaptoethane sulphonate (Brock et al., 1979; Bryant et al., 1980).

No information was available on the possible long-term sequelae of this drug.

Effects on reproduction and prenatal toxicity

No data were available to the Working Group.

Absorption, distribution, excretion and metabolism

The metabolic activation of isophosphamide in man has been proposed to be analogous to that of cyclophosphamide, with ring hydroxylation leading to the formation of isophosphoramide mustard, the active metabolite, and acrolein (Norpoth, 1976; Bryant et al., 1980). An i.v. dose is excreted in the urine mainly as one or both dechlorethylated metabolites (~ 50%), the intact drug (~ 20%) and carboxyisophosphamide (~ 2%), although these percentages vary widely among individuals (Norpoth, 1976; Norpoth et al., 1975). The pharmacokinetics of the intact drug in the plasma of man are reported to be biphasic with a secondary half-life of 15 hours (Allen et al., 1976) when high doses are given, and monophasic with a half-life of 7 hours when lower doses are used (Nelson et al., 1976).

Mutagenicity and chromosomal effects

No data were available to the Working Group.

3.3 Case reports and epidemiological studies of carcinogenicity in humans

No data were available to the Working Group.

4. SUMMARY OF DATA REPORTED AND EVALUATION

4.1 Experimental data

Isophosphamide was tested in four studies in mice and in one in rats by subcutaneous or intraperitoneal administration. In one study in mice with intraperitoneal injection it produced an increased incidence of lung adenomas. The other four studies, although indicating a carcinogenic effect, could not be evaluated.

Isophosphamide can induce teratogenic effects in mice and embryolethality at doses nontoxic to the mother. Isophosphamide is mutagenic in bacteria and produced chromosomal aberrations in Chinese hamster bone-marrow cells.

4.2 Human data

Isophosphamide has been used to a limited but increasing extent since the early 1970s as an antineoplastic and immunosuppressive drug.

No data were available to evaluate the teratogenic or mutagenic potential or chromosomal effects of isophosphamide in humans.

No case report or epidemiological study on isophosphamide was available to the Working Group.

4.3 Evaluation

There is *limited evidence*[1] for the carcinogenicity of isophosphamide in mice and rats.

In the absence of data on humans, no evaluation can be made of the carcinogenic risk of isophosphamide to man.

---

[1] See preamble, p. 19.

5. REFERENCES

Alarcon, R.A., Meienhofer, J. & Atherton, E. (1972) Isophosphamide as a new acrolein-producing anti-neoplastic isomer of cyclophosphamide. *Cancer Res., 32,* 2519-2523

Allen, L.M. & Creaven, P.J. (1972a) Gas chromatographic method for the determination of plasma iso-phosphamide (NSC-109724). *Cancer Chemother. Rep., Part 1, 56,* 721-723

Allen, L.M. & Creaven, P.J. (1972b) Effect of microsomal activation on interaction between isophos-phamide and DNA. *J. pharm. Sci., 61,* 2009-2011

Allen, L.M., Creaven, P.J. & Nelson, R.L. (1976) Studies on the human pharmacokinetics of isophos-phamide (NSC-109724). *Cancer Treat. Rep., 60,* 451-458

Asta-Werke AG (1968) Cyclic derivatives of phosphorodiamidic and phosphorodiamidothionic acids. *French Patent* 1,530, 962, 28 June (*Chem. Abstr., 71,* 49998m)

Benedict, W.F., Baker, M.S., Haroun, L., Choi, E. & Ames, B.N. (1977) Mutagenicity of cancer chemo-therapeutic agents in the *Salmonella*/microsome test. *Cancer Res., 37,* 2209-2213

Bremner, D.N., McCormick, J. StC. & Thomson, J.W.W. (1974) Clinical trial of isophosphamide (NSC-109724) - Results and side effects. *Cancer Chemother. Rep., Part 1, 58,* 889-893

Brock, N., Stekar, J. & Pohl, J. (1979) Antidote against the urotoxic effects of oxazaphosphorin deri-vatives, cyclophosphamide, iphosphamide and trophosphamide (Ger.). *Naturwissenschaften, 66,* 60

Bryant, B.M., Jarman, M., Ford, H.T. & Smith, I.E. (1980) The prevention of isophosphamide-induced urothelial toxicity by 2-mercaptoethane sulphonate sodium (mesnum) in patients with advanced carcinoma. *Lancet, ii,* 657-659

Bus, J.S. & Gibson, J.E., (1973) Teratogenicity and neonatal toxicity of ifosfamide in mice (37450). *Proc. Soc. exp. Biol. Med., 143,* 965-970

Carter, S.K. & Slavik, M. (1977) Current investigational drugs of interest in the chemotherapy program of the National Cancer Institute. *Natl Cancer Inst. Monogr., 45,* 116-117

Creaven, P.J., Allen, L.M., Cohen, M.H. & Nelson, R.L. (1976) Studies on the clinical pharmacology and toxicology of isophosphamide (NSC-109724). *Cancer Treat. Rep., 60,* 445-449

van Dyk, J.J., Falkson, H.C., van der Merwe, A.M. & Falkson, G. (1972) Unexpected toxicity in patients treated with iphosphamide. *Cancer Res., 32,* 921-924

Falkson, G. & Falkson, H.C. (1976) Further experience with isophosphamide. *Cancer Treat. Rep., 60,* 955-957

Greco, C., Corsi, A., Caputo, M., Cavallari, A. & Calabresi, F. (1979) Cyclophosphamide and iphospha-mide against Lewis lung carcinoma: evaluation of toxic and therapeutic effects. *Tumori, 65,* 169-180

Handelsman, H., Goldsmith, M.A. & Slavik, M. (1974) *Isophosphamide NSC-109724, Clinical Brochure,* Bethesda, MD, Division of Cancer Treatment, National Cancer Institute

Hill, D.L., Laster, W.R., Jr, Kirk, M.C., El Dareer, S. & Struck, R.F. (1973) Metabolism of iphosphamide [2-(2-chloroethylamino)-3-(2-chloroethyl)tetrahydro-2H-1,3,2-oxazaphosphorine-2-oxide] and production of a toxic iphosphamide metabolite. *Cancer Res., 33,* 1016-1022

IARC (1979) *IARC Monographs on the Evaluation of the Carcinogenic Risk of Chemicals to Humans,* Vol. 19, *Some Monomers, Plastics and Synthetic Elastomers, and Acrolein,* Lyon, pp. 479-494

Marcy, R., Semont, H. & Prost, R. (1977) Comparative leucotoxic effects of the two isomeric anti-cancer agents cyclophosphamide and ifosfamide. *Int. Res. Commun. Syst. med. Sci. Cancer, 5,* 427

Mitrou, P.S., Fischer, M., Mitrou, G., Röttger, P. & Holtz, G. (1979a) The oncogenic effect of immunosuppressive (cytotoxic) agents in (NZB x NZW) mice. I. Long-term treatment with azathioprine and ifosfamide. *Arzneimittel-Forsch./Drug Res., 29,* 483-488

Mitrou, P.S., Fischer, M., Mitrou, G. & Röttger, P. (1979b) The oncogenic effect of immunosuppressive (cytotoxic) agents in (NZB x NZW) mice. II. Emergence of tumors in young animals treated with azathioprine and ifosfamide, including a histologic assessment of the neoplasms. *Arzneimittel-Forsch./ Drug Res., 29,* 662-667

National Cancer Institute (1977) Bioassay of isophosphamide for possible carcinogenicity. *NCI Carcinog. tech. Rep. Ser., No. 32*

Nelson, R.L., Allen, L.M. & Creaven, P.J. (1976) Pharmacokinetics of divided-dose ifosphamide. *Clin. Pharmacol. Ther., 19,* 365-370

Norpoth, K. (1976) Studies on the metabolism of isophosphamide (NSC-109724) in man. *Cancer Treat. Rep., 60,* 437-443

Norpoth, K., Raidt, H., Witting, U., Müller, G. & Norpoth, R. (1975) Side chain oxidation of ifosphamide in man. *Klin. Wochenschr., 53,* 1075-1076

Rohrborn, G. & Basler, A. (1977) Cytogenetic investigations of mammals. Comparison of the genetic activity of cytostatics in mammals. *Arch. Toxicol., 38,* 35-43

Stoner, G.D., Shimkin, M.B., Kniazeff, A.J., Weisburger, J.H., Weisburger, E.K. & Gori, G.B. (1973) Test for carcinogenicity of food additives and chemotherapeutic agents by the pulmonary tumor response in strain A mice. *Cancer Res., 33,* 3069-3085

Takamizawa, A., Matsumoto, S., Iwata, T., Tochino, Y., Katagiri, K., Yamaguchi, K. & Shiratori, O. (1974) Synthesis and metabolic behavior of the suggested active species of isphosphamide having cytostatic activity. *J. med. Chem., 17,* 1237-1239

1. CHEMICAL AND PHYSICAL DATA

1.1 Synonyms and trade names

Chem. Abstr. Services Reg. No.: 50-44-2

Chem. Abstr. Name: 6*H*-Purine-6-thione, 1,7-dihydro-

IUPAC Systematic Name: Purine-6-thiol

Synonyms: 6-Mercaptopurin; mercaptopurine; mercapto-6-purine; 6-mercapto-1*H*-purine; mercaptopurinum; 7-mercapto-1,3,4,6-tetrazaindene; 6-MP; purinethiol; 6-purinethiol; 3*H*-purine-6-thiol; thiohypoxanthine; 6-thiopurine; 6-thioxopurine

Trade names: IND 1226; Ismipur; Leukerin; Leupurin; Mercaleukin; Mercapurin; Mern; NSC 755; Purinethol

1.2 Structural and molecular formulae and molecular weight

$C_5H_4N_4S$ Mol. wt: 152.19

1.3 Chemical and physical properties of the pure substance (monohydrate)

From Windholz (1976) or Weast (1977), unless otherwise specified

(a) *Description:* Yellow, odourless, crystalline powder (Benezra & Foss, 1978)

(b) *Melting-point:* 313-314°C (dec.); becomes anhydrous at 140°C

(c) *Spectroscopy data:* λ_{max} 327 nm, A_1^1 = 1400 (at pH 1.0); 312 nm, A_1^1 = 1288 (at pH 11) *(d)* *Solubility:* Soluble in boiling water (1 in 100), alkaline solutions (with decomposition), hot ethanol and ethanol (1 in 950); slightly soluble in dilute sulphuric acid; almost insoluble in water, acetone, chloroform and diethyl ether (Wade, 1977)

(e) *Stability:* Sensitive to oxidation and light

1.4 Technical products and impurities

Various national and international pharmacopoeias give specifications for the purity of 6-mercaptopurine in pharmaceutical products. For example, it is available in the US as a USP grade measured as containing 97.0 - 102.0% active ingredient calculated on the anhydrous basis, 12% max. moisture content, and 0.010% max. phosphorus. It is also available in tablets measured as containing 93.0 - 110.0% active ingredient calculated as the monohydrate (US Pharmacopeial Convention, Inc., 1980).

6-Mercaptopurine is available in western Europe as 50-mg tablets (Wade, 1977) and in Japan as a powder.

2. PRODUCTION, USE, OCCURRENCE AND ANALYSIS

2.1 Production and use

(a) Production

Synthesis of 6-mercaptopurine was first reported in 1951 by the reaction of hypoxanthine with phosphorus pentasulphide (Windholz, 1976). Several alternative synthesis routes have subsequently been described (Benezra & Foss, 1978), but the method used for its commercial production is not known.

Commercial production of 6-mercaptopurine in the US was first reported in 1965 (US Tariff Commission, 1967). In 1978, one US company reported the production of an undisclosed amount (see, preamble, p. 20) (US International Trade Commission, 1979).

6-Mercaptopurine is produced by two companies in Finland, and one company each in the Federal Republic of Germany, Italy and the UK. About 100 kg are used annually in western Europe.

The drug has never been produced commercially in Japan; there is evidence that it has been imported and used since 1973, although no quantitative data are available.

(b)   Use

6-Mercaptopurine is used in human medicine as an antineoplastic agent, primarily for the treatment of acute lymphoblastic (or stem-cell) leukaemia. It has also been used in the treatment of acute myeloblastic leukaemia and chronic myelocytic leukaemia (Harvey, 1975; Wade, 1977).

It is an immunosuppressive agent and has been used in the treatment of ulcerative colitis (Harvey, 1975).

The usual initial dose of 6-mercaptopurine is 2.5 mg/kg bw per day in single or divided doses (Goodman & Gilman, 1975; Harvey, 1975; Wade, 1977). Intermittent i.v. therapy is used in the US at a dose of 500 - 800 mg/m^2 body surface area per day for 5 days every 2 weeks (Anon., 1978).

2.2 Occurrence

6-Mercaptopurine is not known to be produced in Nature.

2.3 Analysis

Analytical methods for the determination of 6-mercaptopurine based on titrimetric analysis, spectrophotometry, polarography, mass spectrometry and various chromatographic methods have been reviewed (Benezra & Foss, 1978).

Typical methods for the analysis of 6-mercaptopurine in various matrices are summarized in Table 1.

3. BIOLOGICAL DATA RELEVANT TO THE EVALUATION
OF CARCINOGENIC RISK TO HUMANS

3.1 Carcinogenicity studies in animals

(a)   Skin application

Mouse: Groups of 25 'S' strain mice received 10 mg 6-mercaptopurine in polyethylene glycol by skin application in 10 divided doses given 3 times weekly. Twenty-three days after the first administration of 6-mercaptopurine, a course of croton oil treatment was begun (2 weekly applications of a 0.1% solution in acetone followed by 16 weekly applications of a 0.17% solution). One week after the end of the treatment period (about 29 weeks after the

Table 1. Methods for the analysis of 6-mercaptopurine

Sample matrix	Sample preparation	Assay procedure[a]	Limit of detection	Reference
Formulations	Dissolve in dimethylformamide; add thymol blue solution	T	not given	US Pharmacopeial Convention, Inc. (1980)
Tablets	Powder sample; add aqueous sodium hydroxide; filter; dilute with hydrochloric acid	S	not given	US Pharmacopeial Convention, Inc. (1980)
Blood plasma	Add 9-methylmercaptopurine as internal standard; add dithioerythritol and sodium acetate; extract with ethyl acetate; evaporate; add buffer	HPLC-UV	5 ng/ml	Ding & Benet (1979)
	Add 6-methylthio-2-hydroxy-purine as internal standard; deproteinize with trichloro-acetic acid; centrifuge; add sodium hydroxide	HPLC-UV	0.2 µg/ml	Day et al. (1978)
	Add sulphuric acid; centrifuge; add sodium hydroxide; wash with diethyl ether; treat with tetrahexylammonium hydroxide; extract with iodo-methane and dichloromethane	GC-MS	20 ng/ml	Rosenfeld et al. (1977)

[a] Abbreviations: T, titrimetric analysis; S, spectrophotometry; HPLC-UV, high-performance liquid chromatography with ultra-violet detection; GC-MS, gas chromatography with mass spectrometry

first 6-mercaptopurine administration), 18 surviving mice had no skin tumours (Salaman & Roe, 1956). [The Working Group noted that the duration of the experiment was relatively short.]

(b) Subcutaneous and/or intramuscular administration

Rat: Two groups of 15 female Wistar rats were given s.c. injections of 5 or 2.5 mg 6-mercaptopurine in 0.5% carboxymethylcellulose weekly for 26 weeks. None of 11 rats that received the higher dose developed tumours; however, 1/15 rats given the lower dose developed a tumour at the site of inoculation within 15 months as did 4/180 vehicle control rats (Sugiura *et al.*, 1970). [The tumour types were not specified.]

In a related study, groups of 15 female Wistar and 15 female Sprague-Dawley rats were given s.c. injections of 50 mg 6-mercaptopurine 3-*N*-oxide hydrate in 0.5% carboxymethylcellulose weekly for 26 weeks. It was estimated that each 50-mg dose of 6-mercaptopurine 3-*N*-oxide is reduced *in vivo* to at least 2.5 mg 6-mercaptopurine. Three treated Wistar rats developed fibrosarcomas at the inoculation sites within 461 days, compared with 4/180 vehicle control rats. Of the Sprague-Dawley rats, 0/15 treated rats and 2/45 vehicle control rats developed tumours at the inoculation sites by 15 months (Sugiura & Brown, 1967, Sugiura *et al.*, 1970).

(c) Intraperitoneal administration

Mouse: A group of 35 C57BL mice were given i.p. injections of 20 mg/kg bw 6-mercaptopurine 4 times at weekly intervals, beginning at 1-3 days of age. A total of 10 (29%) developed thymic lymphomas within a mean latent period of 4.8 months. Untreated animals of the same sublines were reported to have fewer than 2% thymic lymphomas at 1 year of age (Doell *et al.*, 1967). [The length of the experiment and matched control data were not given.]

Mouse and rat: In two abstracts (Griswold *et al.*, 1971; Prejean *et al.*, 1972), a study was reported in which groups of Swiss mice and Sprague-Dawley rats of both sexes were administered 6-mercaptopurine intraperitoneally at the maximum tolerated dose and at half that dose. After an observation period of 1 year, 6-mercaptopurine was reported to have caused an increased incidence of haematopoietic tumours in male and female mice and in male rats. In a later publication by the same authors on the same experiment (Weisburger *et al.*, 1975), it was stated that 'Preliminary information indicates that in our test series, 6-mercaptopurine (NSC-755) may have induced lymphosarcomas in mice, a species in which it is a known immunosuppressant .'

Weisburger (1977) reported that in the same study 18/28 male and 35/54 female mice treated with 15 - 30 mg/kg bw 6-mercaptopurine by i.p. injection 3 times per week for 6 months and observed for life developed 12 and 22 lymphosarcomas and 5 and 23 leukaemias, respectively. 6-Mercaptopurine was included in a list of chemotherapeutic agents which caused a 2- to 3-fold increase in tumour incidence over that in controls.

Rat: Of female rats given i.p. injections of 25-50 mg/kg bw 6-mercaptopurine 3 times per week for 6 months and observed for life, 9/24 developed malignant tumours, including 7 in the pituitary, 3 in the mammary gland, 2 in the skin and 2 sarcomas (unspecified). 6-Mercaptopurine was included in a list of compounds which caused a 1.5- to 2-fold increase in tumour incidence over that in controls (Weisburger, 1977).

[Unpublished National Cancer Institute data on the occurrence of lymphoreticular tumours in the same study are as follows (Table 2):

Table 2. Lymphoreticular tumours in mice and rats
given i.p. injections of 6-mercaptopurine

	Males					Females				
untreated control	vehicle control	low dose	mid-dose	high dose	untreated control	vehicle control	low dose	mid-dose	high dose
	Mice						Mice			
1/100	1/14	8/20	-	4/7	3/153	6/28	18/36	-	13/18
	Rats						Rats			
0/179	0/34	6/21	5/10	3/4	1/182	0/39	7/18	0/2	0/2

It was concluded that because of small group sizes, incomplete pathological examination and variability in spontaneous occurrence of these tumours, they cannot be clearly related to administration of the compound.]

(d) Intravenous administration

Rat: A group of 48 male BR 46 strain rats, 100 days old, were given i.v. injections of 16.5 mg/kg bw 6-mercaptopurine (7% of the LD_{50}) once weekly for 52 weeks to give a total dose of 858 mg/kg bw. At the time of appearance of the first tumour, 25 animals were still alive; of these 12% had benign tumours and none had a malignancy, compared with 5% and 6%, respectively, in controls (Schmähl & Osswald, 1970). [The Working Group noted the small number of surviving animals.]

(e) Effects of combinations

Mouse and rat: Doses of 20, 10 or 5 mg/kg bw 6-mercaptopurine plus the same doses of 6-methylmercaptopurine riboside were reported to increase the incidence of lymphoreticular tumours in mice. No such effect was seen in rats given 6 or 3 mg/kg bw of each drug (Weisburger, 1977).

3.2 Other relevant biological data

(a) Experimental systems

Toxic effects

The i.p. LD_{50} of 6-mercaptopurine in male Swiss mice was 100 mg/kg bw given in 5 daily doses and 240 mg/kg bw given as a single injection. The i.p. LD_{50} in rats was 250 mg/kg bw as a single injection (Phillips et al., 1954; Scherf & Schmähl, 1975) and about 70 mg/kg bw as 5 daily doses (Phillips et al., 1954). In dogs, 4 daily i.v. injections of 25 mg/kg bw killed 1/4 animals, while 9 daily injections of 10 mg/kg bw were nonlethal. Oral administration for 9 consecutive days of 12.5 mg/kg bw killed all 4 treated animals, while 10 daily oral doses of 6.3 mg/kg bw were nonlethal (Phillips et al., 1954).

After a single lethal dose of 6-mercaptopurine, the majority of rats survive 2 - 3 days, and deaths do not occur in mice until at least 5 days after injection. In rats, early deaths are due to lung damage, a toxic effect not seen in other species such as mouse, cat or dog. In rats and mice, the predominant toxicity of 6-mercaptopurine is damage to the bone-marrow and intestinal epithelium and hepatic necrosis. Major toxic symptoms in dogs were marked damage to the small intestinal mucosa and bone-marrow depletion. Biochemical evidence of liver damage was present, and jaundice was apparent in treated animals, although livers had only relatively insignificant microscopic foci of necrosis (Phillips et al., 1954).

Effects on reproduction and prenatal toxicity

Female mice were treated subcutaneously with 3 mg/kg bw 6-mercaptopurine daily, starting 3 days before mating with untreated males and up through day 18 of pregnancy. Many of the surviving female offspring, although they had normal body weight, development and general appearance, were either sterile or, if they became pregnant, had smaller litters and more dead fetuses as compared with controls. Histological study of the ovaries of offspring exposed to 6-mercaptopurine in utero revealed that there were few oocytes and ovarian follicles; many ovaries were completely devoid of oocytes (Reimers & Sluss, 1978).

When 6-mercaptopurine was given orally to rats on days 7 and 8 of pregnancy (two doses), 5 mg/kg bw induced death and resorption of about 50% of fetuses, and 10 mg/kg bw caused 90% fetal resorptions. Only 5% resorptions (controls, 2%) were seen when the same doses were given on days 12 and 13 of pregnancy. No gross malformation was noted in any of the fetuses, even in single survivors of otherwise destroyed litters (Thiersch, 1954).

Malformations (anophthalmia, microphthalmia) were observed in the fetuses of rats treated with 50 - 75 mg/kg bw 6-mercaptopurine from day 5 to 9 of pregnancy (Zunin & Borrone, 1955).

Doses of 1 mg/kg bw or more given to Wistar rats on days 6 - 12 of pregnancy were lethal to 100% of embryos; doses of 0.5 - 0.75 mg/kg bw induced anomalies of the central nervous system or of the eyes in 12 - 14% of surviving fetuses. With 50 mg/kg bw given on day 12 of pregnancy, almost 50% of the surviving fetuses had malformations of the limbs. Similar results were obtained using Swiss albino mice: anomalies of the nervous system were seen when 0.5 - 1 mg/kg bw 6-mercaptopurine was given on days 6 - 8 of pregnancy, anomalies of the mandible with 50 mg/kg bw given on day 12, and limb defects when 60 mg/kg bw were given on day 11 of pregnancy. Of the species tested, the rabbit proved to be the most susceptible to the teratogenic action of 6-mercaptopurine: doses of 1 mg/kg bw were sufficient to induce various anomalies in about 50% of surviving fetuses when given on days 6 - 9 or 10 - 14 of pregnancy (Tuchmann-Duplessis & Mercier-Parot, 1958, 1966, 1968; Mercier-Parot & Tuchmann-Duplessis, 1967).

6-Mercaptopurine was found to be embryolethal in rats when given on day 7 of pregnancy and teratogenic when applied on day 12 of pregnancy (Vishniakov, 1968, 1969).

A close analysis of the types of teratogenic effects produced in rats revealed that a large variety of abnormalities can be produced by a single i.p. dose of 6-mercaptopurine given on day 11 of pregnancy. The lowest dose that induced 100% abnormal survivors was found to be 63 mg/kg bw. 6-Mercaptopurine riboside proved to be as teratogenic, with a much lower maternal toxicity (LD$_{50}$, 2 - 3 g/kg bw) (Kury et al., 1968).

Malformations of the gut, limbs, palate, mandible and tongue were observed in a high percentage of the offspring of Syrian golden hamsters given 5 - 9 mg/animal 6-mercaptopurine as a single i.p. injection on day 9 of pregnancy. A much smaller teratogenic effect was induced when the drug was given on day 8 or days 10 - 11 of pregnancy (Shah & Burdett, 1979).

Ochotona rufescens, a small hare, was also sensitive to the teratogenic action of 6-mercaptopurine given i.p. at a dose of 5 - 10 mg/kg bw on days 7 - 12 of pregnancy (Puget et al., 1975).

In NMRI mice, a single s.c. injection of 30 mg/kg bw 6-mercaptopurine riboside induced cleft palates in 100%, malformations of the upper or lower extremities in 95 - 99%, and malformations of the vertebrae in 85% of surviving (71%) fetuses when given on day 10 of pregnancy. Embryos were less suceptible to the drug when it was given on day 11 of pregnancy. No embryotoxic effect was observed with 60 mg/kg bw 6-methylmercaptopurine riboside, a metabolite of 6-mercaptopurine (Neubert et al., 1977).

Results of light- and electron microscopic examinations of the teratogenic action of 6-mercaptopurine have been reported in a number of papers (Adhami & Noack, 1975; Asisi & Merker, 1975; Merker *et al.*, 1975; Adhami, 1979).

Histological studies of rabbit blastocysts indicated that s.c. administration of 25 - 250 mg/kg bw 6-mercaptopurine 24 - 48 hours before autopsy, when given to the mother shortly after mating or on days 4 - 5 of pregnancy, exerted a strongly deleterious effect on the embryo (Adams *et al.*, 1961).

In organ culture studies, typical skeletal abnormalities could be induced during limb development (limb buds from 11-day-old NMRI or C57BL mice) when 6-mercaptopurine or 6-mercaptopurine riboside was added to the culture medium. The smallest effective concentrations were found to be 10 μg/ml 6-mercaptopurine and 3 μg/ml 6-mercaptopurine riboside (Neubert *et al.*, 1974, 1977; Lessmöllmann *et al.*, 1975).

Absorption, distribution, excretion and metabolism

Mice given a single i.p. dose of 10 mg/kg bw ^{35}S-labelled 6-mercaptopurine excreted 21.4% of the dose as unchanged drug in the 24-hour urine, 18.9% as 6-thiouric acid and 29.5% as inorganic sulphate (Elion *et al.*, 1963). Soon after i.p. injection of ^{35}S-labelled material to mice, the concentration of radioactivity was highest in the gut and lowest in the brain. Three hours after injection, radioactive material had been incorporated into both the RNA and DNA fractions of the pooled tissues (Elion *et al.*, 1954). After i.v. administration of 6-mercaptopurine, the half-life for disappearance from the blood was about 9 min in rats and 14 min in mice (Donelli *et al.*, 1972). The concentration of drug after i.p. or i.v. injection is high in many organs, especially liver, soon after injection but falls off rapidly (Esposito *et al.*, 1974; Tterlikkis *et al.*, 1977).

6-Thiouric acid is the major metabolite of 6-mercaptopurine and is formed from this drug by the action of xanthine oxidase (Elion *et al.*, 1963; Chalmers *et al.*, 1967).

As a free base, 6-mercaptopurine competitively inhibits hypoxanthine-guanine phosphoribosyltransferase and xanthine oxidase, but it is not likely that it acts in this way *in vivo*. The major action of 6-mercaptopurine is inhibition of purine ribonucleotide synthesis and interconversions after its anabolism to 6-methylthioinosinate and 6-thioinosinate (Paterson & Tidd, 1975).

Mutagenicity and other short-term tests

6-Mercaptopurine was mutagenic without metabolic activation in *Salmonella typhimurium* tester strains *his* G46 and TA1535 (Herbold & Buselmaier, 1976; Benedict *et al.*, 1977a).

It produced dominant lethal effects *in vivo* in the premeiotic and early meiotic germ cells of male mice (Generoso *et al.*, 1975; Schencking & Frohberg, 1975) and an increase in the number of micronuclei in mouse bone marrow (Maier & Schmid, 1976).

Chromosomal aberrations were observed in the bone-marrow cells of rats and Chinese hamsters following i.p. administration of 6-mercaptopurine (Frohberg & Schencking, 1974, 1975) and in mice after oral or parenteral administration (Frohberg & Bauer, 1973; Holden *et al.*, 1973; Frohberg & Schencking, 1974, 1975). Increases in chromosomal aberrations were also found in human peripheral lymphocytes exposed *in vitro* (Nasjleti & Spencer, 1966; Fedortzeva *et al.*, 1973a, b).

6-Mercaptopurine did not produce morphological transformation in mouse C3H/ 10T½ clone 8 cells at cytotoxic concentrations (Benedict *et al.*, 1977b).

(b) Humans

Toxic effects

The major toxic effect of 6-mercaptopurine is on the haematopoietic system; chiefly the white cells are depressed. The higher doses (2.5 - 5 mg/kg bw per day) used in the past to induce remission in leukaemia also frequently caused reversible jaundice due to hepatocellular toxicity (Greenwald *et al.*, 1973): this occurred in 16/38 patients studied in one series (Einhorn & Davidsohn, 1964). Less common side effects are nausea, mucosal ulceration, skin rash and fever.

Effects on reproduction and prenatal toxicity

Transient profound oligospermia was observed in a young man who was treated with 150 mg/day 6-mercaptopurine and 80 mg/day prednisone for acute leukaemia; he had a normal sperm count 2 years after cessation of the chemotherapy and fathered a normal female child (Hinkes & Plotkin, 1973).

No birth defects were observed in 4 infants whose mothers were treated throughout pregnancy with 25 - 175 mg/day 6-mercaptopurine as the only chemotherapeutic agent (Sokal & Lessmann, 1960).

A mother treated during pregnancy with 100 mg/day 6-mercaptopurine and 400 roentgens to the spleen gave birth to a normal, premature baby. A second infant born to the same mother, who had been treated during pregnancy with the same dose of 6-mercaptopurine, then with 4-6 mg/day busulfan and with one treatment of 200 roentgens to the spleen, had severe multiple anomalies. These included microphthalmia, corneal opacities, cleft palate and hypoplasia of the thyroid and of the ovaries (Diamond *et al.*, 1960).

Microangiopathic haemolytic anaemia but no birth defects were found in an infant whose mother had received 100 mg/day 6-mercaptopurine and prednisone throughout pregnancy (McConnell & Bhoola, 1973).

Absorption, distribution, excretion and metabolism

Approximately 40% of an oral dose of 6-mercaptopurine was absorbed (Elion, 1972). The plasma half-life of ^{35}S-6-mercaptopurine is approximately 1.5 hours. 6-Mercaptopurine penetrates the blood-brain barrier only poorly: cerebrospinal fluid levels are approximately 10% of those in the plasma (Hamilton & Elion, 1954).

After an i.v. dose of ^{35}S-labelled drug, 71% of the radioactivity was recovered in the urine over 24 hours, in contrast to 46% of an oral dose. The urinary excretion products are: (i) 6-mercaptopurine; (ii) 6-thiouric acid; (iii) inorganic sulphate; (iv) 6-methylsulphi-nyl-8-hydroxypurine; (v) 6-methylthio-2,8-dihydroxypurine; and (vi) 6-methylthio-8-hydroxypurine glucuronide. After i.v. administration, (i) and (ii) predominate; while (iii) and (iv) are found in larger quantities following oral administration (Elion *et al.*, 1963; Elion, 1967). Metabolic activation of the drug in man is similar to that in animals, involving conversion to 6-thionucleotides. The methylated derivatives, 6-methylmercaptopurine ribonucleoside mono-, di- and triphosphates, have been shown to be intracellular metabolites (Zimmerman *et al.*, 1974).

Mutagenicity and chromosomal effects

Increases in chromosomal aberrations were observed in the peripheral lymphocytes of most of 14 patients with leukaemia who received cumulative doses of 0.2 - 1.1 g (Fedortzeva *et al.*, 1973a) and of a patient with hypernephroma who received an unstated dose of 6-mercaptopurine (Nasjleti & Spencer, 1966).

3.3 Case reports and epidemiological studies of carcinogenicity in humans

In 3 reported cases, acute nonlymphocytic leukaemia developed following the administration of 6-mercaptopurine to patients with nonmalignant disorders. The underlying disorder was primary renal disease in one case (Blanc *et al.*, 1977), pyoderma gangrenosum in one case (Maldonado *et al.*, 1968) and rheumatoid arthritis in the other (Sheibani *et al.*, 1980). One of these patients had received 6-mercaptopurine as the sole chemotherapeutic agent (Maldonado *et al.*, 1968).

Acute myelogenous leukaemia developed in a patient with Hodgkin's disease treated with 6-mercaptopurine and multiple additional cytotoxic agents (Hollard *et al.*, 1966).

There is no epidemiological study of malignant disease in patients following treatment with 6-mercaptopurine.

4. SUMMARY OF DATA REPORTED AND EVALUATION

4.1 Experimental data

6-Mercaptopurine was tested by intraperitoneal administration and by skin painting (followed by croton oil) in mice and by intraperitoneal, subcutaneous and intravenous routes of administration in rats. Limitations to the data in all the reports precluded evaluation of the possible carcinogenicity of 6-mercaptopurine.

6-Mercaptopurine and 6-mercaptopurine riboside were proven to cause embryolethality at doses nontoxic to the mother and to induce severe teratogenic effects in several animal species. 6-Mercaptopurine is mutagenic in bacteria and in mice. It also produces chromosomal aberrations in various mammalian cells, including human peripheral lymphocytes tested in culture.

4.2 Human data

6-Mercaptopurine has been used commonly since the 1960s in the treatment of acute leukaemias.

It produces chromosomal aberrations in peripheral lymphocytes. No data were available to evaluate the mutagenic potential of the drug in humans. The available data are not sufficient to establish whether 6-mercaptopurine can induce a teratogenic effect.

A small number of case reports document the occurrence of acute nonlymphocytic leukaemia in patients who received 6-mercaptopurine for both non-neoplastic and neoplastic disorders. No epidemiological study was available to the Working Group.

4.3 Evaluation

There was no evidence for the carcinogenicity of 6-mercaptopurine in the limited studies in experimental animals. The data from case reports in humans were insufficient to arrive at a conclusion.

On the basis of the available data, no evaluation could be made of the carcinogenic risk of 6-mercaptopurine to humans.

5. REFERENCES

Adams, C.E., Hay, M.F. & Lutwak-Mann, C. (1961) The action of various agents upon the rabbit embryo. *J. Embryol. exp. Morphol., 9,* 468-491

Adhami, H. (1979) Influence of 6-mercaptopurine on the prenatal development of the rat cortex. *Z. mikrosk.-anat. Forsch., Leipzig, 93,* 21-32

Adhami, H. & Noack, W. (1975) Histological effects of 6-mercaptopurine on the fetal rat central nervous system: a light-microscopic study. *Teratology, 11,* 297-312

Anon. (1978) *Annual Report to the Food and Drug Administration. 6-Mercaptopurine (IV formulation), NSC 755, IND 1226,* Bethesda, MD, Investigational Drug Branch, Cancer Therapy Evaluation Program, Division of Cancer Treatment, National Cancer Institute

Asisi, A. & Merker, H.-J. (1975) A specific malformation of the extremities in rats following administration of 6-mercaptopurine on day 12 of gestation (Ger.). *Arzneimittel-Forsch./Drug Res., 25,* 1924-1926

Benedict, W.F., Baker, M.S., Haroun, L., Choi, E. & Ames, B.N. (1977a) Mutagenicity of cancer chemotherapeutic agents in the *Salmonella*/microsome test. *Cancer Res., 37,* 2209-2213

Benedict, W.F., Banerjee, A., Gardner, A. & Jones, P.A. (1977b) Induction of morphological transformation in mouse C3H/10T½ clone 8 cells and chromosomal damage in hamster A(T_1)C1-3 cells by cancer chemotherapeutic agents. *Cancer Res., 37,* 2202-2208

Benezra, S.A. & Foss, P.R.B. (1978) *6-Mercaptopurine.* In: Florey, K., ed., *Analytical Profiles of Drug Substances,* Vol. 7, New York, Academic Press, pp. 343-357

Blanc, A.-P., Gastaut, J.A., Dalivoust, P. & Carcassonne, Y. (1977) Malignant haemopathies occurring after immunosuppressive treatment. Four new observations (Fr.). *Nouv. Presse méd., 6,* 2503-2509

Chalmers, A.H., Knight, P.R. & Atkinson, M.R. (1967) Conversion of azathioprine into mercaptopurine and mercaptoimidazole derivatives *in vitro* and during immunosuppressive therapy. *Aust. J. exp. Biol. med. Sci., 45,* 681-691

Day, J.L., Tterlikkis, L., Niemann, R., Mobley, A. & Spikes, C. (1978) Assay of mercaptopurine in plasma using paired-ion high-performance liquid chromatography. *J. pharm. Sci., 67,* 1027-1028

Diamond, I., Anderson, M.M. & McCreadie, G.R. (1960) Transplacental transmission of busulfan (myleran) in a mother with leukemia. Production of fetal malformation and cytomegaly. *Pediatrics, 25,* 85-90

Ding, T.L. & Benet, L.Z. (1979) Determination of 6-mercaptopurine and azathioprine in plasma by high-performance liquid chromatography. *J. Chromatogr., 163,* 281-288

Doell, R.G., de Vaux St Cyr, C. & Grabar, P. (1967) Immune reactivity prior to development of thymic lymphoma in C57BL mice. *Int. J. Cancer, 2,* 103-108

Donelli, M.G., Colombo, T., Forgione, A. & Garattini, S. (1972) Distribution of 6-mercaptopurine in tumor-bearing animals. *Pharmacology, 8,* 311-320

Einhorn, M. & Davidsohn, I. (1964) Hepatotoxicity of mercaptopurine. *J. Am. med. Assoc., 188,* 802-806

Elion, G.B. (1967) Biochemistry and pharmacology of purine analogues. *Fed. Proc., 26,* 898-904

Elion, G.B. (1972) Significance of azathioprine metabolites. *Proc. R. Soc. Med., 65,* 257-260

Elion, G.B., Bieber, S. & Hitchings, G.H. (1954) The fate of 6-mercaptopurine in mice. *Ann. N. Y. Acad. Sci., 60,* 297-303

Elion, G.B., Callahan, S., Rundles, R.W. & Hitchings, G.H. (1963) Relationship between metabolic fates and antitumor activities of thiopurines. *Cancer Res., 23,* 1207-1217

Esposito, M., Rosso, R. & Santi, L. (1974) Comparative distribution of some antineoplastic drugs in mouse brain, liver and kidney. *Int. Res. Commun. Syst. Cancer, 2,* 1404

Fedortzeva, R.F., Dygin, V.P., Mamaeva, S.E. & Goroshchenks, Y.L. (1973a) Cytogenetical analysis of the effect of 6-mercaptopurine on human chromosomes. I. Effects on blood cells of acute leukemia patients (Russ.). *Cytologia, 15,* 1172-1176

Fedortzeva, R.F., Dygin, V.P., Mamaeva, S.E. & Goroshchenks, Y.L. (1973b) Cytogenetical analysis of the effect of 6-mercaptopurine on human chromosomes. II. The action of 6-mercaptopurine on cultured human lymphocytes (Russ.). *Cytologia, 15,* 1339-1404

Frohberg, H. & Bauer, A. (1973) Mutagenicity trials under toxicological aspects. *Arzeimittel-Forsch./ Drug Res., 23,* 230-236

Frohberg, H. & Schencking, M.S. (1974) Recent findings concerning dose response relationship in muta-genicity testing of chemicals. *Arch. Toxicol., 32,* 1-17

Frohberg, H. & Schencking, M.S. (1975) *In vivo* cytogenetic investigations in bone marrow cells of rats, Chinese hamsters and mice treated with 6-mercaptopurine. *Arch. Toxicol., 33,* 209-224

Generoso, W.M., Preston, R.J. & Brewen, J.G. (1975) 6-Mercaptopurine, an inducer of cytogenic and dominant-lethal effects in premeiotic and early meiotic germ cells of male mice. *Mutat. Res., 28,* 437-447

Goodman, L.S. & Gilman, A., eds (1975) *The Pharmacological Basis of Therapeutics,* 5th ed., New York, MacMillan, pp. 1282-1283

Greenwald, E.S., Goldstein, M. & Barland, P. (1973) *Cancer Chemotherapy Medical Outline Series,* 2nd ed., Flushing, NY, Medical Examination Publishing Co., pp. 186-197

Griswold, D.P., Prejean, J.O., Casey, A.E., Weisburger, J.H., Weisburger, E.K., Wood, H.B., Jr & Falk, H.L. (1971) Carcinogenicity studies of clinically used anticancer agents (Abstract no. 259). *Proc. Am. Assoc. Cancer Res., 12,* 65

Hamilton, L. & Elion, G.B. (1954) The fate of 6-mercaptopurine in man. *Ann. N.Y. Acad. Sci., 60,* 304-314

Harvey, S.C. (1975) *Antineoplastic and immunosuppressive drugs.* In: Osol, A., ed., *Remington's Pharmaceutical Sciences,* 15th ed., Easton, PA, Mack Publishing Co., p. 1081

Herbold, B. & Buselmaier, W. (1976) Induction of point mutations by different chemical mechanisms in the liver microsomal assay. *Mutat. Res., 40,* 73-84

Hinkes, E. & Plotkin, D. (1973) Reversible drug-induced sterility in a patient with acute leukemia. *J. Am. med. Assoc., 223,* 1490-1491

Holden, H.E., Ray, V.A., Wahrenburg, M.G. & Zelenski, J.D. (1973) Mutagenicity studies with 6-mercaptopurine: I. Cytogenetic activity *in vivo. Mutat. Res., 20,* 257-263

Hollard, D., Morel, P. & Revol, L. (1966) Hodgkin's disease terminating in acute leukosis (Fr.). *Lyon méd., 215,* 1373-1377

Kury, G., Chaube, S. & Murphy, M.L. (1968) Teratogenic effects of some purine analogues on fetal rats. *Arch. Pathol., 86,* 395-402

Lessmöllmann, U., Neubert, D. & Merker, H.-J. (1975) *Mammalian limb buds differentiating* in vitro *as a test system for the evaluation of embryotoxic effects.* In: Neubert, D. & Merker, H.-J., eds, *New Approaches to the Evaluation of Abnormal Embryonic Development,* Stuttgart, Georg Thieme, pp. 99-113

Maier, P. & Schmid, W. (1976) Ten model mutagens evaluated by the micronucleus test. *Mutat. Res., 40,* 325-338

Maldonado, N., Torres, V.M., Mendez-Cashion, D., Perez-Santiago, E. & de Costas, M.C. (1968) Pyoderma grangrenosum treated with 6-mercaptopurine and followed by acute leukemia. *J. Pediatr., 72,* 409-414

McConnell, J.B. & Bhoola, R. (1973) A neonatal complication of maternal leukaemia treated with 6-mercaptopurine. *Postgrad. med. J., 49,* 211-213

Mercier-Parot, L. & Tuchmann-Duplessis, H. (1967) Production of limb malformations by 6-mercaptopurine in three species: rabbit, rat and mouse (Fr.). *C.R. Soc. Biol. Paris, 161,* 762-768

Mercker, H.J., Pospisil, M. & Mewes, P. (1975) Cytotoxic effects of 6-mercaptopurine on the limb-bud blastemal cells of rat embryos. *Teratology, 11,* 199-218

Nasjleti, C.E. & Spencer, H.H. (1966) Chromosome damage and polyploidization induced in human peripheral leukocytes *in vivo* and *in vitro* with nitrogen mustard, 6-mercaptopurine, and A-649. *Cancer Res., 26,* 2437-2443

Neubert, D., Tapken, S. & Merker, H.-J. (1974) Induction of skeletal malformations in organ cultures of mammalian embryonic tissues. *Naunyn-Schmiedeberg's Arch. Pharmacol., 286,* 271-282

Neubert, D., Lessmollmann, U., Hinz, N., Dillmann, I. & Fuchs, G. (1977) Interference of 6-mercapto-purine riboside, 6-methylmercaptopurine riboside and azathioprine with the morphogenetic differen-tiation of mouse extremities *in vivo* and in organ culture. *Naunyn-Schmiedeberg's Arch. Pharmacol., 298,* 93-105

Paterson, A.R.P. & Tidd, D.M. (1975) *6-Thiopurines.* In: Eichler, O., Farah, A., Herken, H. & Welch, A.D., eds, *Handbook of Experimental Pharmacology,* Vol. 38, Berlin, Springer, pp. 384-403

Phillips, F.S., Sternberg, S.S., Hamilton, L. & Clarke, D.A. (1954) The toxic effects of 6-mercaptopurine and related compounds. *Ann. N. Y. Acad. Sci., 60,* 283-296

Prejean, J.D., Griswold, D.P., Casey, A.E., Peckham, J.C., Weisburger, E.K. & Wood, H.B., Jr (1972) Car-cinogenicity studies of clinically used anticancer agents (Abstract no. 447). *Proc. Am. Assoc. Cancer Res., 13,* 112

Puget, A., Cros, S., Oreglia, J. & Tollon, Y. (1975) Study on the embryonal sensitivity of the Afghan pika (*Ochotona rufescens rufescens*) to two teratogenic agents, azathioprine and 6-mercaptopurine (Fr.). *Zbl. Veterinarmed. A, 22,* 38-56

Reimers, T.J. & Sluss, P.M. (1978) 6-Mercaptopurine treatment of pregnant mice: effects on second and third generation. *Science, 201,* 65-67

Rosenfeld, J.M., Taguchi, V.Y., Hillcoat, B.L. & Kawai, M. (1977) Determination of 6-mercaptopurine in plasma by mass spectrometry. *Anal. Chem., 49,* 725-727

Salaman, M.H. & Roe, F.J.C. (1956) Further tests for tumour-initiating activity: *N,N*-di(2-chloroethyl)-*p*-aminophenylbutyric acid (CB1348) as an initiator of skin tumour formation in the mouse. *Br. J. Cancer, 10,* 363-378

Schenking, M.S. & Frohberg, H. (1975) Dominant lethal test in mice with 6-mercaptopurine. *Arch. Toxicol., 34,* 71-75

Scherf, H.R. & Schmähl, D. (1975) Experimental investigations on immunodepressive properties of car-cinogenic substances in male Sprague-Dawley rats. *Recent Results Cancer Res., 52,* 76-87

Schmähl, D. & Osswald, H. (1970) Experimental studies on carcinogenic effects of anticancer chemo-therapeutics and immunodepressives (Ger.). *Arzneimittel-Forsch./Drug Res., 20,* 1461-1467

Shah, R.M. & Burdett, D.N. (1979) Development abnormalities induced by 6-mercaptopurine in the hamster. *Can. J. Physiol. Pharmacol., 57,* 53-58

Sheibani, K., Bukowski, R.M., Tubbs, R.R., Savage, R.A., Sebek, B.A. & Hoffman, G.C. (1980) Acute nonlymphocytic leukemia in patients receiving chemotherapy for nonmalignant diseases. *Hum. Pa-thol., 11,* 175-179

Sokal, J.E. & Lessmann, E.M. (1960) Effects of cancer chemotherapeutic agents on the human fetus. *J. Am. med. Assoc., 172,* 1765-1771

Sugiura, K. & Brown, G.B. (1967) Purine *N*-oxides. 19. On the oncogenic *N*-oxide derivatives of guanine and xanthine and a nononcogenic isomer of xanthine *N*-oxide. *Cancer Res., 27,* 925-931

Sugiura, K., Teller, M.N., Parham, J.C. & Brown, G.B. (1970) A comparison of the oncogenicities of 3-hydroxyxanthine, guanine 3-*N*-oxide, and some related compounds. *Cancer Res., 30,* 184-188

Thiersch, J.B. (1954) The effect of 6-mercaptopurine on the rat fetus and on reproduction of the rat. *Ann. N.Y. Acad. Sci., 60,* 220-227

Tterlikkis, L., Ortega, E., Solomon, R. & Day, J.L. (1977) Pharmacokinetics of mercaptopurine. *J. pharm. Sci., 66,* 1454-1457

Tuchmann-Duplessis, H. & Mercier-Parot, L. (1958) On the teratogenic action of several antimitotic substances in the rat (Fr.). *C.R. Hebd. Acad. Sci., 247,* 152-154

Tuchmann-Duplessis, H. & Mercier-Parot, L. (1966) Production of limb malformations in the rabbit by administration of azathioprine and 6-mercaptopurine (Fr.). *C.R. Soc. Biol. Paris, 160,* 501-507

Tuchmann-Duplessis, H. & Mercier-Parot, L. (1968) Experimental production of limb malformations (Fr.). *Union méd. Can., 97,* 283-288

US International Trade Commission (1979) *Synthetic Organic Chemicals, US Production and Sales, 1978,* USITC Publication 1001, Washington DC, US Government Printing Office, p. 173

US Pharmacopeial Convention, Inc. (1980) *The US Pharmacopeia,* 20th rev., Rockville, MD, pp. 485-486

US Tariff Commission (1967) *Synthetic Organic Chemicals, US Production and Sales, 1965,* TC Publication 206, Washington DC, US Government Printing Office, p. 119

Vishniakov, Y.S. (1968) The specificity of the damaging effect produced by 6-mercaptopurine at different stages of embryogenesis in rats (Russ.). *Farmakol. Toksikol., 31,* 480-481

Vishniakov, Y.S. (1969) Teratogenous effect of 6-mercaptopurine on albino rat embryos (Russ.). *Arkh. Anat., 57,* 37-41

Wade, A., ed. (1977) *Martindale, The Extra Pharmacopoeia,* 27th ed., London, The Pharmaceutical Press, pp. 154-156

Weast, R.C., ed. (1977) *Handbook of Chemistry and Physics,* 58th ed., Cleveland, OH, The Chemical Rubber Company, p. C-469

Weisburger, E.K. (1977) Bioassay program for carcinogenic hazards of cancer chemotherapeutic agents. *Cancer, 40,* 1935-1949

Weisburger, J.H., Griswold, D.P., Prejean, J.D., Casey, A.E., Wood, H.B. & Weisburger, E.K. (1975) The carcinogenic properties of some of the principal drugs used in clinical cancer chemotherapy. *Recent Results Cancer Res., 52,* 1-17

Windholz, M., ed. (1976) *The Merck Index,* 9th ed., Rahway, NJ, Merck & Co., p. 763

Zimmerman, T.P., Chu, L.-C., Buggé, J.L., Nelson, D.J., Lyon, G.M. & Elion, G.B. (1974) Identification of 6-methylmercaptopurine ribonucleoside 5'-diphosphate and 5'-triphosphate as metabolites of 6-mercaptopurine in man. *Cancer Res., 34,* 221-224

Zunin, C. & Borrone, C. (1955) The teratogenic effect of 6-mercaptopurine (Ital.). *Minerva Pediatr., 7,* 66-71

1. CHEMICAL AND PHYSICAL DATA

1.1 Synonyms and trade names

Chem. Abstr. Services Reg. No.: 59-05-2

Chem. Abstr. Name: L-Glutamic acid, *N*-(4-{[(2,4-diamino-6-pteridinyl)methyl] - methylamino} benzoyl-

IUPAC Systematic Name: L-(+)-*N*-(*p*-{[(2,4-Diamino-6-pteridinyl)methyl] methyl-amino} benzoyl)glutamic acid

Synonyms: Amethopterin;   4-amino-10-methylfolic acid;   4-amino-*N*[10]-methyl-pteroylglutamic acid;   *N*-{*para*[(2,4-diamino-6-pteridinyl)methyl] methylamino} -benzoyl L-(+)-glutamic acid; *N*-(4-{[(2,4-diamino-6-pteridinyl)methyl] methylamino} -benzoyl)-L-glutamic   acid;   methotrexatum;   *N*- {*para*-[(2,4-diaminopteridin-6-yl-methyl)methylamino] benzoyl} -L-glutamic acid; α-methopterin; methylaminopterin

Trade names: A-Methopterin;   Antifolan;   CL-14377;   Ledertrexate;   Methotrexate specia; MEXATE; MTX; NSC-740; R 9985

1.2 Structural and molecular formulae and molecular weight

$C_{20}H_{22}N_8O_5$ Mol. wt: 454.4

1.3 Chemical and physical properties of the pure substance

From Wade (1977) or Windholz (1976), unless otherwise specified

(a) *Description:* Bright yellow-orange, odourless (Chamberlin *et al.*, 1976), crys-talline powder

(b) *Melting-point:* 185-204°C (monohydrate)

(c) *Optical rotation:* $[\alpha]_{589}^{21}$ = 20.4 ± 0.6° (c = 1; 0.1 N NaOH) Chamberlin et al., 1976)

(d) *Spectroscopy data:* λ_{max} 243 nm, A^1 = 388; 307 nm, A^1 = 475 (in 0.1N HCl). λ_{max} 258 nm, A^1_1 = 544; 303 nm, A^1_1 = 546; 372 nm, A^1_1 = 177 (in 0.1 N NaOH). Infra-red, mass and nuclear magnetic resonance spectra have been tabulated (Chamberlin et al., 1976).

(e) *Solubility:* Practically insoluble in water, ethanol, chloroform and diethyl ether; freely soluble in dilute solutions of alkaline hydroxides and carbonates; soluble in dilute hydrochloric acid

(f) *Stability:* Sensitive to hydrolysis, oxidation and light

1.4 Technical products and impurities

Various national and international pharmacopoeias give specifications for the purity of methotrexate in pharmaceutical products. For example, it is available in the US as a USP grade containing not less than 94.0% methotrexate and closely related compounds calculated on the dried basis, with 8.0% max. loss on drying and 0.1% max. residue on ignition. Methotrexate is available in 2.5 mg tablets measured as containing 90.0-110.0% of the stated amount (US Pharmacopeial Convention, Inc., 1980). In the US, the sodium salt is available for injection as a lyophilized powder in vials containing the equivalent of 20, 50 or 100 mg methotrexate without preservative (Baker, 1980). It is also available in vials containing the equivalent of 5 or 50 mg in 2.0 ml solvent with a preservative. Ampoules containing the equivalent of 5 or 50 mg methotrexate in 2.0 ml solvent without preservative are available in the UK (Wade, 1977).

Methotrexate is available in Japan as 2.5 mg tablets and in vials containing 5 or 50 mg.

2. PRODUCTION, USE, OCCURRENCE AND ANALYSIS

2.1 Production and use

(a) Production

The synthesis of methotrexate was first reported (Seeger et al., 1949) by the following steps: condensation of 2,3-dibromopropionaldehyde with 2,4,5,6-tetraaminopyrimidine to produce 6-bromomethyl-2,4-diaminopteridine and further condensation of this with N-[para-

(methylamino)benzoyl] glutamic acid to yield methotrexate. It is not known whether this is the process used for its commercial production.

Commercial production of methotrexate in the US was first reported in 1977 (US International Trade Commission, 1978). Only one US company currently manufactures an undisclosed amount (see preamble, p. 20) (US International Trade Commission, 1979a). US imports of methotrexate through the principal customs districts amounted to 7.2 kg in 1978 (US International Trade Commission, 1979b).

The drug is believed to be produced by a single company in the Federal Republic of Germany. Annual consumption in western Europe is approximately 40 kg.

Methotrexate has been used in Japan since 1968 but has never been produced there. Japanese imports (all from the US) in recent years have been as follows: 13.5 kg in 1976, 20.5 kg in 1977 and 31.5 kg in 1978.

(b) Use

Methotrexate is an antineoplastic agent used in the treatment of acute lymphoblastic leukaemia, non-Hodgkin's lymphoma, osteogenic and chondro- and synovial sarcomas, choriocarcinoma, breast cancer, embryonal rhabdomyosarcoma, testicular tumours, carcinomas of the lung and uterine cervix, squamous-cell carcinoma of the head and neck, various soft-tissue sarcomas, mycosis fungoides, histiocytosis and solitary plasmacytoma (Harvey, 1975; Wade, 1977).

It is used to condition patients for bone-marrow transplantation. It is also used in the treatment of psoriasis.

Methotrexate is administered orally, intravenously, intramuscularly, intra-articularly or intrathecally at a wide variety of dose levels and dosage regimens. For instance, in the treatment of testicular tumours, 5 mg/day methotrexate are given orally for 10 days, every 30 days. In combination chemotherapy for breast cancer (e.g., CMF: cyclophosphamide, methotrexate, 5-fluorouracil), 40 mg/m^2 body surface area of methotrexate are given on days 1 and 8 of a 4-week cycle. In treatment by high i.v. doses of methotrexate, with blood level monitoring and leucovorin rescue, the initial dose is as high as 5 g/m^2. When given intrathecally in the treatment or prophylaxis of meningeal leukaemia (Wade, 1977), the dose is often approximately 12 mg/m^2 once a month.

2.2 Occurrence

Methotrexate is not known to be produced in Nature.

2.3 Analysis

Analytical methods for the determination of methotrexate based on titrimetry, polarography, spectrometry, paper chromatography, column chromatography, high-speed liquid chromatography and proton magnetic resonance have been reviewed (Chamberlin *et al.*, 1976).

Typical methods for the analysis of methotrexate in various matrices are summarized in Table 1.

Table 1. Methods for the analysis of methotrexate

Sample matrix	Sample preparation	Assay procedure[a]	Limit of detection	Reference
Formulations	Inject sample; elute with tetra-butylammonium phosphate/acetonitrile (80/20)	HPLC-UV	not given	Wisnicki *et al.* (1978)
	Dissolve sample in buffer/acetonitrile (90/10); filter through 0.45 μ membrane filter; elute with buffer/acetonitrile (90/10)	HPLC-UV	not given	US Pharmacopeial Convention, Inc. (1980)
	Add 2-amino-4-methylpyridine as internal standard	HPLC-UV	1 μg/ml	Chamberlin *et al.* (1976)
	Dissolve sample and internal standard in dimethyl sulphoxide	PMR	not given	Chamberlin *et al.* (1976)
Blood plasma	Add trichloroacetic acid and centrifuge; add acetic acid-sodium acetate buffer; oxidize with aqueous potassium permanganate solution; add hydrogen peroxide	HPLC-F	0.01 μg/ml	Nelson *et al.* (1977)
Blood serum	Dilute sample; add NADPH, dihydrofolate buffer and dihydrofolate reductase	EI-CA	not given	Finley & Williams (1977)
	Mix with methanol and phosphate buffer; centrifuge; allow to stand	HPLC-UV	not given	Miller & Tucker (1979)

Table 1 (contd)

Sample matrix	Sample preparation	Assay procedure[a]	Limit of detection	Reference
Blood serum and urine	Add sample to ^{3}H-metho-trexate; add yeast lysate mix; incubate; centrifuge	RBA	450 ng	Weir et al. (1978)
Urine	Filter through 0.45 μ millipore filter prior to injection; elute with tetrabutylammonium phosphate/methanol (70/30)	HPLC-UV	not given	Wisnicki et al. (1978)
Serum, urine, and cerebro-spinal fluid	Incubate with ^{3}H-methotrexate and antiserum	RIA	1 ng/ml	Aherne et al. (1977)
			0.05 ng	Paxton & Rowell (1977)
Plasma	Incubate with ^{3}H-methotrexate and antiserum	RIA	1 ng/ml	Al-Bassam et al. (1979)
Plasma, urine	Incubate with ^{3}H-methotrexate and antiserum	RIA	1 ng/ml	Virtanen et al. (1979)

[a]Abbreviations: HPLC-UV, high-performance liquid chromatography with ultra-violet detection; PMR, proton magnetic resonance; HPLC-F, high-performance liquid chromatography with fluoroescence detection; EI·CA,   enzyme inhibition with centrifugal analysis;   RBA, radiobinding assay;   RIA, radio-immunoassay

3. BIOLOGICAL DATA RELEVANT TO THE EVALUATION OF CARCINOGENIC RISK TO HUMANS

3.1 Carcinogenicity studies in animals

(a) Oral administration

Mouse: Groups of 7-week-old male and female Swiss mice were fed diets containing methotrexate on alternate weeks for life. Groups of 48 males and 48 females received 10 mg/kg diet; groups of 42 animals of each sex, 8 mg/kg; groups of 36, 5 mg/kg; and groups of 36, 3 mg/kg. Control groups consisted of 70 males and 70 females. The median survival time of control and treated animals was about 80-90 weeks; some animals survived up to 120 weeks. The tumours noted most frequently were malignant lymphomas, lung tumours and haemangiomas of the liver. The incidence of tumours in treated mice was, however, not significantly different from that in controls (Rustia & Shubik, 1973).

Male mice of the XVII/Bln strain were given methotrexate in their drinking-water at a daily dose of 0.1 mg/kg bw, providing a total dose of 55 mg/kg bw over 18 months. Of 32 animals, 5 developed lung adenomas and 16 developed lung carcinomas, for an overall incidence of 66%. This was compared with a spontaneous incidence of 5.1% lung tumours in male animals of that strain. One treated animal also developed a hepatoma (Roschlau & Justus, 1971). [The Working Group noted that no matched controls were included in the study.]

Hamster: Groups of 7-week-old male and female Syrian golden hamsters were fed diets containing methotrexate on alternate weeks for life. Groups of 39 females and 40 males received 20 mg/kg of diet; and groups of 42 animals of each sex received 10 or 5 mg/kg. Control groups consisted of 49 males and 49 females. The median survival time of controls was about 60-70 weeks, and more than 20% survived for 90 weeks, survival in the groups fed 20 mg/kg was reduced to a median of about 40 - 50 weeks, and by 70 weeks only 25% were alive; survival in the other treated groups was comparable with that of controls. Only isolated tumours occurred, and the frequency and organ and tissue of origin showed no significant differences from those in control hamsters (Rustia & Shubik, 1973).

(b)   Intraperitoneal administration

Mouse: Two groups, each of 25 male and 25 female outbred Swiss-Webster-derived mice, 6 weeks old, were given i.p. injections of 0.5 or 1.0 mg/kg bw methotrexate dissolved in physiological saline 3 times weekly for 6 months. Animals that survived over 100 days were observed for up to 12 further months, at which time they were killed. A control group of 101 male mice had a median survival time of 9.8 months, while that of 153 female mice was 18 months. The survival times of the treated animals were reported as percentages of that of the controls [no precise definition of the mode of calculation was given] : the survival times of treated males were 39 - 54% that of controls, and survival of treated females was 77 - 100% that of controls. The tumour incidence in treated males was 8/41 (20%), and that in females 9/32 (28%). These did not differ from the 26% incidence observed in both male and female controls (Weisburger, 1977). [The Working Group considered that the inadequate reporting of certain items, such as survival times, the amalgation of various experimental groups and tumour types, as well as the lack of age-adjustment in the analyses precluded a complete evaluation of this study.]

Rat: A group of 36 male and 36 female 12-day-old Sprague-Dawley rats were given weekly i.p. injections of 0.625 mg/kg bw methotrexate (5% of the acute LD_{50} per week); a control group of 36 males and 36 females remained untreated. All animals were kept under observation until death; only animals that lived longer than 200 days were studied. Thirty treated males survived a mean of 90 ± 14 weeks, and 31 treated females survived a mean of

101 ± 15 weeks. No neoplasms were observed in male animals; 1 female (3%) developed a malignant mammary neoplasm. Male controls survived a mean of 96 ± 17 weeks, and females survived a mean of 94 ± 15 weeks. Male controls developed 1 haemangioendothelioma of the liver and female controls 3 malignant mammary neoplasms (Schmähl & Habs, 1976). [The Working Group noted that information was restricted to malignant tumours.]

Two groups, each of 25 male Sprague-Dawley-derived Charles River (CD) rats, 6 weeks of age, were given i.p. injections of 0.15 or 0.3 mg/kg bw methotrexate in saline, and groups of 25 female rats were given 0.15 or 0.6 mg/kg bw, 3 times weekly for 6 months. Animals that survived over 100 days were observed for 12 further months, at which time they were killed. A control group of 179 males and 181 females had an overall survival time of over 18 months. The survival times of the treated animals were reported as percentages of that of the controls [no precise definition of the mode of calculation was given] : the survival times of treated males were 28 - 100% that of controls, and survival of treated females was 18 - 100% that of controls. Eight of 38 (21%) treated male rats that survived longer than 100 days had neoplasms, of which 4 were considered malignant: 7 animals had pituitary tumours, and 1 had a tumour of the testis. Among male controls, 34% had tumours, most of which were found in endocrine organs, including the pituitary, adrenal, thyroid, testis and mammary glands. Of female rats, 26/45 (58%) had neoplasms by 18 months, 4 of which were malignant; the neoplasms were found in the pituitary in 15 animals, in the mammary gland in 9 and in the adrenal in 4. Control females had a 58% incidence of tumours, involving the same organs as the treated females. The tumour incidences in treated males and females were not considered to be greater than those in controls (Weisburger, 1977). [The Working Group considered that the inadequate reporting of certain items, such as survival times, the amalgation of various experimental groups and tumour types, as well as the lack of age-adjustment in the analyses precluded a complete evaluation of this study.]

(c) Intravenous administration

Rat: A group of 48 male BR46 rats, 100 days old, were given i.v. injections of 1 mg/kg bw methotrexate once weekly for 52 weeks (total dose, 52 mg/kg bw). A control group of 89 rats was maintained. Of the exposed group, 26 rats (29%) were alive when the first tumour appeared, while in the control group 65 (73%) survived to this point. The tumour yields in the exposed group, in relation to the number of animals living when the first tumour appeared, were 12% for benign tumours and 8% for malignant tumours. The benign tumours were 2 thymomas and 2 subcutaneous fibromas. The malignancies were a squamous-cell carcinoma of the skin and a haemangioendothelioma of the thorax; the mean latent period of these tumours was 20 months. In the control group, the yield was 5% for benign tumours and 6% for malignant tumours, with a mean latency of 23 months. The benign tumours were 2 thymomas and 1 mammary fibroma, and the malignancies were 3 mammary carcinomas and 1 pheochromocytoma. The yield in treated animals was not considered to be different from that in controls (Schmähl & Osswald, 1970).

(d) Administration with known carcinogens

Oral administration: Two groups of male Swiss *mice* were fed methotrexate in the diet at an approximate daily dosage of 0.2 mg/kg bw. The two groups plus a control group also received biweekly applications of methylcholanthrene for 11 weeks to shaved epidermis of the intrascapular area. Exposure to methotrexate beginning one week prior to methylcholanthrene reduced the incidence of skin tumours to 35.7%; exposure beginning 6 weeks prior to methylcholanthrene had a cocarcinogenic effect, such that 96.3% of mice had skin tumours by 112 days after methylcholanthrene treatment, whereas the incidence was only 74.4% in the control group (Barich *et al.*, 1962).

In studies of animals subjected simultaneously to immunosuppression and immunostimulation, DBA/2 *mice* were given 3 mg/kg bw per day methotrexate in drinking-water. Antigens were also given, consisting of 0.1 mg H37Ra tubercle bacteria given subcutaneously in adjuvant every other week or bovine serum albumin given intraperitoneally daily at a dose of 0.2 ml of a 10% solution. No lymphomas developed in methotrexate-treated animals that did not receive antigen; those given both treatments had a 12% incidence of lymphomas after a latent period of 5 - 8 months (Krueger, 1975).

Topical administration: Syrian golden *hamsters* received topical applications of 7,12-dimethylbenz[a]anthracene (DMBA) to the buccal pouch. Some animals also received topical applications of methotrexate (approximately 0.1 mg) on alternate days. All treatments were continued for 6 or 12 weeks. No enhancement of carcinogenesis by methotrexate occurred, and even some slight inhibition was noted (Levij *et al.*, 1970).

Subcutaneous and/or intramuscular administration: Male and female Syrian golden *hamsters*, 6 months of age, were given s.c. injections of 0.06 mg sodium methotrexate alone or together with painting of the buccal pouch with DMBA. Animals given combined treatment for 8 weeks developed invasive epidermoid carcinomas, whereas in the group given only DMBA for 8 weeks no carcinoma was found. After 12 weeks of combined treatment, most animals had anaplastic carcinomas of average size 10 - 15 mm; whereas treatment with DMBA alone for 12 weeks resulted in well-differentiated carcinomas only 1 - 3 mm in size. The results were considered to show a cocarcinogenic effect of methotrexate (Shklar *et al.*, 1966).

Young adult male and female Syrian *hamsters* received abrasion of their tongues, after which DMBA was applied. Half of the animals also received a s.c. injection of 0.15 mg methotrexate once a week. No enhancement of lingual carcinogenesis was demonstrated (Marefat & Shklar, 1979).

Intraperitoneal administration: A group of female C3Hf/HeN *mice*, 5-6 weeks old, were given i.p. injections of 2.0 mg/kg bw methotrexate 3 times per week for 23 weeks, together with exposures to ultra-violet light 3 times per week to shaved dorsal skin for 60 weeks. A group of 70 control mice were exposed to ultra-violet light only. The pattern of skin tumour development was similar in both groups. A group of 30 mice given methotrexate only developed no skin tumour. In a second experiment, groups of mice received cutaneous application of benzo[a] pyrene to a shaved area of the back for 80 weeks, alone or together with i.p. injections of methotrexate. The median tumour latent periods did not differ significantly (Daynes *et al.*, 1979).

3.2 Other relevant biological data

(a) Experimental systems

Toxic effects

The oral LD_{50} of methotrexate in rats is 180 ± 45 mg/kg bw; the i.p. LD_{50} is 6-25 mg/kg bw in rats and 94 ± 9 mg/kg bw in mice. At these dose levels, only a few animals died within 3 days: the majority died between 3 and 7 days after administration. When the total i.p. dose was divided into 5 equal, consecutive daily fractions, the LD_{50} (total dose) was decreased to 5.6 ± 1.7 mg/kg bw in rats and to 9.7 ± 1.5 mg/kg bw in mice (Ferguson *et al.*, 1950). Sixteen-week-old mice were less sensitive to the toxic effects of methotrexate than five-week-old mice (Freeman-Narrod *et al.*, 1974), which is in contrast to the situation in rats, where liver toxicity has been shown to increase with age (Custer *et al.*, 1977).

The main toxic effects of methotrexate in mice, rats and dogs are bone-marrow depression, increased susceptibility to infections, intestinal lesions and hepatotoxicity (Ferguson *et al.*, 1950; Delmonte & Jukes, 1962; Custer *et al.*, 1977).

Within 15 hours after an i.p. injection of 50 mg/kg bw methotrexate to rats, the marrow became hypocellular, the reduction of cells of the erythroid series being the most pronounced. In peripheral blood, reticulocytopenia and panleucopenia were also evident at this time. These effects progressed in severity up to 72 hours. When rats were treated ohronically with lower doses, similar findings were noted, with particularly significant anaemia and lymphopenia. In addition, the thymus, spleen and lymph nodes showed marked atrophy (Ferguson *et al.*, 1950; Custer *et al.*, 1977). Such effects, in particular those on lymphocytes, are responsible for an increased incidence of infections by a variety of organisms and for a decrease in the production of antibodies (Scherf & Schmähl, 1975).

The gastrointestinal lesions of dogs and rats were usually confined to the mucosa and were most marked in the colon.   After daily injections of 0.1 - 0.4 mg/kg bw to rats or 1 mg/kg bw to dogs, colonic ulceration, sometimes associated with an ileitis and/or intestinal haemorrhage, occurred (Ferguson et al., 1950).

Hepatotoxicity is much less pronounced in mice than in rats.   Chronic administration to rats resulted in serious liver damage, including histological evidence of fatty metamorphosis, necrosis, atrophy of hepatic cords and fibrosis (Custer et al., 1977).

Lung damage (interstitial pneumonitis) has also been observed in rats (Custer et al., 1977) and hair loss in mice (Zaharko et al., 1976).

Effects on reproduction and prenatal toxicity

I.p. administration of 25 and 50 mg/kg bw methotrexate (LD_{10} and LD_{50}) to ICR mice on day 10 of pregnancy induced malformations in 27% and 92% of survivors, respectively, and 43% and 91% increases in the rate of resorptions.   The abnormalites observed included cleft palates and ectrodactylia (Skalko & Gold, 1974).

In rats receiving treatment with methotrexate for longer than 4 months, there was impaired spermatogenesis and seminiferous tubular atrophy in the testes, with frequent reciprocal hyperplasia of interstitial cells (Custer et al., 1977).

It was reported in an abstract that administration of 19.2 mg/kg bw methotrexate to rabbits on days 10 and 11 of pregnancy resulted in facial clefts, cleft palates and defects of the proximal upper limb bones in fetuses.   Similar defects were observed when the drug was given on days 12 and 13 of pregnancy.   The same dose given on day 8 or 9 of pregnancy produced complete resorption of litters (Jordan, 1973).

I.p. administration of 0.2 and 0.3 mg/kg bw methotrexate to Wistar rats on day 9 of pregnancy was teratogenic in 35% and 75% of the fetuses and embryolethal in 63% and 84%, respectively.   Malformations could also be induced by a single dose of 2.5 mg/kg bw given on day 5;   this dose was lethal to all embryos when applied on days 6-9 of pregnancy. Malformations could also be induced with doses of 0.3 mg/kg bw given on days 9 - 11 of pregnancy.   In New Zealand White (NZW) rabbits, i.v. doses of 0.6 - 19.2 mg/kg bw methotrexate induced malformations in the fetuses when given on day 10 of pregnancy; embryolethality was increased with 9.6 or 19.2 mg/kg bw.   With the dose of 19.2 mg/kg bw , all the surviving fetuses were malformed when the drug was given on days 12 - 14 of pregnancy and about 80% of them when the drug was given on day 10 or 11 of pregnancy.   This dose killed all the embryos when applied on day 8 or 9 of pregnancy (Jordan et al., 1977).

I.v. administration of 19.2 mg/kg bw methotrexate to NZW rabbits on day 12 of pregnancy produced cleft palates, hydrocephalus and fore- and hindlimb reduction defects in the fetuses. Histological studies revealed swollen limb buds 16 hours after the injection, with increased intercellular space, and the ectoderm was dislocated from the mesodermal core; mitotic activity appeared to be reduced in both the ectoderm and the mesoderm when compared with controls. After 32 hours, limb bud mesenchyme had its usual appearance (DeSesso & Jordan, 1977).

Methotrexate was given orally to cats as single daily doses of 0.5 mg/kg bw on days 11 - 14, 14 - 17 or 17-20 of pregnancy. Maternal toxicity was seen in 1/20 animals treated on days 11 - 14, 4/7 treated on days 14 - 17 and 3/18 treated on days 17 - 20 of pregnancy. Skeletal and visceral abnormalities were observed in fetuses exposed on days 11 - 14 and 14 - 17 of pregnancy; only a few visceral abnormalities were seen when the drug was given on days 17 - 20 of pregnancy. The abnormalities included umbilical hernia, cleft palates, hydrocephalus, and spina bifida as well as malformed limbs (Khera, 1976).

Of 11 rhesus monkeys treated intravenously with 2.5 - 4 mg/kg bw methotrexate given as a single dose or 2 - 4 times on consecutive days, on days 17 - 45 of pregnancy, 7 produced normal fetuses (as evaluated after hysterotomy on day 100 of gestation), 3 aborted 3 - 37 days after treatment, and the fetus of 1 had moderate gut malrotation (Wilson, 1971).

When 24 rhesus monkeys were given daily injections of 0.5-4 mg/kg bw methotrexate over periods of 1-24 days between days 17 and 45 of pregnancy, 14 offspring (58%) were found to be normal when evaluated on day 100 of gestation by hysterotomy; 8 monkeys aborted; and one fetus had severe growth retardation, abnormal ossification of long bones and 11 thoracic and 8 cervical vertebrae, and another fetus had 13 thoracic vertebrae and ribs. The author concluded that even with very large doses the embryotoxic effects reported to occur with this drug in man cannot be duplicated in monkeys (Wilson, 1974).

Doses of methotrexate that cause roughly comparable embryolethality were given to Wistar rats (0.3 mg/kg bw on day 10 of pregnancy) and rhesus monkeys (3 mg/kg bw per day on days 29 - 32 of pregnancy) in order to study placental transfer in those two species. Concentrations in the embryo were strikingly different during the first 8 hours, ranging from 108 - 209 ng/g tissue in the monkey but from 3.4 - 7.7 ng/g tissue in the rat. Thus, the degree and type of embryotoxicity could not be closely correlated with the level and duration of the drug concentration in the embryo: in the rat, a small dose produced moderate embryotoxicity and a very low embryonic concentration; in the monkey, a large maternal dose produced slight embryotoxicity in spite of high drug concentrations in the embryo (Scott et al., 1978; Wilson et al., 1979).

Absorption, distribution, excretion and metabolism

Methotrexate is incompletely absorbed from the gut (Henderson *et al.*, 1965). High doses in rats resulted in severe mucosal damage, decreased uptake of ^{14}C-L-leucine and ^{14}C-L-phenylalanine, but increased absorption of methotrexate (Robinson *et al.*, 1966; Jolly & Fletcher, 1977). Some percutaneous absorption has also been documented after topical application to mice (Newbold & Stoughton, 1972).

Methotrexate is retained in the liver, to a degree which is in part dependent upon the dose. It is excreted in the urine and bile; partial reabsorption occurs in the gut. Within 24 - 48 hours after administration, a total of approximately 67 - 91% of methotrexate administered to dogs or monkeys was excreted in urine, blood and stools (Henderson *et al.*, 1965). In mice, tissue:plasma distribution ratios have been found to be: muscle, 0.15:1; kidney, 3:1; liver, 10:1 (Bischoff *et al.*, 1970). It was reported in an abstract that in rats given 0.1 - 10 mg/kg bw ^{3}H-methotrexate on day 20 of gestation, transfer to the fetus was found to be very limited but proportional to the applied dose (McClain & Siekierka, 1975).

The hepatic uptake in rats is an active, carrier-mediated saturable process with a K_m of 1.3 mM and V_{max} of 11.1 μmol/hour per g of liver (Strum & Liem, 1977). Binding of methotrexate to membrane transport proteins and to dihydrofolate reductase has been documented (Strum & Liem, 1977; McCormick *et al.*, 1979).

Methotrexate acts by tight binding inhibition of the enzyme dihydrofolate reductase. The consequent depletion of 1 carbon carrying tetrahydrofolate cofactors leads to a reduction of the *de novo* synthesis of thymidylate and purine nucleotides, thus affecting both DNA and RNA synthesis (Jackson & Harrap, 1973).

Methotrexate is rapidly metabolized to 7-hydroxymethotrexate by hepatic aldehyde oxidase in rabbits but more slowly in other species (Johns & Loo, 1967). Other metabolites found in mice and rats are 4-amino-4-deoxy-N^{10}-methyl pteroic acid and various free pteridines. These latter metabolites may be formed by intestinal flora (Zaharko *et al.*, 1969; Valerino, 1972; Valerino *et al.*, 1972; Zaharko & Oliverio, 1970). None of these metabolites was a significant inhibitor of dihydrofolate reductase (Baugh *et al.*, 1973).

Among the parameters which determine tissue sensitivity to methotrexate are the rate of drug entry, the degree of drug binding to dihydrofolate reductase, and the rate of new synthesis of the reductase. In mice, certain organs can adapt to methotrexate by increasing their rate of new enzyme synthesis (Zaharko *et al.*, 1976). This may not be true for other species, e.g., rat, guinea-pig (Bertino *et al.*, 1962; Ngu *et al.*, 1964).

Mutagenicity and other short-term tests

Methotrexate was not mutagenic in *Salmonella typhimurium* tester strains TA1535, TA1536, TA1537, TA1538, TA92, TA98, TA100 or G46, with or without the addition of a mouse or rat liver microsomal fraction (Herbold & Buselmaier, 1976; Seino *et al.*, 1978). The drug was non-mutagenic in host-mediated assays with *Serratia marcescens* and with *Escherichia coli* (Propping *et al.*, 1972).

When tested at one high concentration (1 mg/ml), without exogenous metabolic activation, the agent was mutagenic in the mouse lymphoma cell line L5178Y (Matheson *et al.*, 1978). Methotrexate also produced dominant lethals in mice (Epstein *et al.*, 1972; Propping *et al.*, 1972).

Methotrexate induced chromosomal aberrations in hamster cells in culture (Benedict *et al.*, 1977). In human lymphocytes in culture, the drug was clastogenic in one study at doses of 1 - 10 μg/ml (Voorhees *et al.*, 1969), but not in another study at doses of between 0.1 and 100 μg/ml (Hampel *et al.*, 1966). An increase in sister chromatid exchanges after *in vitro* treatment with methotrexate was observed in both a hamster cell line (Banerjee & Benedict, 1979) and primary mouse-fetal cells (Raffetto *et al.*, 1979).

In mice *in vivo*, methotrexate was positive in a micronucleus test with bone-marrow cells (Maier & Schmid, 1976).

Methotrexate also induced morphological transformation in C3H10T½ clone 8 cells at concentrations of 10 and 100 μg /ml (Benedict *et al.*, 1977).

(b) Humans

Toxic effects

Methotrexate mainly affects tissues with a rapid cell turnover, particularly the bone marrow, the alimentary tract epithelium, the epidermis, fetal tissues and germinal cells (Muller *et al.*, 1969). Severe and even fatal toxic reactions may occur. Factors that play a role in its toxicity are dosage, age of the patient, status of renal function, frequency and duration of therapy, and sometimes idiosyncrasy (Douglas & Price, 1973). In one study involving 380 patients given 3 oral courses of methotrexate totalling 150 mg, stomatitis occurred in 30.6%, leucopenia in 29.1% and alopecia in 13.4%. Bone-marrow depression is often severe and causes leucopenia, anaemia and thrombocytopenia (Kroese, 1975). Septicaemia and bleeding from various sites may occur and may prove fatal. Methotrexate-induced neutropenia was significantly greater in patients who had received craniospinal irradiation (Medical Research Council Working Party on Leukaemia in Childhood, 1975).

Toxicity to the entire alimentary tract is common, particularly mucositis and ulceration, and is aggravated by concomitant irradiation (Shehata & Meyer, 1980). Serial, peroral, small-bowel biopsies have shown extensive but reversible morphological alterations of human small-intestinal mucosa (Trier, 1961).

Hepatic toxicity has been reported in psoriasis patients, and is related not only to dosage but also to the duration of therapy. Hepatotoxicity is greater in patients treated with frequent small doses than in those receiving large intermittent doses. Acute elevations in hepatic enzymes may occur, and there may be abnormal bromsulphthalein retention. Biopsies may show fatty metamorphosis, necrosis, periportal fibrosis and postnecrotic cirrhosis (Epstein & Croft, 1969; Muller *et al.*, 1969; Roenigk *et al.*, 1971; Chabner *et al.*, 1975; Kroese, 1975); but there is no specific pattern or pathological entity that distinguishes hepatotoxicity due to methotrexate. Abnormal results have been obtained in liver function tests performed on women receiving methotrexate for choriocarcinoma (Hersh *et al.*, 1964).

An unusual pulmonary toxicity presents as cough, fever and shortness of breath, accompanied by radiological findings of patchy basilar infiltrates that closely resemble the picture of *Pneumocystis carinii* pneumonia or other interstitial and intra-alveolar pneumonitides (Clarysse *et al.*, 1969; Gutin *et al.*, 1976). The cause of this lesion is unknown. A case of pulmonary fibrosis attributed to methotrexate has also been described (Lewis & Walter, 1979).

Central nervous system symptoms include headaches, drowsiness, blurred vision, aphasia, hemiparesis and convulsions. Rarely, cerebral and cerebellar cortex calcification has occurred (Flament-Durand *et al.*, 1975). There have also been reports of leucoencephalopathy following i.v. administration of methotrexate to patients who have had craniospinal irradiation.

Intrathecal therapy of meningeal neoplasia with methotrexate is complicated by paraplegia (Gagliano & Costanzi, 1976). In prophylaxis of meningeal leukaemia, neurotoxicity occurred in 14 - 61% of patients, depending on dose and schedule (Geiser *et al.*, 1975). The toxic effects that may occur can be classified as chemical arachnoiditis, transient or permanent paraplegia associated with involvement of one or more spinal nerve roots or leucoencephalopathy (Bleyer, 1977). Predisposing factors include craniospinal irradiation, abnormal cerebrospinal fluid dynamics, elevated methotrexate levels in the cerebrospinal fluid and the presence of neurotoxic preservatives in commercially available methotrexate preparations.

Renal damage may occur, possibly as a result of precipitation of the drug or the 7-hydroxy metabolite in the renal tubules (Jacobs *et al.*, 1977). Haematuria, cystitis, azotaemia and renal failure have been reported.

Cutaneous toxicity presents in a variety of ways. Lesions of psoriasis may be aggravated by concomitant exposure to ultra-violet irradiation (Bleyer, 1977).

Complications involving bone include bone pain, fractures and aseptic necrosis of the head of the femur (Roenigk *et al.*, 1971; Malpas & Whitehouse, 1977).

Effects on reproduction and prenatal toxicity

Two case reports relate to use of methotrexate during pregnancy. A woman who took 2.5 mg/day for 5 days at about the 9th week of gestation in an attempt to abort had an infant with no frontal bone, craniosynostosis of the coronal and lambdoid sutures, limb reduction defects, hypertelorism and a flat nasal bridge (Milunsky *et al.*, 1968). A similar case was reported in a woman who took 5 mg/day methotrexate for the first two months of her pregnancy for treatment of psoriasis (Powell & Ekert, 1971). This pattern of malformations is very like that observed in infants exposed to aminopterin (Milunsky *et al.*, 1968).

Women treated previous to pregnancy for trophoblastic neoplasms with methotrexate do not appear to have an increased risk for spontaneous abortions or for offspring with congenital malformations (Van Thiel *et al.*, 1970; Ross, 1976; Walden & Bagshawe, 1976).

Absorption, distribution, excretion and metabolism

These aspects have been reviewed by Bertino & Johns (1972), Huffman *et al.* (1973) and Bleyer (1977), and much of the information below is derived from those sources.

All doses of methotrexate are absorbed erratically from the gut. Physiological availability is rarely higher than 40% (Stuart *et al.*, 1979).

After i.v. administration, methotrexate is distributed rapidly within the total body water. Disappearance is triphasic, with half-lives of 0.75, 2 - 6 and 10 - 12 hours (Bleyer, 1977).

After injection of methotrexate directly into the cerebrospinal fluid, absorption from the central nervous system into the plasma compartment proceeds slowly. This results in prolongation of plasma levels above the cytotoxic threshold level. For example, intrathecal administration of 10 - 15 mg/m^2 results in plasma levels above 10^{-8} M for 2 - 3 times longer than when the same doses are administered intravenously.

Fifty to 70% of the drug is bound to protein, principally albumin, in human plasma. Binding to proteins in interstitial fluid effusions is variable, ranging from 0 - 17% (Bleyer, 1977). Distribution of methotrexate into interstitial fluid spaces occurs slowly and with characteristics that resemble a passive transport system. If these 'third spaces' are patho-logically increased, as in ascites or pleural effusion, they may act as reservoirs and prolong the presence of methotrexate in the plasma compartment.

Small amounts of methotrexate remain bound to dihydrofolate reductase in some tissues for many weeks.

Recent work has shown that methotrexate is significantly metabolized at all doses used clinically. It is extensively metabolized to 7-hydroxymethotrexate in patients receiving conventional doses ($<$10 mg/kg bw) and high doses ($>$10 mg/kg bw). Twelve hours after i.v. administration, plasma levels of this metabolite exceeded those of methotrexate in several patients treated with low doses. No 7-hydroxymethotrexate was found in cerebro-spinal fluid after implantation of methotrexate under the scalp; however, small amounts of the metabolite were found in the cerebrospinal fluid after i.v. infusion of high doses (Chan et al., 1980).

2,4-Diamino-N^{10}-methylpteroic acid is also formed (Donehower et al., 1979). [The presence of unidentified metabolites was implied since urinary recovery was incomplete.] Polyglutamate derivatives of methotrexate have been found in human cells (Hoffbrand et al., 1976).

Excretion is predominantly renal, with up to 80% of an intravenously administered dose excreted in the urine. This correlates with the glomerular filtration rate but is con-sistently 30% lower (Calvert et al., 1977). Only 1 - 2% of the dose is excreted in the faeces as the parent compound and metabolites; most of the drug secreted in the bile is reabsorbed by intestinal mucosa.

Mutagenicity and chromosomal effects

Chromosomal damage was seen in bone-marrow cells of methotrexate-treated patients after an i.m. dose of 25 mg (Krogh Jensen, 1967), an i.m. or oral dose of 25 - 50 mg (Krogh Jensen & Nyfors, 1979) or a cumulative oral dose of 2105 - 2165 mg (Melnyk et al., 1971), but not in peripheral lymphocytes after cumulative doses of 25 - 9000 mg (Voorhees et al., 1969; Melnyk et al., 1971; Krogh Jensen & Nyfors, 1979).

3.3 Case reports and epidemiological studies of carcinogenicity in humans

Case reports of malignancy in patients treated with methotrexate for psoriasis include 4 basal-cell skin cancers (Bailin et al., 1975); 3 squamous-cell skin cancers (Harris, 1971; Bailin et al., 1975); 1 dermatofibrosarcoma (Bailin et al., 1975); 1 cervical cancer *in situ* (Ringrose, 1974); 1 non-Hodgkin's lymphoma (Schröter et al., 1971); 1 acute mye-loid leukaemia (Rees et al., 1967); 1 breast cancer, 2 renal cancers (Molin & Larsen, 1972); and 1 nasopharyngeal cancer (Craig & Rosenberg, 1971).

There have been a number of case reports of second primary tumours developing in patients with previous malignant disease treated with methotrexate. In most of these cases, other cytotoxic or immunosuppressive agents, and in some of them radiation, had also been administered. These include 7 acute nonlymphocytic leukaemias (Kaslow *et al.*, 1972, Davis *et al.*, 1973; Penn & Starzl, 1973; Greenspan & Tung, 1974; Vogl, 1978); 1 astrocytoma (Regelson *et al.*, 1965); 1 thyroid cancer, 1 breast cancer, 1 fibrosarcoma (Li *et al.*, 1975); 1 Hodgkin's disease, 2 cervical cancers *in situ* (Penn & Starzl, 1973); 1 hepatoma (Ruymann *et al.*, 1977); and 1 occult pancreatic cancer (Tavassoli & Lynch, 1974).

Only one case of malignancy, a uterine cervical cancer *in situ*, was observed among more than 400 patients with choriocarcinoma treated with methotrexate (Bagshawe, 1977).

In an epidemiological study of 205 patients with psoriasis treated with methotrexate without other cytotoxic agents and followed for a minimum of 7 years (Bailin *et al.*, 1975), there were 3 deaths from carcinoma compared with 3.39 expected and 1 death from leukaemia compared with 0.13 expected; 8 cases of malignancy, excluding skin cancers, were found compared with 6.80 expected.

4. SUMMARY OF DATA REPORTED AND EVALUATION

4.1 Experimental data

Methotrexate was tested by oral administration in mice and hamsters, by intraperitoneal injection in mice and rats, and by intravenous injection in rats. One study in mice by oral administration reported a high incidence of lung carcinomas, but it did not include matched controls. All other studies failed to reveal a carcinogenic effect, but the significance of several was limited because of deficiencies in experimental design or reporting of data.

Methotrexate can induce teratogenic effects in several species and embrolethality at doses nontoxic to the mother. In monkeys, only embryolethality was observed.

Methotrexate is mutagenic in mice *in vivo*. In various mammalian cells in culture the drug causes chromosomal aberrations and increases in sister chromatid exchanges. Methotrexate also induces morphological transformation in mouse cells.

4.2 Human data

Methotrexate is an antineoplastic agent that has been commonly used since the early 1950s for the treatment of haematological and solid malignancies and as an immunosuppressive agent in bone-marrow transplantation. It is also used in the treatment of psoriasis.

Methotrexate is a human teratogen which causes a variety of malformations. It causes chromosomal aberrations in bone-marrow cells. No data were available to evaluate the mutagenic potential of this drug.

Methotrexate has been associated in case reports with a variety of subsequent neoplasms. One study of a defined group of patients, in which no expected numbers were presented, produced no suggestion of a cancer excess. The only other epidemiological study showed no excess of cancer in patients treated with methotrexate.

4.3 Evaluation

There was no evidence for the carcinogenicity of methotrexate in rats; its carcinogenicity could not be evaluated in mice and hamsters. The available data from studies in humans were inadequate to evaluate its carcinogenicity.

On the basis of the available data, no evaluation could be made of the carcinogenicity of methotrexate to humans.

5. REFERENCES

Aherne, G.W., Piall, E.M. & Marks, V. (1977) Development and application of a radioimmunoassay for methotrexate. *Br. J. Cancer, 36,* 608-617

Al-Bassam, M.N., O'Sullivan, M.J., Bridges, J.W. & Marks, V. (1979) Improved double-antibody enzyme immunoassay for methotrexate. *Clin. Chem., 25,* 1448-1452

Bagshawe, K.D. (1977) Lessons from choriocarcinoma. *Proc. R. Soc. Med., 70,* 303-306

Bailin, P.L., Tindall, J.P., Roenigk, H.H., Jr & Hogan, M.D. (1975) Is methotrexate therapy for psoriasis carcinogenic? A modified retrospective-prospective analysis. *J. Am. med. Assoc., 232,* 359-362

Baker, C.E., Jr, ed. (1980) *Physicians' Desk Reference,* 34th ed., Oradell, NJ, Medical Economics Co., pp. 717-719

Banerjee, A. & Benedict, W.F. (1979) Production of sister chromatid exchanges by various cancer chemo-therapeutic agents. *Cancer Res., 39,* 797-799

Barich, L.L., Schwarz, J. & Barich, D. (1962) Oral methotrexate in mice: a co-carcinogenic as well as an anti-tumor agent to methylcholanthrene-induced cutaneous tumors. *J. invest. Derm., 39,* 615-619

Baugh, C.M., Krumdieck, C.L. & Nair, M.G. (1973) Polygammaglutamyl metabolites of methotrexate. *Biochem. biophys. Res. Commun., 52,* 27-34

Benedict, W.F., Banerjee, A., Gardner, A. & Jones, P.A. (1977) Induction of morphological transformation in mouse C3H/10T½ clone 8 cells and chromosomal damage in hamster A (T^1)C1-3 cells by cancer chemotherapeutic agents. *Cancer Res., 37,* 2202-2208

Bertino, J.R. & Johns, D.G. (1972) *Folate antagonists.* In: Brodsky, I. & Kahn, S.B., eds, *Cancer Chemo-therapy II. The Twenty-Second Hahnemann Symposium,* New York, Grune & Stratton, pp. 9-22

Bertino, J.R., Simmons, B. & Donohue, D. (1962) Distribution and properties of dihydrofolic acid reduc-tase in guinea pig tissues (Abstract no. 372). *Fed. Proc., 21,* 476

Bischoff, K.B., Dedrick, R.L. & Zaharko, D.S. (1970) Preliminary model for methotrexate pharmaco-kinetics. *J. pharm. Sci., 59,* 149-154

Bleyer, W.A. (1977) Methotrexate: clinical pharmacology, current status and therapeutic guidelines. *Cancer Treat Rev., 4,* 87-101

Calvert, A.H., Bondy, P.K. & Harrap, K.R. (1977) Some observations on the human pharmacology of methotrexate. *Cancer Treat. Rep., 61,* 1647-1656

Chabner, B.A., Myers, C.E., Coleman, C.N. & Johns, D.G. (1975) The clinical pharmacology of antineo-plastic agents. (First of two parts.) *New Engl. J. Med., 292,* 1107-1113

Chamberlin, A.R., Cheung, A.P.K. & Lim, P. (1976) *Methotrexate.* In: Florey, K., ed., *Analytical Pro-files of Drug Substances,* Vol. 5, New York, Academic Press, pp. 283-306

Chan, K.K., Nayar, M.S.B., Cohen, J.L., Chlebowski, R.T., Liebman, H., Stolinsky, D., Mitchell, M.S & Farquhar, D. (1980) Metabolism of methotrexate in man after high and conventional doses. *Res. Commun. chem. Pathol. Pharmacol., 28,* 551-561

Clarysse, A.M., Cathey, W.J., Cartwright, G.E. & Wintrobe, M.M. (1969) Pulmonary disease complicating intermittent therapy with methotrexate. *J. Am. med. Assoc., 209,* 1861-1864

Craig, S.R. & Rosenberg, E.W. (1971) Methotrexate-induced carcinoma? *Arch. Dermatol., 103,* 505-506

Custer, R.P., Freeman-Narrod, M. & Narrod, S.A. (1977) Hepatotoxicity in Wistar rats following chronic methotrexate administration: a model of human reaction. *J. natl Cancer Inst., 58,* 1011-1017

Davis, H.L., Jr, Prout, M.N., McKenna, P.J., Cole, D.R. & Korbitz, B.C. (1973) Acute leukemia complicating metastatic breast cancer. *Cancer, 31,* 543-546

Daynes, R.A., Harris, C.C., Connor, R.J. & Eichwald, E.J. (1979) Skin cancer development in mice exposed chronically to immunosuppressive agents. *J. natl Cancer Inst., 62,* 1075-1081

Delmonte, L. & Jukes, T.H. (1962) Folic acid antagonists in cancer chemotherapy. *Pharmacol. Rev., 14,* 91-135

DeSesso, J.M. & Jordan, R.L. (1977) Drug-induced limb dysplasias in fetal rabbits. *Teratology, 15,* 199-212

Donehower, R.C., Hande, K.R., Drake, J.C. & Chabner, B.A. (1979) Presence of 2,4-diamino-N^{10}-methyl-pteroic acid after high-dose methotrexate. *Clin. Pharmacol. Ther., 26,* 63-72

Douglas, I.D.C. & Price, L.A. (1973) Bone-marrow toxicity of methotrexate: a reassessment. *Br. J. Haematol., 24,* 625-631

Epstein, E.H. & Croft, J.D., Jr (1969) Cirrhosis following methotrexate administration for psoriasis. *Arch. Dermatol., 100,* 531-534

Epstein, S.S., Arnold, E., Andrea, J., Bass, W. & Bishop, Y. (1972) Detection of chemical mutagens by the dominant lethal assay in the mouse. *Toxicol. appl. Pharmacol., 23,* 288-325

Ferguson, F.C., Jr, Thiersch, J.B. & Philips, F.S. (1950) The action of 4-amino-N^{10}-methyl-pteroylglutamic acid in mice, rats, and dogs. *J. Pharmacol. exp. Ther., 98,* 293-299

Finley, P.R. & Williams, R.J. (1977) Methotrexate assay by enzymatic inhibition, with use of the centrifugal analyzer. *Clin. Chem., 23,* 2139-2141

Flament-Durand, J., Ketelbant-Balasse, P., Maurus, R., Regnier, R. & Spehl, M. (1975) Intracerebral calcifications appearing during the course of acute lymphocytic leukemia treated with methotrexate and X rays. *Cancer, 35,* 319-325

Freeman-Narrod, M., Narrod, S. & Custer, R.P. (1974) Toxicity of methotrexate in C57/Bl mice: influence of tolerance and age (Abstract no. 2093). *Fed. Proc., 33,* 582

Gagliano, R.G. & Costanzi, J.J. (1976) Paraplegia following intrathecal methotrexate. Report of a case and review of the literature. *Cancer, 37,* 1663-1668

Geiser, C.F., Bishop, Y., Jaffe, N., Furman, L., Traggis, D. & Frei, E., III (1975) Adverse effects of intrathecal methotrexate in children with acute leukemia in remission. *Blood, 45,* 189-195

Greenspan, E.M. & Tung, B.G. (1974) Acute myeloblastic leukemia after cure of ovarian cancer. *J. Am. med. Assoc., 230,* 418-420

Gutin, P.H., Green, M.R., Bleyer, W.A., Bauer, V.L., Wiernik, P.H. & Walker, M.D. (1976) Methotrexate pneumonitis induced by intrathecal methotrexate therapy. A case report with pharmokinetic data. *Cancer, 38,* 1529-1534

Hampel, K.E., Kober, B., Rösch, D., Gerhartz, H. & Meinig, K.-H. (1966) The action of cytostatic agents on the chromosomes of human leukocytes *in vitro* (preliminary communication). *Blood, 27,* 816-823

Harris, C.C. (1971) Malignancy during methotrexate and steroid therapy for psoriasis. *Arch. Dermatol., 103,* 501-504

Harvey, S.C. (1975) *Antineoplastic and immunosuppressive drugs.* In: Osol, A., ed., *Remington's Pharmaceutical Sciences,* 15th ed., Easton, PA, Mack Publishing Co., pp. 1081-1082

Henderson, E.S., Adamson, R.H., Denham, C. & Oliverio, V.T. (1965) The metabolic fate of tritiated methotrexate. I. Absorption, excretion, and distribution in mice, rats, dogs and monkeys. *Cancer Res., 25,* 1008-1017

Herbold, B. & Buselmaier, W. (1976) Induction of point mutations by different chemical mechanisms in the liver microsomal assay. *Mutat. Res., 40,* 73-84

Hersh, E.M., Wong, V., Henderson, E.S. & Rubin, R. (1964) The acute hepatotoxic effects of methotrexate (MTX) therapy (Abstract no. 101). *Proc. Am. Assoc. Cancer Res., 5,* 26

Hoffbrand, A.V., Tripp, E. & Lavoie, A. (1976) Synthesis of folate polyglutamates in human cells. *Clin. Sci. mol. Med., 50,* 61-68

Huffman, D.H., Wan, S.H., Azarnoff, D.L. & Hoogstraten, B. (1973) Pharmokinetics of methotrexate. *Clin. Pharmacol. Ther., 14,* 572-579

Jackson, R.C. & Harrap, K.R. (1973) Studies with a mathematical model of folate metabolism. *Arch. Biochem. Biophys., 158,* 827-841

Jacobs, S.A., Stoller, R.G., Chabner, B.A. & Johns, D.G. (1977) Dose-dependent metabolism of methotrexate in man and rhesus monkeys. *Cancer Treat. Rep., 61,* 651-656

Johns, D.G. & Loo, T.L. (1967) Metabolite of 4-amino-4-deoxy-N^{10}-methylpteroylglutamic acid (methotrexate). *J. pharm. Sci., 56,* 356-359

Jolly, L.E., Jr & Fletcher, H.P. (1977) The effect of repeated oral dosing of methotrexate on its intestinal absorption in the rat. *Toxicol. appl. Pharmacol., 39,* 23-32

Jordan, R.L. (1973) Response of the rabbit embryo to methotrexate (Abstract). *Teratology, 7,* A-19

Jordan, R.L., Wilson, J.G. & Schumacher, H.J. (1977) Embryotoxicity of the folate antagonist metho-trexate in rats and rabbits. *Teratology, 15,* 73-80

Kaslow, R.A., Wisch, N. & Glass, J.L. (1972) Acute leukemia following cytotoxic chemotherapy. *J. Am. med. Assoc., 219,* 75-76

Khera, K.S. (1976) Teratogenicity studies with methotrexate, aminopterin, and acetylsalicylic acid in domestic cats. *Teratology, 14,* 21-28

Kroese, W.F.S. (1975) *Cytostatic drugs.* In: Dukes, M.N.G., ed, *Meyler's Side Effects of Drugs. A Survey of Unwanted Effects of Drugs Reported in 1972-1975,* Vol. 8, Amsterdam, Excerpta Medica, pp. 939-999

Krogh Jensen, M. (1967) Chromosome studies in patients treated with azathioprine and amethopterin. *Acta med. scand., 182,* 445-455

Krogh Jensen, M. & Nyfors, A. (1979) Cytogenetic effect of methotrexate on human cells *in vivo.* Com-parison between results obtained by chromosome studies on bone-marrow cells and blood lympho-cytes and by the micronucleus test. *Mutat. Res., 64,* 339-343

Krueger, G. (1975) The significance of immunosuppression and antigenic stimulation in the development of malignant lymphomas. *Recent Results Cancer Res., 52,* 88-95

Levij, I.S., Rwomushana, J.W. & Polliack, A. (1970) Effect of topical cyclophosphamide, methotrexate and vinblastine on 9,10-dimethyl-1,2-benzanthracene (DMBA)-carcinogenesis in the hamster cheek pouch. *Eur. J. Cancer, 6,* 187-193

Lewis, W.J. & Walter, J.F. (1979) Methotrexate-induced pulmonary fibrosis. *Arch. Dermatol., 115,* 1169-1170

Li, F.P., Cassady, J.R. & Jaffe, N. (1975) Risk of second tumors in survivors of childhood cancer. *Cancer, 35,* 1230-1235

Maier, P. & Schmid, W. (1976) Ten model mutagens evaluated by the micronucleus test. *Mutat. Res., 40,* 325-388

Malpas, J.S. & Whitehouse, J.M.A. (1977) *Cytostatic and immunosuppressive drugs.* In: Dukes, M.N.G., ed., *Side Effects of Drugs Annual I. A Worldwide Yearly Survey of New Data and Trends,* Amster-dam, Excerpta Medica, pp. 336-351

Marefat, P. & Shklar, G. (1979) The effect of methotrexate on chemical carcinogenesis of hamster tongue. *J. dent. Res., 58,* 1748

Matheson, D., Brusick, D. & Carrano, R. (1978) Comparison of the relative mutagenic activity for eight antineoplastic drugs in the Ames *Salmonella*/microsome and TK$^{+/-}$ mouse lymphoma assays. *Drug chem. Toxicol., 1,* 277-304

McClain, R.M. & Siekierka, J.J. (1975) The placental transfer of methotrexate in rats (Abstract no. 114). *Toxicol. appl. Pharmacol., 33,* 168

McCormick, J.I., Susten, S.S., Rader, J.I. & Freisheim, J.H. (1979) Studies of a methotrexate binding protein fraction from L1210 lymphocyte plasma membranes. *Eur. J. Cancer, 15,* 1377-1386

Medical Research Council Working Party on Leukaemia in Childhood (1975) Analysis of treatment in childhood leukaemia. I. Predisposition to methotrexate-induced neutropenia after craniospinal irradiation. *Br. med. J., iii,* 563-566

Melnyk, J., Duffy, D.M. & Sparkes, R.S. (1971) Human mitotic and meiotic chromosome damage following *in vivo* exposure to methotrexate. *Clin. Genet., 2,* 28-31

Miller, J.M. & Tucker, E. (1979) Use of HPLC for multicomponent serum analysis. Initial experiences in a hospital laboratory. *Am. Lab.,* January, 17-34

Milunsky, A., Graef, J.W. & Gaynor, M.F., Jr (1968) Methotrexate-induced congenital malformations. With a review of the literature. *J. Pediatr., 72,* 790-795

Molin, L. & Larsen, T.E. (1972) Psoriasis, methotrexate, and cancer. *Arch. Dermatol., 105,* 292

Muller, S.A., Farrow, G.M. & Martalock, D.L. (1969) Cirrhosis caused by methotrexate in the treatment of psoriasis. *Arch. Dermatol., 100,* 523-530

Nelson, J.A., Harris, B.A., Decker, W.J. & Farquhar, D. (1977) Analysis of methotrexate in human plasma by high-pressure liquid chromatography with fluorescence detection. *Cancer Res., 37,* 3970-3973

Newbold, P.C.H. & Stoughton, R.B. (1972) Percutaneous absorption of methotrexate. *J. invest. Dermatol., 58,* 319-322

Ngu, V.A., Roberts, D. & Hall, T.C. (1964) Studies on folic reductase. I. Levels in regenerating rat liver and the effect of methotrexate administration. *Cancer Res., 24,* 989-993

Paxton, J.W. & Rowell, F.J. (1977) A rapid, sensitive and specific radioimmunoassay for methotrexate. *Clin. chim. Acta, 80,* 563-572

Penn, I. & Starzl, T.E. (1973) *The effect of immunosuppression on cancer.* In: *Proceedings of the 7th National Cancer Conference,* Philadelphia, Lippincott, pp. 943-947

Powell, H.R. & Ekert, H. (1971) Methotrexate-induced congenital malformations. *Med. J. Aust., 2,* 1076-1077

Propping, P., Röhrborn, G. & Buselmaier, W. (1972) Comparative investigations on the chemical induction of point mutations and dominant lethal mutations in mice. *Mol. gen. Genet., 117,* 197-209

Raffetto, G., Parodi, S., Faggin, P. & Maconi, A. (1979) Relationship between cytotoxicity and induction of sister-chromatid exchanges in mouse foetal cells exposed to several doses of carcinogenic and non-carcinogenic chemicals. *Mutat. Res., 63,* 335-343

Rees, R.B., Bennett, J.H., Maibach, H.I. & Arnold, H.L. (1967) Methotrexate for psoriasis. *Arch. Dermatol., 95,* 2-11

Regelson, W., Bross, I.D., Hananian, J. & Nigogosyan, G. (1965) Incidence of second primary tumors in children with cancer and leukemia. A seven-year survey of 150 consecutive autopsied cases. *Cancer, 18,* 58-72

Ringrose, C.A.D. (1974) Carcinoma *in situ* of the cervix after amethopterin therapy. *Am. J. Obstet. Gynecol., 119,* 1132-1133

Robinson, J.W.L., Antonioli, J.-A. & Vannotti, A. (1966) The effect of oral methotrexate on the rat intestine. *Biochem. Pharmacol., 15,* 1479-1489

Roenigk, H.H., Jr, Bergfeld, W.F., St Jacques, R., Owens, F.J. & Hawk, W.A. (1971) Hepatotoxicity of methotrexate in the treatment of psoriasis. *Arch. Dermatol., 103,* 250-261

Roschlau, G. & Justus, J. (1971) Carcinogenic action of methotrexate and cyclophosphamide in animal experiments (Ger.). *Dtsch. Gesundheitswes., 26,* 219-222

Ross, G.T. (1976) Congenital anomalies among children born to mothers receiving chemotherapy for gestational trophoblastic neoplasm. *Cancer, 37,* 1043-1047

Rustia, M. & Shubik, P. (1973) Life-span carcinogenicity tests with 4-amino-N^{10}-methylpteroylglutamic acid (methotrexate) in Swiss mice and Syrian golden hamsters. *Toxicol. appl. Pharmacol., 26,* 329-338

Ruymann, F.B., Mosijczuk, A.D. & Sayers, R.J. (1977) Hepatoma in a child with methotrexate-induced hepatic fibrosis. *J. Am. med. Assoc., 238,* 2631-2633

Scherf, H.R. & Schmähl, D. (1975) Experimental investigations on immunodepressive properties of carcinogenic substances in male Sprague-Dawley rats. *Recent Results Cancer Res., 52,* 76-87

Schmähl, D. & Habs, M. (1976) Life-span investigations for carcinogenicity of some immune-stimulating, immunodepressive and neurotropic substances in Sprague-Dawley rats. *Z. Krebsforsch., 86,* 77-84

Schmähl, D. & Osswald, H. (1970) Experimental studies on carcinogenic effects of anticancer chemotherapeutics and immunosuppressives (Ger.). *Arzneimittel-Forsch./Drug Res., 20,* 1461-1467

Schröter, R., Kelleter, R. & Kuhn, D. (1971) Reticulosis as a long-term side-effect of methotrexate therapy in a patient with generalized psoriasis and psoriatic arthritis. *Dermatologica, 143,* 131-136

Scott, W.J., Wilson, J.G., Ritter, E.J. & Fradkin, R. (1978) *Further studies on distribution of teratogenic drugs in pregnant rats and rhesus monkeys.* In: Neubert, D., Merker, H.-J., Nau, H. & Langman, J. eds, *Role of Pharmacokinetics in Prenatal and Perinatal Toxicology,* Stuttgart, Georg Thieme, pp. 499-505

Seeger, D.R., Cosulich, D.B., Smith, J.M. & Hultquist, M.E. (1949) Analogs of pteroylglutamic acid. III. 4-Amino derivatives. *J. Am. chem. Soc., 71,* 1753-1758

Seino, Y., Nagao, M., Yahagi, T., Hoshi, A., Kawachi, T. & Sugimura, T. (1978) Mutagenicity of several classes of antitumor agents to *Salmonella typhimurium* TA98, TA100, and TA92. *Cancer Res., 38,* 2148-2156

Shehata, W.M. & Meyer, R.L. (1980) The enhancement effect of irradiation by methotrexate. Report of three complications. *Cancer, 46,* 1349-1352

Shklar, G., Cataldo, E. & Fitzgerald, A.L. (1966) The effect of methotrexate on chemical carcinogenesis of hamster buccal pouch. *Cancer Res., 26,* 2218-2224

Skalko, R.G. & Gold, M.P. (1974) Teratogenicity of methotrexate in mice. *Teratology, 9,* 159-164

Strum, W.B. & Liem, H.H. (1977) Hepatic uptake, intracellular protein binding and biliary excretion of amethopterin. *Biochem. Pharmacol., 26,* 1235-1240

Stuart, J.F.B., Calman, K.C., Watters, J., Paxton, J., Whiting, B., Lawrence, J.R., Steele, W.H. & McVie, J.G. (1979) Bioavailability of methotrexate: implications for clinical use. *Cancer Chemother. Pharmacol., 3,* 239-241

Tavassoli, F.A. & Lynch, R.G. (1974) Occult adenocarcinoma of the pancreas in a 17-year-old patient with immunosuppressed leukemia. *Gastroenterology, 66,* 1054-1057

Trier, J.S. (1961) Morphologic changes in human small intestinal mucosa induced by methotrexate (Abstract no. 282). *Proc. Am. Assoc. Cancer Res., 3,* 273

US International Trade Commission (1978) *Synthetic Organic Chemicals, US Production and Sales, 1978,* USITC Publication 920, Washington DC, US Government Printing Office, p. 180

US International Trade Commission (1979a) *Synthetic Organic Chemicals, US Production and Sales, 1978,* USITC Publication 1001, Washington DC, US Government Printing Office, p. 173

US International Trade Commission (1979b) *Imports of Benzenoid Chemicals and Products, 1978,* USITC Publication 990, Washington DC, US Government Printing Office, p. 86

US Pharmacopeial Convention, Inc. (1980) *The US Pharmacopeia,* 20th rev., Rockville, MD, pp. 508-509

Valerino, D.M. (1972) Studies of the metabolism of methotrexate. II. Isolation and identification of several unconjugated aminopteridines as metabolites in the rat. *Res. Commun. chem. Pathol. Pharmacol., 4,* 529-542

Valerino, D.M., Johns, D.G., Zaharko, D.S. & Oliverio, V.T. (1972) Studies on the metabolism of methotrexate by intestinal flora. I. Identification and study of biological properties of the metabolite 4-amino-4-deoxy-N^{10}-methylpteroic acid. *Biochem. Pharmacol., 21,* 821-831

Van Thiel, D.H., Ross, G.T. & Lipsett, M.B. (1970) Pregnancies after chemotherapy of trophoblastic neoplasms. *Science, 169,* 1326-1327

Virtanen, R., Iisalo, E., Parvinen, M. & Nordman, E. (1979) Methotrexate concentrations in biological fluids: comparison of results obtained by radioimmunoassay and direct ligand binding radioassay. *Acta pharmacol. toxicol., 44,* 296-302

Vogl, S.E. (1978) Acute leukemia complicating treatment of glioblastoma multiforme. *Cancer, 41,* 333-336

Voorhees, J.J., Janzen, M.K., Harrell, E.R. & Chakrabarti, S.G. (1969) Cytogenetic evaluation of methotrexate-treated psoriatic patients. *Arch. Dermatol., 100,* 269-274

Wade, A., ed. (1977) *Martindale, The Extra Pharmacopoeia,* 27th ed., London, The Pharmaceutical Press, pp. 156-161

Walden, P.A.M. & Bagshawe, K.D. (1976) Reproductive performance of women successfully treated for gestational trophoblastic tumors. *Am. J. Obstet. Gynecol., 125,* 1108-1114

Weir, E.E., Kaizer, H., Rosenberg, J. & Ludlum, D.B. (1978) A simplified assay for methotrexate in biological fluids using a crude yeast lysate. *Clin. chim. Acta, 88,* 207-213

Weisburger, E.K. (1977) Bioassay program for carinogenic hazards of cancer chemotherapeutic agents. *Cancer, 40,* 1935-1949

Wilson, J.G. (1971) Use of rhesus monkeys in teratological studies. *Fed. Proc., 30,* 104-109

Wilson, J.G. (1974) *Teratologic causation in man and its evaluation in non-human primates.* In: Motulsky, A.G. & Lenz, W., eds, *Birth Defects,* Amsterdam, Excerpta Medica, pp. 191-203

Wilson, J.G., Scott, W.J., Ritter, E.J. & Fradkin, R. (1979) Comparative distribution and embryotoxicity of methotrexate in pregnant rats and rhesus monkeys. *Teratology, 19,* 71-80

Windholz, M., ed. (1976) *The Merck Index,* 9th ed., Rahway, NJ, Merck & Co., p. 782

Wisnicki, J.L., Tong, W.P. & Ludlum, D.B. (1978) Analysis of methotrexate and 7-hydroxymethotrexate by high-pressure liquid chromatography. *Cancer Treat. Rep., 62,* 529-532

Zaharko, D.S. & Oliverio, V.T. (1970) Reinvestigation of methotrexate metabolism in rodents. *Biochem. Pharmacol., 29,* 2923-2925

Zaharko, D.S., Bruckner, H. & Oliverio, V.T. (1969) Antibiotics alter methotrexate metabolism and excretion. *Science, 166,* 887-888

Zaharko, D.S., Dedrick, R.L., Young, D.M. & Peale, A.L. (1976) Tolerance of long-term methotrexate infusions by mice. *Biochem. Pharmacol., 25,* 1317-1321

1. CHEMICAL AND PHYSICAL DATA

1.1 Synonyms and trade names

Chem. Abstr. Services Reg. No.: 53-03-2

Chem. Abstr. Name: Pregna-1,4-diene-3,11,20-trione, 17,21-dihydroxy-

IUPAC Systematic Name: 17,21-Dihydroxy-pregna-1,4-diene-3,11,20-trione

Synonyms: Dehydrocortisone; 1-dehydrocortisone; 1,2-dehydrocortisone; 17,21-dehydrocortisone; deidrocortisone; deltacortisone; Δ-cortisone; $\Delta(1)$-cortisone; $\Delta(1)$-dehydrocortisone; 17α,21-dihydroxy-1,4-pregnadiene-3,11,20-trione; 17,21-dihydroxypregna-1,4-diene-3,11,20-trione; 17α,21-dihydroxypregna-1,4-diene-3,11,-20-trione; 17,21-dihydroxypregn-1,4-diene-3,11,20-trione; intalsone; 1,4-pregna-diene-17α,21-diol-3,11,20-trione; prednison; prednizon

Trade names: Adasone; Alto-Pred; Ancortone; Ancotone; Antison; Benison; Bicortone; Bi-Delta; Buffacort; Co-Deltra; Colisone; Cortancyl; Cortane, Cortialer; Corticor; Cortidelt; Cortinter; Cortiol; Cortisid; Dabroson; Dacortin; Decortancyl; Decortin; Decortisyl; Decorton; Dekortin; Delco-Cortex; Delcort; Delcortin; Delta-Corlin; Delta-Cortelan; Deltacortene; Deltacortisyl; Deltacortone; Delta-Dome; Delta E; Deltalone; Delta-Prenovis; Delta-Scheroson; Deltasone; Deltasson; Deltastendiolo; Deltatrione; Deltison; Deltisone; Deltra; Di-Adreson; Dispersona; Ejizon; Encorton; Encortone; Enkorton; Erftopred; Fernisone; Fernisone Buffered; Fiasone; Hicorton; Homozol; Hostacortin; Idrosone; Inocortyl; In-sone; Juvason; Keteocort; Keysone; Kolpisone; Leocortine-D; Lisacort; Marnisonal; Marsone; Marvidiene; Marvisona; Mediasone; Me-Korti; Meprison; Metacortandracin; Meta-cortin; Metasone; Meticortem; Meticorten; Meticortene; Metisone; Metreton; Neoaltesona; Nisone; Nizon; Novoprednisone; NSC 10023; Nurison; Orasone; Panafcort; Paracort; Parmenison; Precortal; Predeltin; Predni-Artrit; Prednicen-M; Prednicorm; Prednifor; Prednilong; Prednilonga; Predniment; Predniseguer; Pred-nisol; Predni-Tablinen; Prednital; Predni-Wolner; Prednovister; Predorgasona; Predsol; Predsone; Presone; Pronison; Propred; Rectodelt; Retrocortin; Ropred;

Servisone; Solisone; Sone; Sterapred; Supercortil; Supernisona; Supopred; Tara-corten; Ultracorten; Ultracortene; Ultrilone; Urtilone; Vitazon; Wescopred; Win-pred; Xynisone; Zenidrid

1.2 Structural and molecular formulae and molecular weight

$$C_{21}H_{26}O_5$$

Mol. wt: 358.4

1.3 Chemical and physical properties of the pure substance

From Wade (1977) or Windholz (1976)

(a) *Description:* White or almost white, odourless, crystalline powder, with a persis-tent bitter after-taste

(b) *Melting-point:* 233-235°C (dec.)

(c) *Optical rotation:* $[\alpha]_D^{25} = +172°$ (in dioxane)

(d) *Spectroscopy data:* λ_{max} 238 nm, $A_1^1 = 433$ (in methanol)

(e) *Solubility:* Practically insoluble in water; soluble in ethanol (1 in 190) and chloroform (1 in 200); slightly soluble in dioxane and methanol

(f) *Stability:* Sensitive to oxidation and light

1.4 Technical products and impurities

Various national and international pharmacopoeias give specifications for the purity of prednisone in pharmaceutical products. For example, it is available in the US as a USP grade measured as containing 97.0 - 102.0% active ingredient on a dried basis, 1.0% max. moisture content, 0.003% max. selenium, negligible residue on ignition, and a specific rotation between +167° and +175° (US Pharmacopeial Convention, Inc., 1980). It is also available in 2.5-, 5-, 10-, 20- and 50-mg tablets (Baker, 1980) measured as containing 90.0 - 110.0% of the labelled amount of prednisone (US Pharmacopoeial Convention, Inc., 1980). In the UK, prednisone is available as 1-,2.5-,5-,10-,20- and 25-mg tablets (Wade, 1977); and in Japan in 1- and 5-mg tablets, in powder (1% per g) and in vials for injection (5 - 25 mg/ml per vial).

2. PRODUCTION, USE, OCCURRENCE AND ANALYSIS

2.1 Production and use

(a) Production

Chemical synthesis of prednisone was first reported (Herzog *et al.*, 1955) by introduction of the two double bonds in ring A by 2,4-dibromination of the 3-ketone and dehydrobromination, but the yields were only 10-15%. Prednisone is prepared more efficiently microbiologically by the dehydrogenation of cortisone: a pure culture of *Corynebacterium simplex* is grown in a sterilized nutrient medium of yeast extract, and cortisone is added. The *C. simplex* selectively dehydrogenates the cortisone. When the reaction is complete, the fermentation broth is extracted and purifed to give prednisone in good yield (Nobile *et al.*, 1955).

Commercial production of prednisone in the US was first reported in 1955 (US Tariff Commission, 1956). In 1966, 3 companies reported a combined production of 8172 kg (US Tariff Commission, 1968). Only one US company reported production, of an undisclosed amount (see preamble, p. 20), in 1978 (US International Trade Commission, 1979). Data on US imports and exports were not available.

Prednisone is manufactured by one company each in the Federal Republic of Germany, France and The Netherlands, and by two companies each in Italy and the UK. No data were available on the amounts produced.

Commercial production of prednisone in Japan started in 1956. Two companies presently produce about 200 kg per year; Japanese imports have amounted to 150 kg per year, for a total consumption of about 350 kg during the last 3 years.

(b)   Use

Prednisone is a synthetic glucocorticoid used in human medicine for its potent anti-inflammatory effects in disorders of many organ systems.   It also modifies some immunological responses.   Prednisone is thus used in almost every branch of medicine.   Particular applications include the treatment of allergic, autoimmune and rheumatological complaints, and lymphoproliferative neoplastic diseases, and its use in immunosuppressive therapy for organ transplantation.

The daily recommended dose varies widely for different diseases.   Initially, 5 - 50 mg per day are given orally in 2 - 4 divided doses until a satisfactory response occurs;   the usual maintenance dose is 10 - 20 mg per day (Harvey, 1975).   For special cases, a daily oral dose of as high as 250 mg has been recommended (Wade, 1977).   In the treatment of acute lymphoblastic leukaemia, the dose for adults is initially 60 mg daily;   for children, it is 1 - 2.2 mg/kg bw daily in 3 divided doses.   Administration is continued for 4 - 6 weeks, when the dose is reduced or completely withdrawn for patients in remission (Anon., 1977).

Prednisone is one of the components of MOPP (nitrogen mustard, vincristine sulphate, procarbazine hydrochloride, prednisone), a combination drug regimen used in the treatment of advanced Hodgkin's disease, and in POMP (vincristine sulphate, methotrexate, 6-mercaptopurine, prednisone), a combination used for treatement of acute leukaemia.

2.2   Occurrence

Prednisone is not known to be produced in Nature.

2.3   Analysis

Typical methods for the analysis of prednisone in various matrices are summarized in Table 1.

Table 1. Methods for the analysis of prednisone

Sample matrix	Sample preparation	Assay procedure[a]	Limit of detection	Reference
Formulations	Dissolve in chloroform and ethanol; develop with dichloromethane-methanol mixture	TLC-UV	not given	US Pharmacopoeial Convention, Inc. (1980)
Tablets	Powder sample; dissolve in water and methanol; extract with chloroform; add prednisone as internal standard	HPLC-UV	not given	Bunch (1968)
Tablets	Powder sample; dissolve in ethanol; add phosphate buffer	DPP	5 μg/ml	Yadav & Teare (1978)
Blood plasma	Extract with diethyl ether; purify on magnesium silicate column; derivatize with trimethylsilyl-imidazole	GC-CIMS	10 ng/ml	Matin & Amos (1978)
Serum	Purify on Lipidex column; incubate with [^{3}H]-prednisone and antiserum	RIA	25 pg	Caffin et al. (1978)

[a]Abbreviations: TLC-UV, thin-layer chromatography with ultra-violet detection; HPLC-UV, high-performance liquid chromatography with ultra-violet detection; DPP, differential pulse polarography; GC-CIMS, gas chromatography with chemical ionization mass spectrometry; RIA, radioimmunoassay

3. BIOLOGICAL DATA RELEVANT TO THE EVALUATION OF CARCINOGENIC RISK TO HUMANS

3.1 Carcinogenicity studies in animals

(a) Intraperitoneal administration

Mouse: Two groups, each of 25 male and 25 female 6-week-old outbred Swiss-Webster-derived mice were given i.p. injections of 6 or 12 (females, 6 or 25) mg/kg bw prednisone at a concentration of 0.1 ml/10 g bw in saline 3 times weekly for 6 months. Animals that survived over 100 days were observed for 12 further months, at which time they were killed. Untreated mice served as controls: spontaneous tumours were reported in 28/101 (28%) male and 38/153 (25%) female controls. The survival times of the treated animals were reported as percentages of that of the controls [no precise definition of the mode of calculation was given]: the survival time of treated males of both dose groups was 34% that of controls and that of females was 34% and 100%, respectively. The tumour incidence in treated males was 4/19 (21%), with 2 lymphosarcomas and 2 lung tumours, and that in treated females was 8/27 (30%), with 4 lung tumours, 2 lymphosarcomas and 2 uterine tumours. These incidences were not significantly greater than those in controls (Weisburger, 1977). [The Working Group considered that the inadequate reporting of certain items, such as survival times, the amalgation of various experimental groups and tumour types, as well as the lack of age-adjustment in the analyses precluded a complete evaluation of this study.]

Rat: Two groups, each of 25 male and 25 - 28 female 6-week-old Sprague-Dawley-derived Charles River (CD) rats, were given i.p. injections of 11 or 22 (males, 11 or 45) mg/kg bw prednisone at a concentration of 0.25 ml/100 g bw in saline 3 times weekly for 6 months. Animals that survived over 100 days were observed for 12 further months, at which time they were killed. Untreated rats served as controls: spontaneous tumours were reported in 60/179 (34%) male and 105/181 (58%) female controls. The survival times of the treated animals were reported as percentages of that of the controls [no precise definition of the mode of calculation was given]: the survival times of treated males were 23 and 100%, respectively, that of controls; and treated females of both dose groups had the same survival time as controls, i.e., 100%. Of treated males, 7/20 developed tumours, among which were 3 pituitary tumours and 1 tumour of the breast; 16/18 (89%) female rats developed tumours, 8 of the breast, 5 of the pituitary, 2 of the adrenal and 1 of the liver. The authors reported that the overall tumour incidence in females was 1.5 - 2-fold higher than that in controls (Weisburger, 1977). [The Working Group considered that inadequate reporting of certain items, such as survival times, the amalgation of various experimental groups and tumour types, as well as the lack of age-adjustment in the analyses precluded a complete evaluation of this study.]

(b) Effects of combinations

Mouse: Groups of 20 hr/hr hairless female albino mice, 5 - 8 weeks old, were either (i) fed 30 mg/kg of diet prednisone for 4 months (at which time the dose was reduced to 20 mg/kg of diet), (ii) remained untreated, (iii) received ultra-violet radiation on 5 days a week, or (iv) received a combined treatment with radiation and prednisone. The study was terminated after 220 days. Tumours were seen in 3/17 (18%) mice that were irradiated only; histologically, the observed skin tumours proved to be squamous-cell carcinomas. No tumour occurred in untreated controls, nor in animals subjected to prednisone treatment or to prednisone plus radiation (Koranda et al., 1975). [See also monograph on azathioprine, p. 55.]

3.2 Other relevant biological data

(a) Experimental systems

Toxic effects

Extensive studies in laboratory animals have demonstrated that glucocorticoids, including prednisone, significantly enhance susceptibility to infection by a large variety of organisms (Kass & Finland, 1958; Sidransky & Friedman, 1959; Louria *et al.*, 1960; Miller & Hedberg, 1965).

Although the toxicity of such glucocorticoids is less severe in axenic than in holo-xenic mice, several complications, leading occasionally to death, were noted in axenic mice with high dosages. These toxic effects include severe atrophy of lymphoid organs, especially the thymus and the spleen, hypotrophy of adrenal glands, disappearance of sub-cutaneous fat and moderate haematological and biochemical alterations (Branceni *et al.*, 1968). Lymphopenia with increased numbers of eosinophils and polymorphonuclear leucocytes has been observed consistently in treated mice and rats (Tolksdorf *et al.*, 1956; Branceni *et al.*, 1968). Several of the changes induced by prolonged administration of prednisone are, however, reversible after cessation of treatment (Tolksdorf *et al.*, 1956).

Effects on reproduction and prenatal toxicity

The glucocorticoids, including prednisone, are well known to induce teratogenic effects, predominantly cleft palate, in mice and rats and less frequently in rabbits. The effect varies considerably with the mouse strain used and depends on the glucocorticoid potency of the respective drug. A review of the embryotoxic potential of such drugs is given by Frohberg (1975).

Prednisone given to rats from the 11th day of pregnancy until parturition at daily doses of 2.5 or 5 mg was reported to inhibit the growth of the fetal thymus and spleen (Angervall & Lundin, 1964).

Absorption, distribution, excretion and metabolism

Prednisone is readily absorbed from the gut. Serum concentrations of prednisone and prednisolone, its active metabolite, have been found to be maximal 1 hour after oral administration of a 5-mg tablet of prednisone to beagle dogs (Colburn *et al.*, 1976). Follow-ing both i.p. and oral administration of prednisone to mice, serum levels of prednisone, prednisolone and other metabolites were maximal at l5 min. These levels were higher in mice given i.p. injections of prednisone than in those receiving the same doses by the oral route. Oral administration of prednisone to dogs and monkeys led to serum levels comparable with those following i.v. injections, but individual variations were relatively large (El Dareer *et al.*, 1977).

Use of radioimmunoassays for glucocorticoids (Colburn & Buller, 1973) has facilitated the study of interconversion of steroids *in vivo*. Prednisolone (11β,17α,21-trihydroxy-pregn-1,4-diene-3,20-dione), the product of an enzymatic reduction of the 11-carbonyl of prednisone, is the biologically active form of this agent (Jenkins & Sampson, 1967). When either prednisone or prednisolone is administered to dogs, both compounds shortly appear in the serum, indicating that the biological interconversion is very rapid; however, the concentration of the administered drug is highest during the first few hours (Colburn *et al.*, 1976). Prednisone gives rise to several other metabolites, some of which have not yet been identified (El Dareer *et al.*, 1975, 1977). Metabolism takes place primarily in the liver.

Thirty minutes after i.v. administration of ^{3}H-prednisone to a monkey, the concentration of prednisone was highest in the kidney. The drug was also found in the liver, spleen, lung, small intestine, serum and bile. The concentration of prednisolone was highest in the liver. It was also found in the kidney, pancreas, spleen, lung, small intestine, serum and bile (El Dareer *et al.*, 1977).

In vitro, prednisone is converted to prednisolone by liver, lung and renal tissue. Conversely, prednisolone is converted to prednisone by renal tissue (Hajós *et al.*, 1970).

In mice given an i.p. injection of 10 mg/kg bw ^{3}H-prednisone, 57% of the injected dose was bound to serum proteins (El Dareer *et al.*, 1975).

Specific receptors for the various corticosteroids (Feldman *et al.*, 1972) are present in both cytosol and nucleus (Lang & Stevens, 1970).

Mutagenicity and other short-term tests

Prednisone was not mutagenic in *Escherichia coli* (Szybalski, 1952), and it caused no chromosomal damage when administered to Wistar rats (Steflea *et al.*, 1977).

(b) Humans

Toxic effects

Prednisone causes profound and varied metabolic effects when used at therapeutic doses, given on a continuous basis. When given in large doses it can induce cardiac complications (David *et al.*, 1970). In addition, it modifies the body's immune response to diverse stimuli; among the changes that occur are lymphopenia, monocytopenia and suppression of delayed hypersensitivity skin tests (Dujovne & Azarnoff, 1973). Fluid and electrolyte disturbances may occur, including sodium and fluid retention, which may lead to congestive heart failure and hypertension. With large doses, potassium loss, hypokalaemic alkalosis, and increased calcium excretion may occur (David *et al.*, 1970).

Musculoskeletal disturbances may manifest, with muscle wasting and weakness (steroid myopathy). This is due in large part to catabolic effects, with loss of tissue, especially from muscle (Cope, 1972). Osteoporosis may be severe and may lead to vertebral compression fractures or to pathological fractures of long bones. Aseptic necrosis of the femoral and humeral heads and of other bones may occur (David *et al.*, 1970; Cope, 1972; Dujovne & Azarnoff, 1973).

The use of prednisone has been associated with peptic ulceration, although this has been questioned seriously by Conn & Blitzer (1976); existing ulceration may be aggravated by steroid therapy. Pancreatitis has also been described as a complication of corticosteroid therapy (Carone & Liebow, 1957; Riemenschneider *et al.*, 1968).

Corticosteroids may also contribute to colonic complications observed in organ transplant recipients. Massive bleeding from ulceration may occur. Perforation is seen in 2-4% of patients; it may result from diverticular disease (Perloff *et al.*, 1976; Penn, 1980).

Prednisone may also cause fatty infiltration of the liver and may account for some of the abnormalities in hepatic function that occur. Other gastrointestinal disturbances include abdominal distension and ulcerative oesophagitis (Penn, 1980).

Dermatological disturbances include delayed wound healing, thin, fragile skin, petechiae and ecchymoses, facial erythema and increased sweating (David *et al.*, 1970; Dujovne & Azarnoff, 1973).

Pseudo tumour cerebri (benign intracranial hypertension) occurs mainly in children as a rare reaction following reduction or withdrawal of corticosteroids (Cope, 1972; Dujovne & Azarnoff, 1973).

There are numerous endocrine side effects. Most frequent is development of the Cushingoid state (David *et al.*, 1970). Fatty deposits in the mediastinum causing mediastinal widening may simulate mediastinal lymphadenopathy (Strother, 1975). Menstrual irregularities, including amenorrhoea, may occur. There may be secondary adrenocortical and pituitary unresponsiveness, particularly in times of stress, as in trauma, surgery or illness (David *et al.*, 1970; Dujovne & Azarnoff, 1973). The processes of recovery of normal pituitary and adrenal function require about 1 year in some patients (Penn, 1980). There may be stunted growth and delayed skeletal maturation in children (David *et al.*,

1970; Dujovne & Azarnoff, 1973). Prednisone causes decreased carbohydrate tolerance and may unmask the features of latent diabetes (David *et al.*, 1970; Cope, 1972; Dujovne & Azarnoff, 1973).

Ophthalmic complications include the development of posterior subcapsular cataracts, and increased intraocular pressure which may lead to glaucoma (David *et al.*, 1970; Dujovne & Azarnoff, 1973; Penn, 1980). In patients with ocular herpes simplex, it may cause corneal perforation.

Psychiatric reactions have been reported in 4-36% of patients. These disturbances may take various forms, for example, insomnia, changes in mood or psyche, and psychopathies of the manic-depressive or schizophrenic type (Dujovne & Azarnoff, 1973).

The profound effects of prednisone on the immune system place patients at increased risk of developing infections of various types. Prednisone may mask some of the signs of infection, and may decrease host resistance and interfere with the ability to localize infections. During prednisone therapy, a polymorphonuclear leucocytosis may develop and may give rise to confusion in the diagnosis of infection. This elevation is dose-related (Floyd *et al.*, 1969).

Effects on reproduction and prenatal toxicity

Prednisone has been widely used during pregnancy, and many instances of first trimester exposure to this drug have been recorded in the literature.

Among women who received 10 mg/day of prednisone throughout their entire pregnancy, a statistically significant decrease in the birth weight of term infants (36 - 40 weeks' gestation) was observed: among the control group of infants, 1 out of 67 had a birth weight below 2500 g; while among the infants whose mothers were treated with prednisone, the birth weights of 16 out of 119 were below 2500 g (Fisher exact test, $P < 0.01$; odds ratio = 10.3). Thus, the prednisone-treated group was 10 times more likely to have had a term infant with a low birth weight (Reinisch *et al.*, 1978).

A series of 56 pregnancies among 37 women who had received a renal homograft and were taking azathioprine (37.5 - 150 mg/day) and prednisone (0 - 35 mg/day) during the entire pregnancy was reported. Forty-four live infants were born. Four had major congenital anomalies: 2 had pulmonary arterial stenosis, 1 had a deformed hand, and 1 had bilateral inguinal hernias. Another infant had seizures of unknown etiology. Ten out of 44 live-born infants (23%) were premature (gestational age < 36 weeks), and 8/34 (24%) full-term infants weighed less than 2500 g. The mean birth weight was 3030 g, with no significant difference between males and females (Penn *et al.*, 1980).

In a series of 13 pregnancies in 8 women treated with prednisone (5 - 60 mg/day) for systemic lupus erythematosus, no malformations were observed among 8 live-births. There were 2 spontaneous and 3 therapeutic abortions; one of the women who had a spontaneous abortion had also received azathioprine. Two of the 8 live-born infants were small for gestational age (Devoe & Taylor, 1979).

No birth defects were reported in 22 infants who were exposed *in utero* to prednisone during the first trimester (Frohberg, 1975).

Adrenocortical failure was reported in a premature infant whose mother had received a total dose of 0.348 mg prednisone; the child died after 4 hours (Oppenheimer, 1964). Two similar cases were reported by Penn *et al.* (1980).

Absorption, distribution, excretion and metabolism

Prednisone is readily absorbed from the gut. In a series of 22 normal subjects, the mean peak serum concentration was 930 μg/l (range, 508-1579) following oral adminis- tration of a 50-mg tablet. The overall mean serum half-life was 2.95 hours (Disanto & DeSante, 1975). Reduction of the 11-oxo to the 11β-hydroxyl group by the enzyme 11β-hydroxyde-hydrogenase converts prednisone to prednisolone, its biologically active form. This reaction takes place mainly in the liver, and may proceed satisfactorily even in the presence of liver disease (Jenkins & Sampson, 1967).

Orally administered prednisone produces lower circulating concentrations of pred- nisolone than prednisolone itself given by the same route (Tse & Welling, 1979). Considerable variation in plasma concentrations may occur in a single subject, with peak drug values varying almost 2-fold. A wide intersubject variation in prednisolone concen- tration is evident after administration of either drug, which suggests impaired drug absorp- tion in some individuals (Hsueh *et al.*, 1979).

In one study after an oral dose of prednisone, the plasma prednisolone concentration peaked between 60 and 120 min and then declined exponentially. After rapid i.v. injection of steroid, the plasma prednisolone concentration peaked within 10 to 20 min. An initial rapid distribution phase succeeded by a slower decay phase was expressed by a biphasic exponential disappearance curve of the plasma prednisolone concentration *versus* time. Plasma prednisolone concentrations achieved with an oral dose of prednisone were in the same range as those obtained during the second phase after i.v. administration (Hsueh *et al.*, 1979).

Prednisolone is bound in serum to albumin and transcortin (corticosteroid-binding globulin), the latter showing high affinity for the steroid but low capacity, whereas albumin shows low affinity but high capacity for binding (Pickup, 1979). Reduced doses are necessary in patients with hypoalbuminaemia, otherwise the incidence of side effects is increased (Lewis *et al.*, 1971).

Pharmacokinetic drug interactions occur: particularly accelerated clearance of prednisolone is caused by enzyme-inducing agents such as barbiturates, phenytoin, rifampicin and other corticosteroids. On the other hand, oral contraceptives have been reported to increase the half-life and to decrease distribution volume and clearance of prednisolone, due to increased levels of transcortin. No apparent relationship has been demonstrated between blood level (total or non-protein bound concentration) and therapeutic effect (Pickup, 1979).

Urinary excretion is greater after i.v. administration than after oral dosage. At the end of 12 hours the percentage of the dose excreted in the urine was higher after i.v. administration by a factor of 1.41; between 14.6 and 24.30% of an i.v. dose is excreted in this time (Hsueh *et al.*, 1979).

The corresponding 20β-alcohols are present in smaller amounts (Gray *et al.*, 1956). Whereas the dog excretes large amounts of 20-dihydroprednisolone in the urine (El Dareer *et al.*, 1977), humans excrete only small amounts of this derivative. Other uncommon metabolites are mentioned by Bush & Mahesh (1964).

Mutagenicity and chromosomal effects

No chromosomal damage was detected in peripheral lymphocytes of patients treated with 3 mg/kg bw per day prednisone alone for 28 days and then with 0.5 - 1 mg/kg bw per day for 18 - 120 months (Fischer *et al.*, 1977). Krogh Jensen (1967) also found no chromosomal damage in the lymphocytes of patients treated with an unstated dose.

3.3 Case reports and epidemiological studies of carcinogenicity in humans

There are many case reports of cancer, too numerous to cite, that include a mention of previous treatment with prednisone, as would be expected by chance alone in view of the very wide use of this drug in many different disorders [see Section 2.1(*b*)]. No epidemiological study on prednisone alone was available to the Working Group.

4. SUMMARY OF DATA REPORTED AND EVALUATION

4.1 Experimental data

Prednisone was tested in mice and rats by intraperitoneal administration. Little or no carcinogenic effect was observed, but the studies suffered from limitations in design and reporting.

Prednisone can induce teratogenic effects (predominantly cleft palate) in rodents. The available data do not indicate that the agent produces mutations or chromosomal damage.

4.2 Human data

Prednisone is a common anti-inflammatory and immunosuppressive agent frequently used in the therapy of a great variety of non-neoplastic and neoplastic conditions.

Use of prednisone during pregnancy may have a significant effect on reducing birth weight. The data are not sufficient to evaluate whether this drug can induce teratogenic effects in humans. There are no data available indicating that prednisone is mutagenic or clastogenic.

In view of its wide use, the many references to previous administration of prednisone in patients with cancer are to be expected by chance alone. There is no epidemiological evidence suggesting an etiological relationship between prednisone and neoplasia.

4.3 Evaluation

The available data from studies in experimental animals and in humans were inadequate to evaluate the carcinogenicity of prednisone to humans.

5. REFERENCES

Angervall, L. & Lundin, P.M. (1964) Corticosteroid action on the fetal thymus and spleen. *Endocrinology, 74,* 986-989

Anon. (1977) *AMA Drug Evaluations,* 3rd ed., Littleton, MA, PSG Publishing Company, Inc., pp. 1141-1142, 1144-1145

Baker, C.E., Jr, ed. (1980) *Physicians' Desk Reference,* 34th ed., Oradell, NJ, Medical Economics Co., pp. 564, 812, 1388-1389, 1392, 1399, 1407

Branceni, D., Benveniste, J. & Salomon, J.-C. (1968) Effects of continuous massive administration of a glucocorticoid in the axenic mouse. Anatomicopathological, haematological and biochemical studies (Fr.). *Ann. Inst. Pasteur, 114,* 828-845

Bunch, E.A. (1968) *Determination of Related Foreign Steroids and Assay - Prednisone, Prednisolone, Hydrocortisone and Cortisone Acetate (Techn. Rep. 3),* Washington DC, US Food and Drug Administration, Executive Director of Regional Operations - Science Advisor Research Associate Programs, pp. 117-180

Bush, I.E. & Mahesh, V.B. (1964) Metabolism of 11-oxygenated steroids. 3. Some 1-dehydro and 9α-fluoro steroids. *Biochem. J., 93,* 236-255

Caffin, J.A., Halliday, J.W. & Powell, L.W. (1978) Specific assays for prednisolone and prednisone in serum: lipidex chromatography followed by radioimmunoassay. *J. pharmacol. Methods, 3,* 223-231

Carone, F.A. & Liebow, A.A. (1957) Acute pancreatic lesions in patients treated with ACTH and adrenal corticoids. *New Engl. J. Med., 257,* 690-697

Colburn, W.A. & Buller, R.H. (1973) Radioimmunoassay for prednisolone. *Steroids, 21,* 833-846

Colburn, W.A., Sibley, C.R. & Buller, R.H. (1976) Comparative serum prednisone and prednisolone concentrations following prednisone or prednisolone administration to beagle dogs. *J. pharm. Sci., 65,* 997-1001

Conn, H.O. & Blitzer, B.L. (1976) Nonassociation of adrenocorticosteroid therapy and peptic ulcer. *New Engl. J. Med., 294,* 473-479

Cope, C.L. (1972) *Adrenal Steroids and Disease,* 2nd ed., London, Pitman, pp. 533-556

David, D.S., Grieco, M.H. & Cushman, P., Jr (1970) Adrenal glucocorticoids after twenty years. A review of their clinically relevant consequences. *J. chronic Dis., 22,* 637-711

Devoe, L.D. & Taylor, R.L. (1979) Systemic lupus erythematosus in pregnancy. *Am. J. Obstet. Gynecol., 135,* 473-479

Disanto, A.R. & DeSante, K.A. (1975) Bioavailability and pharmokinetics of prednisone in humans. *J. pharm. Sci., 64,* 109-112

Dujovne, C.A. & Azarnoff, D.L. (1973) Clinical complications of corticosteroid therapy. A selected review. *Med. Clin. N. Am., 57,* 1331-1342

El Dareer, S.M., Mellett, L.B. & White, V.M. (1975) The metabolic disposition of ^{3}H-prednisone in BDF$_1$ mice (Abstract no. 495). *Pharmacologist, 17,* 226

El Dareer, S.M., Struck, R.F., White, V.M., Mellett, L.B. & Hill, D.L. (1977) Distribution and metabolism of prednisone in mice, dogs and monkeys. *Cancer Treat. Rep., 61,* 1279-1289

Feldman, D., Funder, J.W. & Edelman, I.S. (1972) Subcellular mechanisms in the action of adrenal steroids. *Am. J. Med., 53,* 545-560

Fischer, P., Vetterlein, M., Pohl-Rühling, J. & Krepler, P. (1977) Cytogenetic effects of chemotherapy and cranial irradiation on the peripheral blood lymphocytes of children with malignant disease. *Oncology, 34,* 224-228

Floyd, M., Muckle, T.J. & Kerr, D.N.S. (1969) Prednisone-induced leucocytosis in nephrotic syndrome. *Lancet, i,* 1192-1193

Frohberg, H. (1975) *Embryotoxic Action of Glucocorticoids in Animals and Humans. Inaugural Dissertation* (Ger.). Ph D Thesis, Medical Faculty, University of Heidelberg, Heidelberg

Gray, C.H., Green, M.A.S., Holness, N.J. & Lunnon, J.B. (1956) Urinary metabolic products of prednisone and prednisolone. *J. Endocrinol., 14,* 146-154

Hajós, G.T., Szporny, L. & Tuba, Z. (1970) 11-Oxido reduction of some natural and synthetic glucocorticoids in rat tissue *in vitro. Steroids, 15,* 449-458

Harvey, S.C. (1975) *Hormones.* In: Osol, A., ed., *Remington's Pharmaceutical Sciences,* 15th ed., Easton, PA, Mack Publishing Co., p. 897

Herzog, H.L., Payne, C.C., Jevnik, M.A., Gould, D., Shapiro, E.L., Oliveto, E.P. & Hershberg, E.G. (1955) 11-Oxygenated steroids. XIII. Synthesis and proof of structure of $\Delta^{1,4}$-pregnadiene-17α,21-diol-3,11,20-trione and $\Delta^{1,4}$-pregnadiene-11β,17α, 21-triol-3,20-dione. *J. Am. chem. Soc., 77,* 4871-4874

Hsueh, W.A., Paz-Guevara, A. & Bledsoe, T. (1979) Studies comparing the metabolic clearance rate of 11β-17,21-trihydroxypregn-1,4-diene-3,20-dione (prednisolone) after oral 17,21-dehydroxypregn-1,4-diene--3,11,20-trione and intravenous prednisolone. *J. clin. Endocrinol. Metab., 48,* 748-752

Jenkins, J.S. & Sampson, P.A. (1967) Conversion of cortisone to cortisol and prednisone to prednisolone. *Br. med. J., ii,* 205-207

Kass, E.H. & Finland, M. (1958) Corticosteroids and infections. *Adv. intern. Med., 9,* 45-80

Koranda, F.C., Loeffler, R.T., Koranda, D.M. & Penn, I. (1975) Accelerated induction of skin cancers by ultraviolet radiation in hairless mice treated with immunosuppressive agents. *Surg. Forum, 26,* 145-146

Krogh Jensen, M. (1967) Chromosome studies in patients treated with azathioprine and amethopterin. *Acta med. scand., 182,* 445-455

Lang, R.F. & Stevens, W. (1970) Evidence for intranuclear receptor sites for cortisol in lymphatic tissue. *J. reticuloendothel. Soc., 7,* 294-304

Lewis, G.P., Jusko, W.J., Burke, C.W. & Graves, L. (1971) Prednisone side-effects and serum-protein levels. A collaborative study. *Lancet, ii,* 778-781

Louria, D.B., Fallon, N. & Browne, H.G. (1960) The influence of cortisone on experimental fungus infections in mice. *J. clin. Invest., 39,* 1435-1449

Matin, S.B. & Amos, B. (1978) Quantitative determination of prednisone and prednisolone in human plasma using GLC and chemical-ionization mass spectrometry. *J. pharm. Sci., 67,* 923-926

Miller, J.K. & Hedberg, M. (1965) Effects of cortisone on susceptibility of mice to *Listeria monocytogenes. Am. J. clin. Pathol., 43,* 248-250

Nobile, A., Charney, W., Perlman, P.L., Herzog, H.L., Payne, C.C., Tully, M.E., Jevnik, M.A. & Hershberg, E.B. (1955) Microbiological transformation of steroids. I. $\Delta^{1,4}$-Diene-3-ketosteroids. *J. Am. chem. Soc., 77,* 4184

Oppenheimer, E.H. (1964) Lesions in the adrenals of an infant following maternal corticosteroid therapy. *Bull. John's Hopkins Hosp., 114,* 146-151

Penn, I. (1980) *Transplantation.* In: Hill, G.J., II, ed., *Outpatient Surgery,* 2nd ed., Philadelphia, W.B. Saunders Co., pp. 1223-1263

Penn, I., Makowski, E.L. & Harris, P. (1980) Parenthood following renal transplantation. *Kidney Int., 18,* 221-233

Perloff, L.J., Chon, H., Petrella, E.J., Grossman, R.A. & Barker, C.F. (1976) Acute colitis in the renal allograft recipient. *Ann. Surg., 183,* 77-83

Pickup, M.E. (1979) Clinical pharmacokinetics of prednisone and prednisolone. *Clin. Pharmacokinet., 4,* 111-128

Reinisch, J.M., Simon, N.G., Karow, W.G. & Gandelman, R. (1978) Prenatal exposure to prednisone in humans and animals retards intrauterine growth. *Science, 202,* 436-438

Riemenschneider, T.A., Wilson, J.F. & Vernier, R.L. (1968) Glucocorticoid-induced pancreatitis in children. *Pediatrics, 41,* 428-437

Sidransky, H. & Friedman, L. (1959) The effect of cortisone and antibiotic agents on experimental pulmonary aspergillosis. *Am. J. Pathol., 35,* 169-179

Steflea, D., Cilievici, O., Tone, P. & Popescu, L. (1977) Chromosomal aberrations induced in animals with imuran and prednisone (Rum.). *Med. intern., 29,* 379-384

Strother, C.M. (1975) Corticosteroid-induced mediastinal widening in myasthenia gravis. *Arch. Neurol.,* *32,* 702-703

Szybalski, W. (1952) Special microbiological systems. II. Observations on chemical mutagenesis in micro-organisms. *Ann. N.Y. Acad. Sci., 76,* 475-489

Tolksdorf, S., Battin, M.L., Cassidy, J.W., MacLeod, R.M., Warren, F.H. & Perlman, P.L. (1956) Adreno-cortical properties of $\Delta^{1,4}$-pregnadiene-17α,21-diol-3,11,20-trione (meticorten) and $\Delta^{1,4}$-pregnadiene-11β, 17α,21-triol-3,20-dione (meticortelone). *Proc. Soc. exp. Biol. Med., 92,* 207-214

Tse, F.L.S. & Welling, P.G. (1979) Relative bioavailability of prednisone and prednisolone in man. *J. pharm. Pharmacol., 31,* 492-493

US International Trade Commission (1979) *Synthetic Organic Chemicals, US Production and Sales, 1978,* USITC Publication 1001, Washington DC, US Government Printing Office, p. 170

US Pharmacopeial Convention, Inc. (1980) *The US Pharmacopeia,* 20th rev., Rockville, MD, pp. 655-656

US Tariff Commission (1956) *Synthetic Organic Chemicals, US Production and Sales, 1955,* 2nd series, Report No. 198, Washington DC, US Government Printing Office, p. 111

US Tariff Commission (1968) *Synthetic Organic Chemicals, US Production and Sales, 1966,* TC Publication 248, Washington DC, US Government Printing Office, pp. 33, 126

Wade, A., ed. (1977) *Martindale, The Extra Pharmacopoeia,* 27th ed., London, The Pharmaceutical Press, pp. 430-432

Weisburger, E.K. (1977) Bioassay program for carcinogenic hazards of cancer chemotherapeutic agents. *Cancer, 40,* 1935-1949

Windholz, M., ed. (1976) *The Merck Index,* 9th ed., Rahway, NJ, Merck & Co., p. 999

Yadav, R.N. & Teare, F.W. (1978) Determination of fluoxymesterone, norethandrolone, prednisolone, and prednisone in tablets by differential pulse polarography. *J. pharm. Sci., 67,* 436-438

1. CHEMICAL AND PHYSICAL DATA

1.1 Synonyms and trade names

Chem. Abstr. Services Reg. No.: 366-70-1

Chem. Abstr. Name: Benzamide, N-(1-methylethyl)-4-[(2-methylhydrazino)methyl]-, monohydrochloride

IUPAC Systematic Name: N-Isopropyl-α-(2-methylhydrazino)-para-toluamide monohydrochloride

Synonyms: Ibenzmethyzin hydrochloride; ibenzmethyzine hydrochloride; IBZ; N-4-isopropylcarbamoylbenzyl-N'-methylhydrazine hydrochloride; 2-[para-(isopropylcarbamoyl)benzyl]-1-methylhydrazine hydrochloride; N-isopropyl-para-(2-methylhydrazinomethyl)benzamide hydrochloride; MBH; para-(N[1]-methylhydrazinomethyl)-N-isopropylbenzamide hydrochloride; 1-methyl-2-[para-(isopropylcarbamoyl)benzyl]hydrazine hydrochloride; 1-methyl-2-para-(isopropylcarbamoyl)benzylhydrazine hydrochloride; MIH

Trade names: Matulane; Natulanar; Natulan; NSC 77213; PRO; Ro 4-6467; Ro 46467/1

1.2 Structural and molecular formulae and molecular weight

$C_{12}H_{19}N_3O.HCl$ Mol. wt: 257.8

1.3 Chemical and physical properties of the pure substance

From Wade (1977) or Rucki (1976), unless otherwise specified

(a) Description: A white to pale-yellow crystalline powder with a slight odour

(b) Melting-point: 223°C (dec.)

(c) Spectroscopy data: λ_{max} 232 nm, A_1^1 = 504 (in 0.1N HCl)

(d) Solubility: Very soluble in water and methanol; freely soluble in chloroform and diethyl ether

(e) Stability: Sensitive to oxidation (Harvey, 1975)

1.4 Technical products and impurities

Various national and international pharmacopoeias give specifications for the purity of procarbazine hydrochloride in pharmaceutical products. For example, it is available in the US as a USP grade measured as containing 98.5 - 100.5% active ingredient, 0.002% max. heavy metals, and 0.1% max. residue on ignition. It is also available in capsules measured as containing 90.0 - 110.0% of the stated amount (US Pharmacopeial Convention, Inc., 1980).

In Japan, the US and western Europe, procarbazine hydrochloride is available as capsules containing 50 mg of the drug (Wade, 1977; Baker, 1980). In certain countries, it is available as an injectable form in vials containing 250 mg.

2. PRODUCTION, USE, OCCURRENCE AND ANALYSIS

2.1 Production and use

(a) Production

Procarbazine hydrochloride was synthesized at the same time as other methylhydrazine derivatives in 1963 (Goodman & Gilman, 1975; Reed, 1975). It can be prepared by reacting 1,2-di(carbobenzoxy)-1-methylhydrazine with 4-(bromoethyl)benzoic acid methyl ester to yield 4-{[2-methyl-1,2-di(carbobenzoxy)hydrazino] methyl} benzoic acid. Thionyl chloride is used to produce the acid chloride, which is then reacted with isopropylamine. Treatment of the resulting amide with 33% hydrobromic acid in glacial acetic acid yields procarbazine hydrobromide, which is then converted to the hydrochloride (Harvey, 1975).

Procarbazine hydrochloride is believed to be supplied by one company in the US; however, the country where it is manufactured is not known and no data were available on the quantities produced.

It has never been produced commercially in Japan; approximately 40 kg were imported in 1978. It was first used there in 1974.

(b)   Use

Procarbazine hydrochloride is used in human medicine as an antineoplastic agent (Goodman & Gilman, 1975; Harvey, 1975; Wade, 1977). A combination of procarbazine hydrochloride, vincristine sulphate, nitrogen mustard and prednisone (MOPP) is used to treat Hodgkin's disease. Procarbazine hydrochloride is also used to treat malignant melanoma, non-Hodgkin's lymphoma and small-cell carcinoma of the lung.

The usual initial dose of procarbazine hydrochloride is 2 - 4 mg/kg bw per day given orally in divided doses for one week, then 4 - 6 mg/kg bw daily, until signs of bone-marrow depression occur. The drug is then discontinued until bone-marrow recovery is obtained, and then treatment is resumed at a dose level of 1 - 2 mg/kg bw per day. In the MOPP regimens, procarbazine hydrochloride is administered in doses of 100 mg/m^2 body surface daily for the first 2 weeks of a 4 - 6 week cycle (Wade, 1977).

2.2 Occurrence

Procarbazine hydrochloride is not known to be produced in Nature.

2.3 Analysis

Analytical methods for the determination of procarbazine hydrochloride based on thin-layer chromatography, spectrophotometry, coulometric analysis, polarography and titrimetric analysis have been reviewed (Rucki, 1976).

Typical methods for the analysis of procarbazine hydrochloride in capsules are summarized in Table 1.

Table 1. Methods for the analysis of procarbazine hydrochloride

Sample matrix	Sample preparation	Assay procedure[a]	Limit of detection	Reference
Formulations	Mix powder with hydrochloric acid; filter	S	not given	Rucki (1976)
	Dissolve in potassium iodide solution; apply current using platinum generating system and polarized platinum indicating system	C	not given	Oliveri-Vigh et al. (1971)
	Dissolve in water; titrate with sodium hydroxide; determine endpoint potentiometrically	T	not given	US Pharmacopeial Convention, Inc. (1980)
	Dissolve in pH12 buffer	P	not given	US Pharmacopeial Convention, Inc. (1980)

[a] Abbreviations: S, spectrophotometry; C, coulometric analysis; T, titrimetric analysis; P, polarography

3. BIOLOGICAL DATA RELEVANT TO THE EVALUATION OF CARCINOGENIC RISK TO HUMANS

3.1 Carcinogenicity studies in animals

(a) Oral administration

Mouse: Groups [size unspecified] of male and female CD_2F_1 mice were given single or multiple administrations of procarbazine hydrochloride. One group received a single administration of 450 - 675 mg/kg bw; another was given 1000 - 1800 mg/kg bw; a third group received 258 mg/kg bw once a week for 8 weeks; and untreated controls were maintained for 38 or 55 weeks. In the single low-dose group, 8/9 had lung tumours 10 - 14 weeks after exposure, and 9/9 at 25 weeks. In the high-dose group, lung tumours were found in 3/4 at 10 - 14 weeks and in 5/5 at 22 - 25 weeks. Multiple administrations produced lung tumours in 7/7 mice by 15 - 22 weeks and, in addition, 3/7 had leukaemia. Among controls, only 2/100 developed lung tumours by 38 weeks and 2/111 by 55 weeks; no leukaemia was found. All of the lung tumours were considered to be benign (Kelly et al., 1964). [The Working Group noted the absence of information on matched controls, group size and survival.]

A group [size unspecified] of male and female general purpose (non-inbred albino) mice were given 300 mg/kg bw procarbazine hydrochloride once a week for 8 weeks. Untreated controls were maintained for 24 or 44 - 55 weeks. By 6 - 11 weeks after first exposure, 9/14 mice had lung tumours (adenomas) and 2/14 had leukaemia; at 12 - 16 weeks, the incidence of lung tumours was 21/21 and of leukaemia 17/21. Of the controls, none out of 70 had a lung tumour or leukaemia at 24 weeks; and 29/144 and 1/144 had lung tumours and leukaemia, respectively, at 44 - 55 weeks (Kelly et al., 1964). [The Working Group noted the absence of information on matched controls, group size and survival.]

Groups of male and female (BALB/c x DBA/2) F_1 (CDF$_1$) mice, 7 - 8 weeks of age, were given 0.2 ml/mouse procarbazine hydrochloride in water by gavage at 3 dose levels: 25 males were given 300 mg/kg bw weekly for 4 weeks followed by 200 mg/kg bw weekly for 4 weeks (low dose); 25 males received 300 mg/kg bw weekly for 8 weeks (medium dose) ; and 30 females were given weekly administrations of 10.24 mg/mouse once, 5.16 mg/mouse twice and 2.58 mg/mouse 5 times over 10 weeks, for a total dose of 33.5 mg/ mouse (high dose). Mortality was 40% in the low-dose group, 16% in the medium-dose group and 73% in the high-dose group. Controls given sodium carboxymethylcellulose or saline survived until the end of the experiment. In the low-dose group, 7/10 developed pulmonary tumours within a median latent period of 25 weeks; and 4/10 had leukaemia (median latent period, 25 weeks) and 2/10 renal adenomas (median latent period, 47 weeks). In the medium-dose group, 9/11 animals had pulmonary tumours within a median latent period of 28 weeks; and 10/11 had leukaemia within a median latent period of 18 weeks. Surviving animals in the high-dose group were killed at 28-33 weeks: 8/8 had developed pulmonary tumours within a median latent period of 16 weeks; and 5/8 animals had leukaemia within a median latent period of 21 weeks. In the control group given sodium carboxymethylcellulose, 1/23 had a pulmonary tumour within a latent period of 54 weeks, none had leukaemia, and 1/23 had an adenoma of the kidney (median latent period, 34 weeks). Of the saline controls, 1/10 had a pulmonary tumour within a latent period of 33 weeks, and none had leukaemia (Kelly et al., 1969). [The Working Group noted the absence of information on matched controls, group size and survival.]

Rat: Groups of 10 young female Sprague-Dawley rats were given procarbazine hydrochloride by gastric intubation: 3 groups received single doses of 50, 100 or 150 mg at 50 days of age; one group received 3 doses of 50 mg each at age 50, 53 and 56 days; and a positive control group was given 20 mg 7,12-dimethylbenz[a]anthracene in 3 doses. By 20 weeks after treatment, 100% of animals in all groups displayed mammary tumours, most of which were carcinomas (Heuson & Heimann, 1966). [The Working Group noted the absence of negative controls and of information on survival.]

Groups of random-bred Osborne-Mendel female rats were given procarbazine hydro-chloride orally once only at 6 weeks of age or once a week for 10 weeks beginning at 4 weeks of age. The single doses administered were 500 or 1000 mg/kg bw; the multiple doses were 50 or 100 mg/kg bw. Rats that lived 11 weeks or more after the initial exposure were evaluated for mammary tumour induction. Of those that received a single low dose, 9/9 females developed mammary adenocarcinomas within a median latent period of 12 weeks. Of those that had a single, high dose, 1/1 female developed a mammary adenocarcinoma at 19 weeks. Of those that received multiple low doses, 17/19 females developed mammary adenocarcinomas within a median latent period of 19 weeks. With multiple high doses, 17/18 females developed mammary adenocarcinomas within a median latent period of 13 weeks (Kelly *et al.*, 1968). [The Working Group noted the absence of information on matched controls, group size and survival.]

Groups of male and female inbred Fischer 344/N rats were given single oral doses of 500 or 1000 mg/kg bw procarbazine hydrochloride at 8 - 10 weeks of age (males) or 8 weeks of age (females). Other groups of females received 100 mg/kg bw once a week for 10 weeks beginning at 6 weeks of age or 250 mg/kg bw once a week for 4 weeks beginning at 9 - 16 weeks of age. Rats that lived 11 weeks or more after the initial exposure were evaluated for mammary tumour induction. Of those given a single low dose, 0/9 male rats but 2/5 females developed adenocarcinomas, 1 a fibroadenoma and 1 an adenocarcinoma plus a fibroadenoma within a median latent period of 43 weeks. Of those given the single high dose, 0/9 male rats but 1/5 females developed a mammary adenocarcinoma at 34 weeks. With multiple low doses, 7/15 females developed mammary adenocarcinomas and 1 a fibro-adenoma within a median latent period of 38 weeks. With multiple high doses, 8/19 females developed mammary adenocarcinomas and 1 a fibroadenoma within a median latent period of 37 weeks (Kelly *et al.*, 1968). [The Working Group noted the absence of information on matched controls, group size and survival.]

(b) Intraperitoneal administration

Mouse: Groups [size unspecified] of male and female CD_2F_1 mice were given weekly i.p. injections of procarbazine hydrochloride for 1, 4 or 8 weeks. The single doses were 300 - 450 mg/kg bw and 740 - 827 mg/kg bw; the doses for 4 injections were 200 - 450 mg/kg bw; and the doses for 8 injections were 200 - 400 mg/kg bw. Two groups of un-treated controls were observed for 38 weeks (100 mice) and 55 weeks (111 mice). Of mice that received a single low dose, 3/10 developed pulmonary tumours by 14 weeks and 10/10 by 25 weeks. With a single high dose, 6/6 mice had pulmonary tumours by 17 weeks. With 4 injections, 3/9 animals had pulmonary tumours by 10 - 12 weeks and 29/32 by 13 - 21 weeks; in addition, 1/9 and 3/32 had leukaemia. With 8 injections, the pulmonary tumour incidences were 1/11 at 6 - 9 weeks, 4/10 at 10 - 12 weeks and 21/21 at 13 - 21 weeks; 11/21 animals in the last group also had leukaemia. Of untreated controls, 2/100 had pul-monary tumours by 38 weeks and 2/111 by 55 weeks; no leukaemia occurred. All of the lung tumours were considered to be benign (Kelly *et al.*, 1964). [The Working Group noted the absence of information on group size and survival.]

A group [size unspecified] of male and female general purpose (non-inbred albino) mice were given i.p. injections of 300 mg/kg bw procarbazine hydrochloride once a week for 8 weeks. Untreated controls were maintained for up to 55 weeks. By 6 - 11 weeks after the first injection, 3/9 mice had pulmonary tumours, and by 12 - 16 weeks the incidence was 12/12; 10/12 of these animals had leukaemia. Among controls, the incidence of pulmonary tumours was 0/70 at 24 weeks and 29/144 at 44 - 55 weeks; leukaemia occurred in only 1/144 animals at 44 - 55 weeks. All of the lung tumours were considered to be benign (Kelly *et al.*, 1964). [The Working Group noted the absence of information on matched controls, group size and survival.]

A group of 30 male (BALB/c x DBA/2) F_1 (CDF$_1$) mice, 7 - 8 weeks of age, were given i.p. injections of 0.1 ml/mouse procarbazine hydrochloride in water once a week for 8 weeks: 3 injections of 5.16 mg/mouse were followed by 5 of 2.58 mg/mouse, for a total dose of 28.4 mg/mouse. Mortality was 30%; that in saline-injected controls was 10%. Surviving mice were killed at 28-33 weeks and evaluated for the induction of pulmonary tumours and leukaemia. Of the treated animals, 17/21 had pulmonary tumours within a mean latent period of 16 weeks, and 10/21 had leukaemia. Of the saline-injected controls, 1/9 had a pulmonary tumour within a mean latent period of 32 weeks, and none had leukaemia (Kelly *et al.*, 1969). [The Working Group noted the absence of information on matched controls, group size and survival.]

Two groups, each of 25 male and 25 female outbred Swiss-Webster-derived mice, 6 weeks old, were given i.p. injections of 12 or 25 mg/kg bw procarbazine hydrochloride dissolved in physiological saline 3 times a week for 6 months. Animals that survived over 100 days were observed for up to 12 further months, at which time they were killed. A control group of 101 male mice had a median survival time of 9.8 months, while that of 153 female control mice was 18 months. The survival times of the treated animals were reported as percentages of that of the controls [no precise definition of the mode of calculation was given]. The incidence of lung tumours in treated males was 15/33, compared with 10/101 in controls. Of treated females, 23/34 developed lung tumours, 9/34 lymphomas, 3/34 renal tumours and 8/34 uterine tumours; the incidences in control females were 21/153 lung tumours, 2/153 lymphomas, 0/153 renal tumours and 3/153 uterine tumours. The increases in tumour incidence at all these sites were reported to be significant (Weisburger *et al.*, 1975; Weisburger, 1977). [The Working Group considered that the inadequate reporting of certain items, such as survival times, the amalgamation of various experimental groups and tumour types, as well as the lack of age-adjustment in the analyses precluded a complete evaluation of this study.]

Groups of 35 male and 35 female B6C3F1 mice, 35 days of age, were given i.p. injections of 6 or 12 mg/kg bw procarbazine hydrochloride dissolved in buffered saline 3 times a week for 52 weeks. Groups of 15 male and 15 female mice were untreated or received the vehicle only and were maintained for 85 weeks, the duration of the study. Of the male mice, 40% of the vehicle controls and 31% of the low-dose group, but none of the high-dose group, lived to the end of the study: their median survival times were 62 weeks, 75 weeks and 56 weeks, respectively. Of the female mice, 80% of the vehicle controls and 21% of the low-dose group, but none of the high-dose group, survived to the end of the study. Of autopsied males, 18/30 in the low-dose group and 20/31 in the high-dose group developed tumours; 5 occurred in 15 untreated males and male vehicle controls. The sites at which tumour incidences were significantly increased in males were lung, haematopoietic system and nervous system. Of autopsied females, 19/23 in the low-dose group and 20/26 in the high-dose group had tumours; no tumours were found in vehicle controls, and only a low incidence was found in the lung, liver and haematopoietic system in untreated male controls. The sites at which tumour incidences were significantly increased in females included lung, haematopoietic system, nervous system and uterus. The neoplasm that occurred most frequently was olfactory neuroblastoma, which was found only in 10/29 high-dose males and 11/25 high-dose females (National Cancer Institute, 1979).

Rat: A group [size unspecified] of female Fischer 344/N rats were given i.p. injections of 50 mg/kg bw procarbazine hydrochloride once a week for 10 weeks beginning at 4 weeks of age. Rats that lived 11 weeks or more were evaluated for induction of mammary tumours: 3/15 treated animals developed adenocarcinomas within a mean latent period of 34 weeks (Kelly *et al.*, 1968). [The Working Group noted the absence of information on matched controls, group size and survival.]

Two groups [size unspecified] of female random-bred Osborne-Mendel rats were given an i.p. injection of 500 mg/kg bw procarbazine hydrochloride once only at 6 weeks of age or weekly i.p. injections of 50 mg/kg bw for 10 weeks starting at 4 weeks of age. Rats that lived more than 11 weeks after the initial injection were evaluated for mammary tumour development. Of females that received a single injection, 4/7 developed mammary adenocarcinomas within a median latent period of 39 weeks. Of the females that received weekly injections, 19/20 developed mammary adenocarcinomas within a median latent period of 17 weeks (Kelly *et al.*, 1968).

A group of 10 6-week-old female R strain rats were given 15 i.p. injections of 15 mg procarbazine dissolved in physiological saline over 7.5 months. All exposed rats developed malignant tumours after a median latent period of 301 days: 8/10 in the mammary gland, 3/10 in the uterus and 2/10 in the ear duct. No tumour was observed in a control group of unspecified size (Deckers *et al.*, 1974). [The Working Group noted the limited reporting of this study.]

Two groups, each of 25 male or 25 female Sprague-Dawley-derived Charles River (CD) rats, 6 weeks of age, were given i.p. injections of 30 or 60 mg/kg bw procarbazine hydrochloride dissolved in physiological saline 3 times weekly for 6 months. Animals that survived over 100 days were observed for up to 12 further months, at which time they were killed. A control group of 179 males and 181 females had an overall survival time of over 18 months. The survival times of the treated animals were reported as percentages of that of the controls [no precise definition of the mode of calculation was given]. In treated males, breast carcinomas occurred in 18/47, lymphomas in 11/47 and leukaemias in 14/47; in control males, breast carcinomas were found in 2/179, lymphomas in 0/179 and leukaemias in 2/179. Of treated females, 20/37 developed breast carcinomas, 4/37 lymphomas and 13/37 leukaemias; the incidences of these tumours in control females were 13/181 breast carcinomas, 1/181 lymphoma and 0/181 leukaemia. The incidences of all these tumour types were considered to be significantly increased in the treated animals ($P < 0.001$ for all tumours except lymphomas in females, $P = 0.003$) (Weisburger et al., 1975; Weisburger, 1977). [The Working Group considered that the inadequate reporting of certain items, such as survival times, the amalgamation of various experimental groups and tumour types, as well as the lack of age-adjustment in the analyses precluded a complete evaluation of this study.]

Groups of 35-day-old male and 42-day-old female Sprague-Dawley rats were given i.p. injections of 15 or 30 mg/kg bw procarbazine hydrochloride in buffered saline 3 times a week for 26 weeks. The low-dose groups comprised 34 males and 36 females, and the high-dose groups comprised 35 animals of each sex. Untreated and vehicle control groups of 10 males and 10 females were maintained for 86 weeks, the duration of the study. The median surivival times were 31 weeks for low-dose males and females, 26 weeks for high-dose males, and 22 weeks for high-dose females. Of the vehicle controls, 80% of males and 89% of females survived to the end of the study. The early mortality among treated animals was due to the occurrence of neoplasms; the incidences in low-dose groups were 19/30 in males and 27/30 in females, and those in the high-dose groups were 30/33 in males and 30/31 in females. Neoplasms seen most frequently were of the neuroepithelial tissues, mammary gland, lymphoreticular tissue and haematopoietic system. Lymphomas occurred in 1/10 male vehicle controls, in 2/31 low-dose males and 9/33 high-dose males, and in 20/31 high-dose females. Leukaemia was found exclusively in 3/33 high-dose males. No adenocarcinoma of the mammary gland occurred in controls; but these tumours occurred in 1/31 low-dose and 7/33 high-dose males and 16/31 low-dose and 25/31 high-dose females. Among males, olfactory neuroblastomas occurred in 12/27 low-dose animals and in 9/33 given the high dose, but in none of the controls. Tumours of the nervous system in males included 1 sarcoma in the low-dose group and 1 oligodendroglioma in the high-dose group; 1 untreated male had an astrocytoma. Among the females, olfactory neuroblastomas occurred in 17/28 low-dose animals and in 2/31 at the high dose, but in none of the controls. The incidences of malignant lymphomas, adenocarcinomas of the mammary gland and olfactory adenocarcinomas or neuroepitheliomas in treated animals were statistically significantly greater than those in pooled male controls and in all female controls (National Cancer Institute, 1979).

(c) Intravenous administration

Rat: A group of 48 male BR46 rats, 100 days old, were given i.v. injections of 24 mg/kg bw of a commercial preparation of procarbazine hydrochloride once weekly for 52 weeks. A control group of 89 rats was maintained. Of the exposed group, 34 (71%) were alive at the appearance of the first tumour; in the control group, 65 (73%) survived to this point. In the exposed group, 1/34 and 14/34 died with benign and malignant neoplasms, respectively. The malignant tumours comprised 3 renal sarcomas and 1 adenocarcinoma, 1 carcinoma of the testis, 1 rectal carcinoma, 2 intra-abdominal spindle-cell sarcomas, 1 squamous-cell carcinoma of the ear duct, 1 neurilemmoma and 1 subaxillary sarcoma. The benign tumours were a prostatic adenoma and subcutaneous fibromas. Three rats had multiple tumours. The average induction time was 14 ± 6 months. Of the control group, 3/65 and 4/65 died with benign and malignant tumours, respectively. The malignancies were 3 mammary sarcomas and 1 pheochromocytoma, and the benign tumours were 2 thymomas and 1 mammary fibroma. The average latent period was 23 ± 5 months (Schmähl & Osswald, 1970).

(d) Perinatal exposure

Rat: Four pregnant BD-IX rats were given i.v. injections of 125 mg/kg bw procarbazine hydrochloride on the 22nd day of pregnancy. Of 26 offspring, 11 died of toxic effects; of the remaining 15, 3 died of pneumonia at 187 - 414 days of age and showed no tumour development. The remaining 12 offspring all developed tumours within a median induction time of 315 days; the tumours included 11 malignant neurinomas, 2 ependymomas, 2 renal adenosarcomas, an ovarian carcinoma and 1 oligodendroglioma of the brain. No controls were mentioned (Ivankovic, 1972).

(e) Multiple routes of exposure

Rat: Groups [size unspecified] of male and female Osborne-Mendel rats were given i.p. injections of 100 mg/kg bw procarbazine hydrochloride as newborns, then 50 mg/kg bw intraperitoneally once a week for the next 4 weeks, followed by 250 mg/kg bw orally once a week for the next 3 weeks, for a total dose of 40 mg/animal. No mammary tumours were found among 5 males and females killed at 5 - 11 weeks; at 12 - 16 weeks, 2/2 males and 10/10 females killed had mammary tumours; at 17 weeks, 2/2 killed males had mammary tumours, and 7 males that were still alive showed no evidence of mammary neoplasms (Kelly *et al.*,1964). [The Working Group noted the absence of information on matched controls, group size and survival.]

A group [size unspecified] of male and female random-bred Osborne-Mendel rats were given an i.p. injection of 100 mg/kg bw procarbazine hydrochloride at birth, followed by 50 mg/kg bw each week for the next 4 weeks and then 250 mg/kg bw orally each week for the next 3 weeks. Rats that lived more than 11 weeks after the initial injection were evaluated for mammary tumour development: 8/13 males developed mammary adenocarcinomas within a mean latent period of 27 weeks, and 10/11 females developed mammary adeno-carcinomas within a mean latent period of 15 weeks. Of the males, 5/13 also had kidney tumours (4 sarcomas, 1 haemangioendothelioma), 3/13 had tumours described as pulmonary septal-cell tumours, 5/13 had splenic angiosarcomas (3 haemangioendotheliomas, 2 haemangiomas), 2/13 had jejunal tumours (1 adenoma, 1 adenocarcinoma), and individual animals had tumours in the liver, duodenum, bone marrow, oral submucosa and subcutaneous tissue. Of the females, 2/11 also had tumours described as pulmonary septal-cell tumours and 1 had a uterine tumour (Kelly et al., 1968). [The Working Group noted the absence of information on matched controls, group size and survival.]

Monkey: A 17-month-old and a 5½-year-old female rhesus monkey developed leukaemia following s.c. and oral administrations of procarbazine hydrochloride. The first had received weekly s.c. injections from birth of 50 mg/kg bw (total, 2.4 g) or oral doses of 10 mg/kg bw (total, 0.29 g). The second had received weekly s.c. injections of 10 - 50 mg/kg bw for the first 35 months of life (5. 2 g) and then oral doses of 10 mg/kg bw (31.1 g) 5 times weekly thereafter. Both animals developed myelogenous leukaemia, which because of its rarity in monkeys was concluded to have been induced by the treatment (O'Gara et al., 1971). [Although this study involved only 2 animals and no controls, the Working Group considered that these results should be included because of the rarity of reports of such studies in nonhuman primates.]

Fifty-five male and female monkeys, including rhesus, cynomolgus and African green monkeys, were given procarbazine hydrochloride by s.c., i.p., i.v. and oral routes. Of 42 animals that were autopsied, 11 (26%) had malignant tumours, whereas only 2/66 (3.1%) untreated or vehicle-exposed controls did so. Of the 11 monkeys with malignancy, 4 were rhesus (3 females, 1 male) and 2 were cynomolgus (1 female, 1 male), whose primary exposure was s.c.; and 2 were rhesus (1 female, 1 male) and 2 cynomolgus (both male), whose primary exposure was i.p. Four rhesus monkeys developed acute myelogenous leukaemia, 1 a renal haemangioendothelial sarcoma and 1 an osteosarcoma. Three cynomolgus had leukaemia or lymphoma, 1 had an osteosarcoma, and the other had multi-ple haemangiosarcomas. The rarity of neoplasms, and in particular leukaemias (none in control monkeys in that colony), strongly suggests that procarbazine induced the tumours (Sieber et al., 1978). [The Working Group noted the absence of information regarding the ancestry and environment of the animals and on controls and survival. The Working Group considered that these results should be included despite these limitations, since few reports of studies in nonhuman primates are available].

3.2 Other relevant biological data

(a) Experimental systems

The antitumour activity, pharmacology, metabolism and mode of action of procarbazine and its hydrochloride have been reviewed (Sartorelli & Creasey, 1969; Reed, 1975).

Toxic effects

The oral LD_{50} of procarbazine hydrochloride was 1320 mg/kg bw in mice, 145 mg/kg bw in rabbits (Reed, 1975), 270 mg/kg bw in newborn rats and 785 mg/kg bw in 40 - 60-day-old rats (Goldenthal, 1971).

In monkeys, single i.v. doses of 400 mg/kg bw were lethal; but 2 animals given 300 mg/kg bw survived. Daily i.v. doses of 28 mg/kg bw administered for 13 days were lethal to 2 monkeys; daily i.v. doses of 16 mg/kg bw given for 28 days or 56 mg/kg bw given twice weekly for 4 weeks were tolerated by 4 animals. The main toxic signs were anaemia and marked decreases in platelet and white blood cell counts. Blood urea nitrogen and biochemical parameters of liver function remained within the normal range (Oliverio et al., 1964).

Effects on reproduction and prenatal toxicity

A group of 252 Wistar (CF) rats were given single i.p. injections of 5 - 550 mg/kg bw procarbazine hydrochloride on the 5th to 17th day of pregnancy, and the fetuses were evaluated on the 21st day of gestation. No maternal toxicity was observed with doses up to 400 mg/kg bw; but 12.5% of the females died when 500 mg/kg bw were injected on the 14th day, and 50% when this dose was given on the 17th day of pregnancy; none of the females survived when 550 mg/kg bw were given on the 14th or 17th day of pregnancy. One hundred percent embryomortality was observed after a single injection of 100 mg/kg bw on day 5 - 8 of pregnancy and with 75, 175, 200, 400, 530 or > 500 mg/kg bw given on day 9, 10, 11, 12, 14 or 17 of pregnancy, respectively. Doses of 25 - 75 mg/kg bw were teratogenic when given as a single dose on day 5, 6 or 9 - 12 of pregnancy, and doses of 100 mg/kg bw were active when given on day 10, 11, 12, 14 or 17. The abnormalities observed included tail and limb defects, cleft palate, exencephaly, encephalocele, omphalocele and short maxilla or mandible (Chaube & Murphy, 1969).

It was reported in an abstract that procarbazine was teratogenic in Sprague-Dawley rats but not clearly so in rabbits when given for 4 or 10 days during the period of organogenesis (Thompson et al., 1978).

Absorption, distribution, excretion and metabolism

The half-life of procarbazine in the plasma of dogs and rats was 12 and 24 min, respectively. As the concentration of procarbazine in plasma fell, the concentration of an azo compound derived from the drug increased   (See Fig. 1.) (Raaflaub & Schwartz, 1965; Reed, 1975).

Within 30 min after i.v. injection of 100 mg/kg bw procarbazine hydrochloride to dogs, the level in the plasma and the cerebrospinal fluid equilibrated. In rodents and in dogs, the main urinary metabolite is *N*-isopropyl terephthalamic acid (Oliverio *et al.*, 1964).

In rats given i.p. injections of 20 or 200 mg/kg bw procarbazine hydrochloride labelled with either ^{14}C or ^{3}H at the methyl group, 7 - 10% of the dose was exhaled as methane and 11 - 22% as CO_2 within 8 hours. Since similar proportions were found after administration of methylhydrazine, it was suggested that the metabolism of procarbazine proceeds *via* formation of methylhydrazine (Dost & Reed, 1967).

Procarbazine has also been shown to be demethylated by rat hepatic microsomal enzymes. The rate of demethylation may be increased up to 3-fold by pretreatment of rodents with enzyme inducers; either procarbazine itself or its metabolite monomethyl-hydrazine may be demethylated (Baggiolini & Bickel, 1966). The formation of the azo and azoxy compounds has been demonstrated *in vivo*. *N*-Isopropyl-*para*-toluamide and methane were also found as metabolites (Weinkam & Shiba, 1978). Procarbazine and the azo compound exhibited similar cytotoxic activity against the L1210 ascites leukaemia *in vivo*, whereas a mixture of the azoxy isomers was substantially more effective (Shiba *et al.*, 1979).

Mutagenicity and other short-term tests

The genetic toxicology of procarbazine hydrochloride has been reviewed (Lee & Dixon, 1978).

Procarbazine was toxic but did not induce reverse mutations in *Salmonella typhimurium* strains TA1535, TA1537, TA98 and TA100 in the presence or absence of mouse or rat liver activation systems (Heddle & Bruce, 1977a; Painter & Howard, 1978; Bronzetti *et al.*, 1979). However, in a forward mutation assay with *S. typhimurium* (to L-arabinose-resistance), the drug induced mutants without metabolic activation (Pueyo, 1979). Procarbazine was active in inducing mitotic crossover, gene conversions and reverse mutations in *Saccharomyces cerevisiae* strain D7 without addition of an exogenous metabolic activation system (Bronzetti *et al.*, 1979).

Fig. 1. Possible metabolic pathways of procarbazine[a]; postulated intermediates are given in square brackets

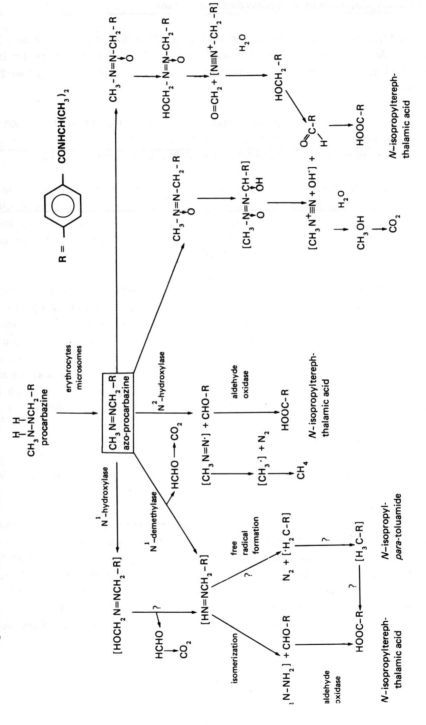

[a]From Reed (1975) and Weinkam & Shiba (1978)

The compound was highly mutagenic in *Drosophila melanogaster*, inducing recessive lethal mutations (in all stages of spermatogenesis), total sex-chromosome loss and dominant lethality, without inducing any breakage events (Blijleven & Vogel, 1977).

In mouse lymphoma cells L5178Y, the drug induced dose-related mutations after metabolic activation by a rat liver microsomal preparation (Clive *et al.*, 1979).

The genetic effects of procarbazine have been studied in a number of assays in mice *in vivo*. It has been found to induce sperm abnormalities (Heddle & Bruce, 1977a,b); micro-nuclei in bone-marrow cells (Heddle & Bruce, 1977a,b; Wild, 1978; Cole *et al.*, 1979); micronuclei in fetal liver and blood cells after transplacental treatment (Cole *et al.*, 1979); increased sister chromatid exchange in bone-marrow cells (Renault *et al.*, 1978); dominant lethal mutations in spermatids, spermatocytes and spermatogonia (Epstein *et al.*, 1972; Ehling, 1976, 1977; Roberts *et al.*, 1979); and specific-locus mutations (Ehling & Neuhäuser, 1979). Specific-locus mutations were also induced in rats *in vivo* (Maier & Zbinden, 1980).

In rabbits administered the drug intravenously, unscheduled DNA synthesis (indicating DNA damage) was induced in spermatids and spermatocytes (Bürgin *et al.*, 1979). An increase in sister chromatid exchanges was also produced in bone-marrow cells of Chinese hamsters following i.p. administration (Bayer, 1978).

(b) Humans

Toxic effects

Procarbazine causes dose-related, reversible depression of peripheral leucocyte and plate-let counts, with a low 2 - 3 weeks after the start of daily oral doses of 250 - 300 mg. Nausea and vomiting are seen in 50 - 70% of patients. Neurological complications are common but minor after oral administration of procarbazine and consist of somnolence, lethargy, hallu-cinations, confusion and agitation; after i.v. injection, these may be aggravated, and cere-bellar ataxia has been reported (DeVita *et al.*, 1966). Peripheral neuropathy is occasional, usually comprising paresthesiae, myalgia and decrease of deep tendon reflexes; all are reversible, sometimes without cessation of the drug (Wade, 1977). Central nervous symptoms are a hazard of concomitant phenothiazine therapy (don Poster, 1979), and optic neuro-retinitis has been reported in one patient treated with BCNU and procarbazine (Lennan & Taylor, 1978). Alcohol may not be tolerated due to a disulfiram-like reaction, *viz* flushing of head and neck, palpitations, sweating, hypotension and dyspnoea. As procarbazine hydro-chloride is a mild monoamine oxidase inhibitor, high doses can lead to hypotension; but it may also accentuate the sympathomimetic effects of drugs like the tricyclic antidepressants and of tyramine-containing foods.

Allergic skin reactions were seen in 4/44 patients with Hodgkin's disease and 8/23 with non-Hodgkin's lymphoma treated repeatedly with procarbazine (Andersen & Videbaek, 1980). Pulmonary eosinophilia resulting from such treatment may be mistaken radiologically for malignant lymphangitis (Jones et al., 1972; Ecker et al., 1978). A single case has been reported of acute myelofibrosis following treatment of Peyronie's disease with procarbazine (Pinedo et al., 1974).

Effects on reproduction and prenatal toxicity

Only case reports are available on prenatal exposure to procarbazine hydrochloride. Most mothers had received combination therapy.

Bilateral absence of the fifth toe and syndactyly of the third and fourth toes on the right foot with absence of the fourth and fifth metatarsi were observed in an infant who had been exposed to nitrogen mustard, vinblastine sulphate and procarbazine during the first trimester of gestation (Garrett, 1974).

A pregnant woman was treated during the first trimester with 4 mg nitrogen mustard and 100 mg vincristine sulphate as single i.v. injections; 100 mg/day procarbazine and 60 mg/day prednisone were then given orally for the next 7 days. Following abortion at 3 months, both kidneys of the fetus were located in the pelvic inlet at the level of the bifurcation of the aorta (Mennuti et al., 1975).

Verrucous and other haemangiomas were observed in an infant whose mother received 150 mg/m^2 procarbazine during the first 38 days of pregnancy. In addition, several doses of 50 - 150 mg/m^2 had been taken prior to the estimated time of conception (Wells et al., 1968).

An infant whose mother took 50 mg/day procarbazine for 30 days from the 12th week of gestation had no recognizable birth defects (Daw, 1970).

Absorption, distribution, excretion and metabolism

Procarbazine hydrochloride is given by mouth, since it is absorbed almost completely from the gut. The half-life of disappearance from the plasma is 7 min (Raaflaub & Schwartz, 1965), due to oxidative metabolism to azo derivatives and hydrogen peroxide (Oliverio, 1973). Using ^{14}C-radiolabelled drug, 70% was shown to appear in urine within 24 hours - less than 5% as the unchanged parent compound and the remainder predominantly as N-isopropyl terephthalaminic acid. Between 10 and 20% of the methyl moiety can be traced to methane and expired CO_2. Faecal excretion is negligible (Bollag, 1965; Schwartz et al., 1967).

The drug and its metabolites equilibrate with cerebrospinal fluid within a short time after i.v. injection, which may account for some of its central nervous toxicity.

Mutagenicity and chromosomal effects

Chromosomal aberrations were observed in bone-marrow and lymph node cells in all of 16 patients who received procarbazine (100 mg/m^2 per day) for the treatment of Hodgkin's disease. No untreated patients were included in this study (Neistadt *et al.*, 1978).

3.3 Case reports and epidemiological studies of carcinogenicity in humans

At least 35 cases of acute nonlymphocytic leukaemia have been reported in patients with Hodgkin's disease treated with procarbazine. All of them also received other cytotoxic drugs and/or radiation (Schaefer & Kanzler, 1972; Wakem & Bennett, 1972; Castro *et al.*, 1973; Veenhof *et al.*, 1973; Kardinal *et al.*, 1974; Mauri & Quaglino, 1974; Sahakian *et al.*, 1974; Armenta *et al.*, 1975; Canellos, 1975; Canellos *et al.*, 1975; Connolly, 1975; Parmley *et al.*, 1976; Rosenberg & Kaplan, 1975; Rosner & Grünwald, 1975; Cadman *et al.*, 1977; Casciato & Scott, 1979; Wolf *et al.*, 1979). Four patients with Hodgkin's disease treated with multiple drug regimens which included procarbazine were reported to have developed solid tumours subsequently: 1 squamous-cell carcinoma of the skin (Poleksic & Yeung, 1978); 1 oat-cell carcinoma of the lung (Cehreli *et al.*, 1979); 1 lung cancer and a renal adenocarcinoma *in situ*; and 1 with multiple squamous-cell carcinomas of the cervix, perineum and vagina (O'Sullivan *et al.*, 1979).

Several authors have described the occurrence of acute nonlymphocytic leukaemia in cohorts of patients with Hodgkin's disease treated with various combinations of multiple chemotherapy and radiation (Ayoub *et al.*, 1978; Auclerc *et al.*, 1979; Papa *et al.*, 1979). The treatment regimens typically included procarbazine, vincristine and/or vinblastine and nitrogen mustard. However, these cohorts were not described in detail, and the relative risk of acute leukaemia in treated patients was not quantified. Taken together, the reports present data on approximately 2400 patients with Hodgkin's disease, in whom 21 cases of acute nonlymphocytic leukaemia were subsequently diagnosed. Seventeen of these leukaemia cases occurred in patients who had received both combination chemotherapy and radiation. The occurrence of solid tumours was not systematically documented.

A cohort of 452 patients with Hodgkin's disease treated at the US National Cancer Institute has been studied with reference to subsequent neoplasms (Arseneau *et al.*, 1972, 1977; Canellos *et al.*, 1974, 1975). The primary chemotherapeutic regimens employed were incompletely described but consisted primarily of procarbazine, vincristine, prednisone plus nitrogen mustard (MOPP) or cyclophosphamide (COPP). [An apparent initial excess of solid tumours, particularly in patients receiving both radiation and chemotherapy, may have been due to the inappropriate inclusion of non-melanoma skin cancers among their observations, when such tumours were not included in the cancer incidence rates used to calculate the expected values.] With additional follow-up, 3 cases of acute nonlymphocytic leukaemia developed among the 65 patients treated with both combination chemotherapy (which included procarbazine) and intensive radiation. This was described as a significant excess, although no expected number was given. The latent periods for development of leukaemia in these 3 patients were 12, 48 and 84 months.

A series of 1028 patients with Hodgkin's disease was reported from the Sloan-Kettering Cancer Center, New York (Brody *et al.*, 1977); in this cohort a significant excess of all cancers was noted among patients receiving various incompletely described regimens including combination chemotherapy (primarily procarbazine, vincristine , prednisone and nitrogen mustard - MOPP) and among patients treated with single-agent chemotherapy. Risk estimates were not provided for specific cancer types, but at least 3 cases of acute non-lymphocytic leukaemia occurred.

At Stanford Univeristy, California, 680 patients with Hodgkin's disease were followed up for at least one year, for a median period of 5 years. Of these, 320 received radiation alone, 30 chemotherapy alone and 330 radiation plus chemotherapy. Chemotherapy consisted of nitrogen mustard, vincristine , prednisone and procarbazine (MOPP). Eight cases of acute nonlymphocytic leukaemia occurred among those treated with chemotherapy plus radiation, whereas none occurred in either of the other two groups. Although no expected number was calculated, the actuarial risk at 7 years was estimated to be 3.9 ± 1.5% (Coleman *et al.*, 1977). An excess risk of non-Hodgkin's lymphoma was also observed among 579 patients with Hodgkin's disease at the same centre, all 5 cases occurring in those 344 patients treated with both radiation and combination chemotherapy. The 10-year actuarial risk was estimated to be 15.2% (Krikorian *et al.*, 1979). The median latent period for development of leukaemia was 52 months, and that for non-Hodgkin's lymphoma was 94 months.

In Denmark, three cases of acute nonlymphocytic leukaemia were observed in a series of 201 consecutive patients with Hodgkin's disease, compared with 0.04 cases expected (Larsen & Brincker, 1977). One patient received radiation and chemotherapy without pro-carbazine, and the other two received both radiation and combination chemotherapy including procarbazine, vincristine, prednisone and nitrogen mustard (MOPP). The latent period ranged from 2 - 8 years. No risk estimate for specific therapeutic subgroups was provided.

Among 232 patients with Hodgkin's disease treated in Manitoba, Canada (Neufeld *et al.*, 1978), 2 cases of acute nonlymphocytic leukaemia developed, while 0.05 were expected. Both patients had received combination drug regimens which included procarbazine and vincristine, with radiation. The latent periods were 37 and 48 months. No risk estimate for specific therapeutic subgroups was provided.

Among 643 patients with Hodgkin's disease (Toland & Coltman, 1975; Toland et al., 1978) treated under the auspices of the Southwest Oncology Group in the US, 11 cases of acute nonlymphocytic leukaemia were reported, compared with 0.04 cases expected. The excess was greatest in patients treated with both radiation and combination chemotherapy (procarbazine, vincristine , prednisone and nitrogen mustard [MOPP] with or without bleomycin), among whom 8 cases of acute nonlymphocytic leukaemia were observed compared with 0.02 cases expected. A smaller excess was noted among patients treated with chemotherapy alone (3 observed, 0.012 expected). No leukaemia was observed among 205 patients who received radiation only.

Pajak et al. (1979) reported in an abstract 9 cases of acute nonlymphocytic leukaemia among 802 patients with Hodgkin's disease who were in complete remission following treatment regimens consisting of procarbazine, vincristine, prednisone and nitrogen mustard (MOPP) or procarbazine, prednisone, vincristine and BCNU (BOP). All patients were subsequently given maintenance therapy with chlorambucil (with or without vincristine and prednisone), and many also received radiation therapy. The median latent period for developing leukaemia was 53 months.

In a series of 764 patients with Hodgkin's disease from Milan (Valagussa et al., 1980), 9 cases of acute nonlymphocytic leukaemia were noted (expected numbers were not calculated). Three combined chemotherapy regimens were employed: procarbazine, vincristine, prednisone and nitrogen mustard (MOPP); vincristine, nitrogen mustard, adriamycin, bleomycin and prednisone (MABOP); and vinblastine, adriamycin, bleomycin and dacarbazine (ABVD). Many patients received radiation therapy as well. Six cases of acute nonlymphocytic leukaemia developed in 350 patients who had received a drug regimen containing both procarbazine and vincristine (plus radiation therapy); two developed in 87 patients who had received a drug regimen containing vincristine (plus radiation therapy), and one developed in 36 patients who had received a drug regimen containing vincristine (without radiation therapy). The frequency of leukaemia was greatest among the 147 patients treated with MOPP plus radiation, among whom 5 cases resulted in an actuarial 5-year risk of leukaemia of 5.4%. The median latent period for developing the leukaemia was 34 months. Patients in this study also developed 15 solid tumours (5 of which arose in an irradiated field), for which the 10-year actuarial risk was 7.3%. No specific chemotherapeutic regimen was implicated in these cases, and no risk estimate was presented for specific tumour types.

A cohort study specifically designed to evaluate the carcinogenicity of treatment for Hodgkin's disease was undertaken in 1553 patients diagnosed between 1940-1975 in Montreal and Boston (Boivin, 1981). Patients were classified as having received intensive chemotherapy, no intensive chemotherapy, intensive radiation or no intensive radiation therapy. No specific data were provided on the drugs used, although the 'intensive' chemotherapeutic regimen generally comprised procarbazine/vincristine, prednisone and nitrogen mustard (MOPP). Procarbazine was used in 32% of patients. Six cases of acute nonlympho-cytic leukaemia (0.36 expected) and 21 other cancers (14.0 expected) were reported. In the subgroup treated with both intensive chemotherapy and intensive radiation (87 patients, 193 person-years of observation), 2 cases of this leukaemia were noted, compared with 0.007 cases expected. All 6 cases had been exposed to both procarbazine and nitrogen mustard. The relative risks for cancers other than leukaemia were not significantly elevated with any treatment category.

The occurrence of second malignancies was evaluated in a series of 438 patients with non-Hodgkin's lymphoma from the State University of New York at Stony Brook (Zarabbi, 1980). Three cases of acute nonlymphocytic leukaemia were observed, compared with 0.3 cases expected. All 3 patients had received both radiation and a combination chemotherapy regimen containing procarbazine and vincristine . Sixteen solid cancers were diagnosed, compared with 15.0 expected; no significant excess of any specific non-haematological malignancy was noted. The excess of leukaemia was not attributed to a specific therapeutic modality.

[The multiple agents, the inadequate description of methods of computation and the different formats of data presentation all preclude comparisons between studies and accurate calculation of the magnitude of risk.

[Nonetheless, the increase in risk of acute nonlymphocytic leukaemia has consistently been very large and cannot be explained by the above factors. This risk has been shown to increase over time in the same institutions (coincident with the introduction and increased use of multiple cytotoxic agents), independent of the effects of age, sex, stage of disease and interval since diagnosis (Brody et al., 1977; Boivin, 1981). The latent period for these leukaemias was consistently 3 - 5 years. Internal comparisons are consistent in implicating the combination of intensive chemotherapy and intensive radiation, and, while solid tumours have tended to occur following radiation, the remaining cases of acute nonlymphocytic leukaemia have tended to occur after intensive chemotherapy alone.

[These studies do not permit distinctions to be made between alkylating agents, vin-cristine and procarbazine as potential causes of acute nonlymphocytic leukaemia.

[An excess of non-Hodgkin's lymphoma after combined chemotherapy for Hodgkin's disease has so far been reported from only one centre. Other centres have sufficient follow-up, and the chemotherapy regimen is a standard one.]

4. SUMMARY OF DATA REPORTED AND EVALUATION

4.1 Experimental data

Procarbazine hydrochloride is carcinogenic in mice and rats after its intraperitoneal administration, producing malignant tumours of the nervous system, haematopoietic system and possibly other organs in both species, and tumours of the mammary gland in rats only. Evidence of carcinogenicity was also found in mice and rats following its oral administration, in rats following its intravenous administration, and in one instance following transplacental exposure. Two studies in two species of nonhuman primates suggest that procarbazine hydrochloride may also produce myelogenous leukaemia when administered by multiple routes in the same animal.

Procarbazine hydrochloride can induce teratogenic effects in rats and embryolethality at doses nontoxic to the mother. This compound is mutagenic in bacteria, yeast, cultured mammalian cells and *Drosophila melanogaster,* and in mice and rats *in vivo*.

4.2 Human data

Procarbazine hydrochloride is used primarily in the treatment of Hodgkin's disease, non-Hodgkin's lymphoma and lung cancer, in combination with other drugs.

The available data are insufficient to evaluate the teratogenicity, mutagenicity or chromosomal effects of procarbazine hydrochloride in humans.

Both case reports and epidemiological studies indicate that acute nonlymphocytic leukaemia is produced in patients with Hodgkin's disease treated with combined therapeutic regimens which include vinca alkaloids, alkylating agents and procarbazine hydrochloride, often in conjunction with radiotherapy. No data were available to the Working Group which permit the assessment of the separate effects of procarbazine hydrochloride.

4.3 Evaluation

There is *sufficient evidence*[1] for the carcinogenicity of procarbazine hydrochloride in mice and rats. There is *limited evidence*[1] of its carcinogenicity in monkeys. There is *sufficient evidence*[2] for the carcinogenicity in humans of intensive chemotherapeutic regimens that include alkylating agents, vinca alkaloids, procarbazine hydrochloride and prednisone. There is inadequate evidence of the carcinogenicity of procarbazine hydrochloride alone in humans.

---

[1]See preamble, p. 18-19.

[2]See preamble, p. 17.

On the basis of the combined experimental and human evidence, this compound should be considered for practical purposes as if it presented a carcinogenic risk to humans.

5. REFERENCES

Andersen, E. & Videbaek, A. (1980) Procarbazine-induced skin reactions in Hodgkin's disease and other malignant lymphomas. *Scand. J. Haematol., 24,* 149-151

Armenta, D., Pretty, H.M., Long, L.A., Neemeh, J.A. & Gosselin, G. (1975) Hodgkin's disease developing into leukaemia. Presentation of 2 cases. (Fr.). *Union méd. Can., 104,* 744-748

Arseneau, J.C., Sponzo, R.W., Levin, D.L., Schnipper, L.E., Bonner, H., Young, R.C., Canellos, G.P., Johnson, R.E. & DeVita, V.T. (1972) Nonlymphomatous malignant tumors complicating Hodgkin's disease. Possible association with intensive therapy. *New Engl. J. Med., 287,* 1119-1122

Arseneau, J.C., Canellos, G.P., Johnson, R.C. & DeVita, V.T. (1977) Risk of new cancers in patients with Hodgkin's disease. *Cancer, 40,* 1912-1916

Auclerc, G., Jacquillat, C., Auclerc, M.F., Weil, M. & Bernard, J. (1979) Post-therapeutic acute leukemia. *Cancer, 44,* 2017-2025

Ayoub, J.I.G., Dubois, A., Cosendal, A.-M., Teitreault, L. & Pretty, H. (1978) Pre- and post-treatment second malignant neoplasms (SMN) in Hodgkin's disease (HD) (Abstract no. C-61). *Proc. Am. Assoc. Cancer Res., 19,* 322

Baggiolini, M. & Bickel, M.H. (1966) Demethylation of ibenzemthyzin (Natulan®), monomethylhydrazine and methylamine by the rat *in vivo* and by the isolated perfused rat liver. *Life Sci., 5,* 795-802

Baker, C.E., Jr, ed. (1980) *Physicians' Desk Reference,* 34th ed., Oradell, NJ, Medical Economics Co., pp. 1468-1469

Bayer, U. (1978) The *in vivo* induction of sister chromatid exchanges in the bone marrow of the Chinese hamster. II. *N*-Nitrosodiethylamine (DEN) and *N*-isopropyl-α-(2-methylhydrazine)-*p*-toluamide (Natulan), two carcinogenic compounds with specific mutagenicity problems. *Mutat. Res., 56,* 305-309

Blijleven, W.G.H. & Vogel, E. (1977) The mutational spectrum of procarbazine in *Drosophila melanogaster. Mutat. Res., 45,* 47-59

Boivin, J.-F. (1981) *Late Side Effects of Treatment for Hodgkin's Disease.* Thesis, Boston, MA, Harvard School of Public Health, pp. 34-79

Bollag, W. (1965) *Experimental studies with a methyl-hydrazine derivative, ibenzymethyzin.* In: Jellife, A.M. & Marks, J., eds, *Natulan,* Bristol, Wright

Brody, R.S., Schottenfeld, D. & Reid, A. (1977) Multiple primary cancer risk after therapy for Hodgkin's disease. *Cancer, 40,* 1917-1926

Bronzetti, G., Zeiger, E. & Malling, H.V. (1979) Genetic toxicity of procarbazine in bacteria and yeast. *Mutat. Res., 68,* 51-58

Bürgin, H., Schmid, B. & Zbinden, G. (1979) Assessment of DNA damage in germ cells of male rabbits treated with isoniazid and procarbazine. *Toxicology, 12,* 251-257

Cadman, E.C., Capizzi, R.L. & Bertino, J.R. (1977) Acute nonlymphocytic leukemia. A delayed complication of Hodgkin's disease therapy: analysis of 109 cases. *Cancer, 40,* 1280-1296

Canellos, G.P. (1975) Second malignancies complicating Hodgkin's disease in remission. *Lancet, i,* 1294

Canellos, G.P., DeVita, V.T., Arseneau, J.C. & Johnson, R.C. (1974) Carcinogenesis by cancer chemotherapeutic agents: second malignancies complicating Hodgkin's disease in remission. *Recent Results Cancer Res., 49,* 108-114

Canellos, G.P., DeVita, V.T., Arseneau, J.C, Whang-Peng, J. & Johnson, R.E. (1975) Second malignancies complicating Hodgkin's disease in remission. *Lancet, i,* 947-949

Casciato, D.A. & Scott, J.L. (1979) Acute leukemia following prolonged cytotoxic agent therapy. *Medicine, 58,* 32-47

Castro, G.A.M., Church, A., Pechet, L. & Snyder, L.M. (1973) Leukemia after chemotherapy of Hodgkin's disease. *New Engl. J. Med., 289,* 103-104

Cehreli, C., Ruacan, S.A., Firat, D. & Kucuksu, N. (1979) Hodgkin's disease terminating in oat cell carcinoma of the lung. *Cancer, 43,* 1507-1512

Chaube, S. & Murphy, M.L. (1969) Fetal malformations produced in rats by *N*-isopropyl-α-(2-methyl-hydrazino)-*p*-toluamide hydrochloride (procarbazine). *Teratology, 2,* 23-32

Clive, D., Johnson, K.O., Spector, J.F.S., Batson, A.G. & Brown, M.M.M. (1979) Validation and characterization of the L5178Y/TK$^{+/-}$ mouse lymphoma mutagen assay system. *Mutat. Res., 59,* 61-108

Cole, R.J., Taylor, N.A., Cole, J. & Arlett, C.F. (1979) Transplacental effects of chemical mutagens detected by the micronucleus test. *Nature, 277,* 317-318

Coleman, C.N., Williams, C.J., Flint, A., Glatstein, E.J., Rosenberg, S.A. & Kaplan, H.S. (1977) Hematologic neoplasia in patients treated for Hodgkin's disease. *New Engl. J. Med., 297,* 1249-1252

Connolly, E. (1975) Hodgkin's disease complicated by acute leukaemia. *J. Ir. med. Assoc., 68,* 6-8

Daw, E.G. (1970) Procarbazine in pregnancy. *Lancet, ii,* 984

Deckers, C., Deckers-Passau, L., Maisin, J., Gauthier, J.M. & Mace, F. (1974) Carcinogenicity of procarbazine. *Z. Krebsforsch., 81,* 79-84

DeVita, V.T., Serpick, A. & Carbone, P.P. (1966) Preliminary clinical studies with ibenzmethyzin. *Clin. Pharmacol. Ther., 7,* 542-546

Dost, F.N. & Reed, D.J. (1967) Methane formation *in vivo* from *N*-isopropyl-α-(2-methylhydrazine)-*p*-toluamide hydrochloride, a tumor-inhibiting methylhydrazine derivative. *Biochem. Pharmacol., 16,* 1741-1746

Ecker, M.D., Jay, B. & Keohane, M.F. (1978) Procarbazine lung. *Am. J. Roentgenol., 131,* 527-528

Ehling, U.H. (1976) Mutagenicity testing and risk estimation with mammals. *Mutat. Res., 41,* 113-122

Ehling, U.H. (1977) Dominant lethal mutations in male mice. *Arch. Toxicol., 38,* 1-11

Ehling, U.H. & Neuhäuser, A. (1979) Procarbazine-induced specific-locus mutations in male mice. *Mutat. Res., 59,* 245-256

Epstein, S.S., Arnold, E., Andrea, J., Bass, W. & Bishop, Y. (1972) Detection of chemical mutagens by the dominant lethal assay in the mouse. *Toxicol. appl. Pharmacol., 23,* 288-325

Garrett, M.J. (1974) Teratogenic effects of combination chemotherapy. *Ann. intern. Med., 80,* 667

Goldenthal, E.I. (1971) A compilation of LD_{50} values in newborn and adult animals. *Toxicol. appl. Pharmacol., 18,* 185-207

Goodman, L.S. & Gilman, A., eds (1975) *The Pharmacological Basis of Therapeutics,* 5th ed., New York, Macmillan, pp. 1382-1383

Harvey, S.C. (1975) *Antineoplastic and immunosuppressive drugs.* In: Osol, A., ed., *Remington's Pharmaceutical Sciences,* 15th ed., Easton, PA, Mack Publishing Co., pp. 1083-1084

Heddle, J.A. & Bruce, W.R. (1977a) *Comparison of tests for mutagenicity or carcinogenicity using assays for sperm abnormalities, formation of micronuclei and mutations in* Salmonella. In: Hiatt, H.H., Watson, J.D. & Winsten, J.A., eds, *Origins of Human Cancer,* Cold Spring Harbor, NY, Cold Spring Harbor Laboratory, pp. 1549-1557

Heddle, J.A. & Bruce, W.R. (1977b) *On the use of multiple assays for mutagenicity, especially the micronucleus,* Salmonella *and sperm abnormality assays.* In: Scott, D., Bridges, B.A. & Sobels, F.H., eds, *Progress in Genetic Toxicology,* Amsterdam, Elsevier/North-Holland Biomedical Press, pp. 265-274

Heuson, J.C. & Heimann, R. (1966) Ibenzmethyzin (Natulan[®]), a highly effective mammary carcinogen in the Huggins system. *Eur. J. Cancer, 2,* 385-386

Ivankovic, S. (1972) Induction of malignancies in rats after transplacental exposure to N-isopropyl-α-2-(methylhydrazino)-p-toluamide·HCl (Ger.). *Arzneimittel-Forsch., 22,* 905-907

Jones, S.E., Moore, M., Blank, N. & Castellino, R.A. (1972) Hypersensitivity to procarbazine (Matulane[®]) manifested by fever and pleuropulmonary reaction. *Cancer, 29,* 498-500

Kardinal, C.G., Barnes, A. & Pugh, R.P. (1974) Acute leukemia: a disease of medical progress? *Missouri Med., 71,* 683-684, 689

Kelly, M.G., O'Gara, R.W., Gadekar, K., Yancey, S.T. & Oliverio, V.T. (1964) Carcinogenic activity of a new antitumor agent, N-isopropyl-α-(2-methylhydrazino)-p-toluamide, hydrochloride (NSC-77213). *Cancer Chemother. Rep., 39,* 77-80

Kelly, M.G., O'Gara, R.W., Yancey, S.T. & Botkin, C. (1968) Induction of tumors in rats with procarbazine hydrochloride. *J. natl Cancer Inst., 40,* 1027-1051

Kelly, M.G., O'Gara, R.W., Yancey, S.T., Gadekar, K., Botkin, C. & Oliverio, V.T. (1969) Comparative carcinogenicity of *N*-isopropyl-α-(2-methylhydrazino)-*p*-toluamide HCl (procarbazine hydrochloride). Its degradation products, other hydrazines, and isonicotinic acid hydrazide. *J. natl Cancer Inst., 42,* 337-344

Krikorian, J.G., Burke, J.S., Rosenberg, S.A. & Kaplan, H.S. (1979) Occurrence of non-Hodgkin's lymphoma after therapy for Hodgkin's disease. *New Engl. J. Med., 300,* 452-458

Larsen, J. & Brincker, H. (1977) The incidence and characteristics of acute myeloid leukaemia arising in Hodgkin's disease. *Scand. J. Haematol., 18,* 197-206

Lee, I.P. & Dixon, R.L. (1978) Mutagenicity, carcinogenicity and teratogenicity of procarbazine. *Mutat. Res., 55,* 1-14

Lennan, R.M. & Taylor, H.R. (1978) Optic neuroretinitis in association with BCNU and procarbazine therapy. *Med. pediatr. Oncol., 4,* 43-48

Maier, P. & Zbinden, G. (1980) Specific locus mutations induced in somatic cells of rats by orally and parenterally administered procarbazine. *Science, 209,* 299-301

Mauri, C. & Quaglino, D. (1974) Hodgkin's disease terminating in acute myeloid leukaemia. *Haematologica (Pavia), 59,* 86-90

Mennuti, M.T., Shepart, T.H. & Mellman, W.J. (1975) Fetal renal malformation following treatment of Hodgkin's disease during pregnancy. *Obstet. Gynecol., 46,* 194-196

National Cancer Institute (1979) Bioassay of procarbazine for possible carcinogenicity. *NCI Carcinog. tech. Rep. Ser., No. 19*

Neistadt, E.L., Gershanovich, M.L., Kolygin, B.A., Ogorodnikova, B.N., Fedoreev, G.A., Chekharina, E.A. & Filov, V.A. (1978) Effect of chemotherapy on the lymph node and bone marrow cell chromosomes in patients with Hodgkin's disease. *Neoplasma, 25,* 91-94

Neufeld, H., Weinerman, B.H. & Kemel, S. (1978) Secondary malignant neoplasms in patients with Hodgkin's disease. *J. Am. med. Assoc., 239,* 2470-2471

O'Gara, R.W., Adamson, R.H., Kelly, M.G. & Dalgard, D.W. (1971) Neoplasms of the hematopoietic system in nonhuman primates: report of one spontaneous tumor and two leukemias induced by procarbazine. *J. natl Cancer Inst., 46,* 1121-1130

Oliverio, V.T. (1973) *Derivatives of triazenes and hydrazines.* In: Holland, J.F. & Frei, E., III, eds, *Cancer Medicine,* Philadelphia, Lea & Febiger, pp. 806-817

Oliverio, V.T., Denham, C., DeVita, V.T. & Kelly, M.G. (1964) Some pharmacologic properties of a new antitumor agent, *N*-isopropyl-α-(2-methylhydrazino)-*p*-toluamide, hydrochloride (NSC-77213). *Cancer Chemother. Rep., 42,* 1-7

Oliveri-Vigh, S., Donahue, J.J., Heveran, J.E. & Senkowski, B.Z. (1971) Coulometric titration of N-iso-propyl-α-(2-methylhydrazino)-p-toluamide hydrochloride. *J. pharm. Sci., 60,* 1851-1853

O'Sullivan, D.D., Raghuprasad, P. & Ezdinli, E.Z. (1979) Solid tumors complicating Hodgkin's disease. A report on two patients with immunoglobulin deficiency. *Arch. intern. Med., 139,* 1131-1134

Painter, R.B. & Howard, R. (1978) A comparison of the HeLa DNA-synthesis inhibition test and the Ames test for screening of mutagenic carcinogens. *Mutat. Res., 54,* 113-115

Pajak, T.F., Nissen, N.I., Stutzman, L., Hoogstraten, B., Cooper, M.R., Glowienka, L.P., Glidewell, O. & Glicksman, A. (1979) Acute myeloid leukemia (AML) occurring during complete remission (CR) in Hodgkin's disease (Abstract no. C-425). *Proc. Am. Soc. clin. Oncol., 20,* 394

Papa, G., Alimena, G., Annino, L., Anselmo, A.P., Ciccone, F., De Luca, A.M., Granati, L., Petti, N. & Mandelli, F. (1979) Acute non lymphoid leukaemia following Hodgkin's disease. Clinical, biological and cytogenetic aspects of 3 cases. *Scand. J. Haematol., 23,* 339-347

Parmley, R.T., Spicer, S.S., Morgan, S.K. & Grush, O.C. (1976) Hodgkin's disease and myelomonocytic leukemia. An ultrastructural and immunochemical study. *Cancer, 38,* 1188-1198

Pinedo, H.M., van Hemel, J.O., Vrede, M.A. & van der Sluys Veer, J. (1974) Acute myelofibrosis and chromosome damage after procarbazine treatment. *Br. med. J., iii,* 525

Poleksic, S. & Yeung, K.-Y. (1978) Rapid development of keratoacanthoma and accelerated transformation into squamous cell carcinoma of the skin. A mutagenic effect of polychemotherapy in a patient with Hodgkin's disease? *Cancer, 41,* 12-16

don Poster, S. (1979) Procarbazine-prochlorperazine interaction: an underreported phenomenon. *J. Med., 9,* 519-524

Pueyo, C. (1979) Natulan induces forward mutations to L-arabinose-resistance in *Salmonella typhimurium. Mutat. Res., 67,* 189-192

Raaflaub, J. & Schwartz, D.E. (1965) Metabolism of a potent cytostatic methylhydrazine derivative (Natu-lan) (Ger.). *Experientia, 21,* 44-45

Reed, D.J., (1975) *Procarbazine.* In: Sartorelli, A.C. & Johns, D.G., eds, *Antineoplastic and Immuno-suppressive Agents,* Part II, New York, Springer, pp. 747-765

Renault, G., Pot-Deprun, J. & Chouroulinkov, I. (1978) Induction of sister chromatid exchanges *in vivo* in bone-marrow cells of AKR mice (Fr.). *C.R. Acad. Sci. Paris, 286,* 887-890

Roberts, G.T., Johnson, F.M., Malling, H.V. & Sharma, R.K. (1979) Action of N-isopropyl-α-(2-methyl-hydrazino)-p-toluamide hydrochloride (procarbazine hydrochloride) in the germ tissue of mice: domi-nant lethal effects. *Arch. Toxicol., 41,* 287-294

Rosner, F. & Grünwald, H. (1975) Hodgkin's disease and acute leukemia. Report of eight cases and review of the literature. *Am. J. Med., 58,* 339-353

Rucki, R.J. (1976) *Procarbazine hydrochloride.* In: Florey, K., ed., *Analytical Profiles of Drug Substances,* Vol. 5, New York, Academic Press, pp. 404-427

Sahakian, G.J., Al-Mondhiny, H., Lacher, M.J. & Connolly, C.E. (1974) Acute leukemia in Hodgkin's disease. *Cancer, 33,* 1369-1375

Sartorelli, A.C. & Creasey, W.A. (1969) Cancer chemotherapy. *Ann. Rev. Pharmacol., 9,* 51-72

Schaefer, U.W. & Kanzler, G. (1972) Leukaemia after Hodgkin's disease. Can it be a consequence of therapy? (Ger.) *Med. klin., 67,* 1024-1028

Schmähl, D. & Osswald, H. (1970) Experimental studies on carcinogenic effects of anticancer chemotherapeutics and immunosuppressives (Ger.). *Arzneimittel-Forsch./Drug Res., 20,* 1461-1467

Schwartz, D.E., Bollag, W. & Obrecht, P. (1967) Distribution and excretion studies of procarbazine in animals and man. *Arzneimittel-Forsch., 17,* 1389-1393

Shiba, D.A., Weinkam, R.J. & Levin, V.A. (1979) Metabolic activation of procarbazine: activity of the intermediates and effects of pretreatment (Abstract no. 562). *Proc. Am. Assoc. Cancer Res., 20,* 139

Sieber, S.M., Correa, P., Dalgard, D.W. & Adamson, R.H. (1978) Carcinogenic and other adverse effects of procarbazine in nonhuman primates. *Cancer Res., 38,* 2125-2134

Thompson, D.J., Molello, J.A. & LeBeau, J.E. (1978) Differential sensitivity of the rat and rabbit to the teratogenic and embryotoxic effects of eleven antineoplastic drugs (Abstract no. 314). *Toxicol. appl. Pharmacol., 45,* 353

Toland, D.M. & Coltman, C.A., Jr (1975) Second malignancies complicating Hodgkin's disease. (Abstract No. 39). *Blood, 46,* 1013

Toland, D.M., Coltman, C.A., Jr & Moon, T.E. (1978) Second malignancies complicating Hodgkin's disease - the Southwest Oncology Group experience. *Cancer clin. Trials, 1,* 27-33

US Pharmacopeial Convention, Inc. (1980) *The US Pharmacopeia,* 20th rev., Rockville, MD, pp. 662-663

Valagussa, P., Santoro, A., Kenda, R., Fossati Bellani, F., Franchi, F., Banfi, A., Rilke, F. & Bonaddona, G. (1980) Second malignancies in Hodgkin's disease: a complication of certain forms of treatment. *Br. med. J., i,* 216-219

Veenhof, C.H.N., van der Meer, J. & Goudsmit, R. (1973) Successfully treated priapism in acute myeloblastic leukemia complicating Hodgkin's disease. *Acta med. scand., 194,* 349-352

Wade, A., ed. (1977) *Martindale, The Extra Pharmacopoeia,* 27th ed., London, The Pharmaceutical Press, pp. 166-167

Wakem, C.J. & Bennett, J.M. (1972) Hodgkin's disease terminating as acute leukaemia: case report and review of the literature. *N.Z. med. J., 76,* 187-194

Weinkam, R.J. & Shiba, D.A. (1978) Metabolic activation of procarbazine. *Life Sci., 22,* 937-946

Weisburger, E.K. (1977) Bioassay program for carcinogenic hazards of cancer chemotherapeutic agents. *Cancer, 40,* 1935-1949

Weisburger, J.H., Griswold, D.P., Prejean, J.D., Casey, A.E., Wood, H.B. & Weisburger, E.K. (1975) The carcinogenic properties of some of the principal drugs used in clinical cancer chemotherapy. *Recent Results Cancer Res., 52,* 1-17

Wells, J.H., Marshall, J.R. & Carbone, P.P (1968) Procarbazine therapy for Hodgkin's disease in early pregnancy. *J. Am. med. Assoc., 205,* 119-121

Wild, D. (1978) Cytogenetic effects in the mouse of 17 chemical mutagens and carcinogens evaluated by the micronucleus test. *Mutat. Res., 56,* 319-327

Wolf, M.M., Cooper, I.A. & Ding, J.C. (1979) Hodgkin's disease terminating in acute leukaemia: report of seven cases. *Aust. N.Z. J. Med., 9,* 398-402

Zarabbi, M.H. (1980) Association of non-Hodgkin's lymphoma (NHL) and second neoplasms. *Semin. Oncol., 7,* 340-351

1. CHEMICAL AND PHYSICAL DATA

1.1 Synonyms and trade names

Chem. Abstr. Services Reg. No.: 299-75-2

Chem. Abstr. Name: 1,2,3,4-Butanetetrol, 1,4-dimethanesulfonate, [S-(R*,R*)]-

IUPAC Systematic Name: L-Threitol 1,4-dimethanesulfonate

Synonyms: 1,4-Bis-O-methanesulphonyl-L-threitol;   dihydroxybusulphan;   1,4-di-O-methanesulfonylbutan-1,2,3,4-tetrole;   1,4-dimethanesulphonate-(L-threitol);   1-threitol-1,4-bis(methanesulphonate);   (2S,3S)-threitol 1,4-bismethanesulphonate;   L-(+)threitol 1,4-dimethanesulphonate;   L-threitol dimethanesulphonate;   treosulfan;   tresulphan

Trade names: NSC-39069; Treosulphan Leo; 40-067

1.2 Structural and molecular formulae and molecular weight

$C_6 H_{14} O_8 S_2$ Mol. wt: 278.3

1.3 Chemical and physical properties of the pure substance

From Wade (1977) or White (1962), unless otherwise specified

(a) *Description:* White, odourless, crystalline powder

(b) *Melting-point:* 102°C

(c) *Optical rotation:* $[\alpha]_D^{20}$ = -5.3° (c = 2, acetone)

(d)   Solubility: Soluble in water (1 in 14), acetone (1 in 8), ethanol (1 in 200) and chloroform (1 in 2000)

(e)   Stability: Sensitive to hydrolysis

(f)   Reactivity: At pH 7.5 and 25°C, it is converted to 1,2:3,4-diepoxybutane (see IARC, 1976) within 3 hours (Matagne, 1967).

2. PRODUCTION, USE, OCCURRENCE AND ANALYSIS

2.1 Production and use

(a)   Production

Synthesis of treosulphan was first reported in 1961 by ring opening of the corresponding stereoisomer of 1,2:3,4-diepoxybutane with methanesulphonic acid (Feit, 1961). It was subsequently produced by treatment of diethyl L-tartrate with acetone to form a diketal, which on reduction with lithium aluminium hydride produced 2,3-*O*-iso-propylideine-L-threitol. Subsequent reaction with methanesulphonyl chloride in pyridine yielded 2,3-*O*-isopropylidene-L-threitol 1,4-bismethanesulphonate, from which treosulphan was obtained by acid-catalysed hydrolysis (Feit, 1964). The method used for commercial production is not known.

Treosulphan is believed to have been produced only by one company in Denmark since 1969 (Sørensen, 1973); no quantitative data were available.

(b)   Use

Treosulphan is used in human medicine, mainly in Denmark, as an antineoplastic agent for the treatment of ovarian cancer. The preferred initial dose, given orally, is 1 - 1.25 g per day for 4 weeks; maintenance doses of 500 mg per day are then used. If radiotherapy is also being given, the initial dose is reduced to 750 mg per day (Wade, 1977).

2.2 Occurrence

Treosulphan is not known to be produced in Nature.

2.3 Analysis

No data on methods of analysis for treosulphan were available to the Working Group.

3. BIOLOGICAL DATA RELEVANT TO THE EVALUATION
OF CARCINOGENIC RISK TO HUMANS

3.1 Carcinogenicity studies in animals

No data were available to the Working Group.

3.2 Other relevant biological data

(a)   Experimental systems

Toxic effects

In Holtzman and Fischer rats, the i.p. LD_{50} of treosulphan was 1.3 g and 745 mg/kg bw daily for 5 days, respectively; by oral administration, it was 973 and 472 mg/kg bw daily for 5 days, respectively. The oral LD_{50} in dogs was between 111 mg/kg bw daily for 18 days and 222 mg/kg bw daily for 11 days; in monkeys it was between 222 and 444 mg/kg bw daily for 13 days. The i.v. LD_{50} in dogs was between 111 mg/kg bw daily for 18 days and 222 mg/kg bw daily for 11 days, that in monkeys was between 111 mg/kg bw daily for 14 days and 222 mg/kg bw daily for 13 days (White, 1962).

In the above study, the following toxic effects were observed in dogs and monkeys given the LD_{50} dose: anorexia and weight loss; depression of bone-marrow activity and accompanying reticulocytopenia, leucopenia and thrombocytopenia, causing haemorrhagic lesions in the gut and soft tissues. These effects were dose-related in severity. The thrombocytopenic effects were more severe in dogs than in monkeys.

Effects on reproduction and prenatal toxicity

No data were available to the Working Group.

Absorption, distribution, excretion and metabolism

No data were available to the Working Group.

Mutagenicity and other short-term tests

The mutagenic activity of treosulphan has been investigated in plants. It induced chromosomal aberrations (probably due to the formation of 1,2:3,4-diepoxybutane) in seeds of *Allium cepa* (onion), *Hordeum sativum* (barley), *Nigella damascena* (love-in-a-mist) and *Vicia faba* (vetch) (Matagne, 1967, 1968, 1969; Moutschen & Reekmans, 1964; Moutschen *et al.*, 1966). It did not produce chlorophyll mutations in *Arabidopsis thaliana* (thale cress) at pH 8 (Matagne, 1969).

(b) Humans

Toxic effects

Treosulphan is an alkylating agent, and predictably depresses leucocyte and platelet counts within 4 weeks of the start of oral therapy with a daily dose of 10 - 25 mg/kg bw (Loeb, 1964). Recovery of blood cell counts after stopping the drug may take about a month. Nausea and vomiting occur in about 20% of patients. Stomatitis may accompany agranulocytosis, but has not been found to be severe (Fennelly, 1977). Jaundice was reported in one patient, and mild exanthemata and pigmentation in a few. Addison's syndrome was associated with treosulphan administration in one case report (Prior & White, 1978).

Effects on reproduction and prenatal toxicity

No data were available to the Working Group.

Absorption, distribution, excretion and metabolism

No data were available to the Working Group.

Mutagenicity and chromosomal effects

No data were available to the Working Group.

3.3 Case reports and epidemiological studies of carcinogenicity in humans

No individual case report of cancer occurring after treatment with treosulphan was available.

Pedersen-Bjergaard *et al.* (1979, 1980) reported on 553 patients with ovarian cancer treated only with treosulphan and followed for 1 - 8 years after treatment (1159 patient-years). Seven patients developed acute nonlymphocytic leukaemia 21 - 58 (median, 50) months after the start of chemotherapy. On the basis of age-specific data from the Danish Cancer Registry, the expected number of cases among the patients was 0.04, giving a relative risk of 175. There was a correlation between cumulative dose of treosulphan and risk of leukaemia, although it was not statistically significant. The relative risk was not affected by tumour stage or radiation therapy (only 2 patients had also received radiation), although no formal analysis of these data has been presented. The authors also cite 3 additional, similar cases that were referred to them.

No excess of acute nonlymphocytic leukaemia has been seen in patients treated for ovarian cancer without chemotherapy (Reimer et al., 1977). [See also monograph on chlorambucil, p. 127.]

4. SUMMARY OF DATA REPORTED AND EVALUATION

4.1 Experimental data

No data on the carcinogenicity or teratogenicity of treosulphan in experimental animals were available to the Working Group.

The only available studies on chromosomal effects showed that it produces chromosomal aberrations in plants.

4.2 Human data

Treosulphan has had limited use since 1969, almost exclusively in the treatment of ovarian cancer.

The only epidemiological study indicates that use of this drug is followed by an increased risk of acute nonlymphocytic leukaemia.

4.3 Evaluation

There is *sufficient evidence*[1] for the carcinogenicity of treosulphan in humans.

---

[1] See preamble, p. 17.

5. REFERENCES

Feit, P.W. (1961) Stereoisomere 1,4-di-O-methansulfonyl-butan-1,2,3,4-tetrole. *Tetrahedron Lett., 20,* 716-717

Feit, P.W. (1964) 1,4-Bismethanesulfonates of the stereoisomeric butanetetraols and related compounds. *J. med. Chem., 7,* 14-17

Fennelly, J. (1977) Treosulfan (dihydroxybusulphan) in the management of ovarian carcinoma. *Br. J. Obstet. Gynaecol., 84,* 300-303

IARC (1976) *IARC Monographs on the Evaluation of Carcinogenic Risk of Chemicals to Man,* Vol. 11, *Cadmium, nickel, some epoxides, miscellaneous industrial chemicals and general considerations on volatile anaesthetics,* Lyon, pp. 115-123

Loeb, V. (1964) Dihydroxybusulfan (NSC-39069) in chronic myelocytic leukemia and miscellaneous malignant neoplasms. *Cancer Chemother. Rep., 42,* 39-43

Matagne, R. (1967) Acitivity of L-threitol-1,4-bismethanesulfonate on barley chromosomes in relation to chemical transformation during treatment. *Mutat. Res., 4,* 621-630

Matagne, R. (1968) Chromosomal aberrations induced by dialkylating agents in *Allium cepa* root-tips and their relation to the mitotic cycle and DNA synthesis. *Radiat. Bot., 8,* 489-497

Matagne, R. (1969) Induction of chromosomal aberrations and mutations with isomeric forms of L-threitol-1,4-bismethanesulfonate in plant materials. *Mutat. Res., 7,* 241-247

Moutschen, J. & Reekmans, M. (1964)   Effects of L-threitol-1,4-bismethanesulfonate on chromosomes. *Caryologia, 17,* 495-508

Moutschen, J., Matagne, R. & Gilot, J. (1966) Chromosome breakage with two isomers of /-threitol 1,4-bismethanesulphonate in plants. *Nature, 210,* 762-763

Pedersen-Bjergaard, J., Sørensen, H.M., Hou-Jensen, K. & Ersbøl, J. (1979) Acute non-lymphocytic leukemia (ANLL) in patients with ovarian carcinoma following long term treatment with treosulfan (= dihydroxybusulfan) (Abstract no. 1164). *Proc. Am. Assoc. Cancer Res., 20,* 287

Pedersen-Bjergaard, J. Nissen, N.I., Sørensen, H.M., Hou-Jensen, K., Larsen, M.S., Ernst, P., Ersbøl, J., Knudtzon,S., & Rose, C. (1980) Acute non-lymphocytic leukemia in patients with ovarian carcinoma following long-term treatment with treosulphan (= dihydroxybusulfan). *Cancer, 45,* 19-29

Prior, J. & White, L. (1978) Addisonian syndrome associated with treosulfan. *Lancet, ii,* 1207-1208

Reimer, R.R., Hoover, R., Fraumeni, J.F., Jr & Young, R.C. (1977) Acute leukemia after alkylating-agent therapy of ovarian cancer. *New Engl. J. Med., 297,* 177-181

Sørensen, H.M. (1973)   Ovarian carcinoma treatment with treosulfan.   *Acta obstet.-gynaecol. scand., Suppl.,* *22,* 18-30

Wade, A. (1977)   *Martindale, The Extra Pharmacopoeia,* 27th ed., London, The Pharmaceutical Press, p. 1824

White, F.R. (1962) L-Threitol dimethanesulfonate. *Cancer Chemother. Rep., 24,* 95-97

VINBLASTINE SULPHATE[1]

1. CHEMICAL AND PHYSICAL DATA

1.1 Synonyms and trade names

Chem. Abstr. Services Reg. No.: 143-67-9

Chem. Abstr. Name: Vincaleukoblastine, sulfate (1:1) (salt)

IUPAC Systematic Name: Vincaleukoblastine sulfate (1:1) (salt)

Synonyms: Vincaleucoblastine sulphate; vincaleukoblastine sulphate

Trade names: Exal; 29060-LE; LE 29060; NSC 49842; Velban; Velbe; VLB sulphate

1.2 Structural and molecular formulae and molecular weight

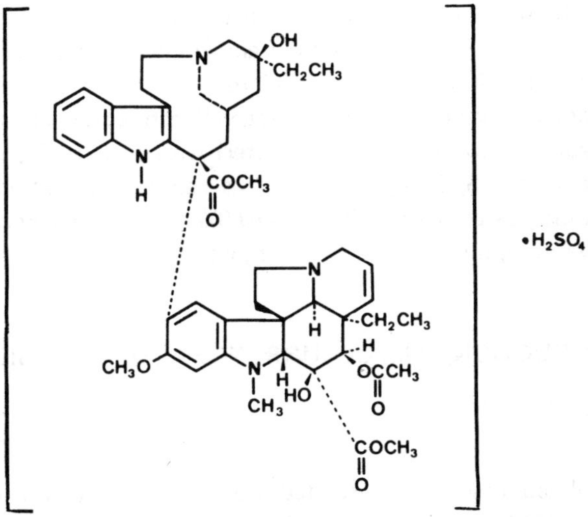

$\cdot H_2SO_4$

$C_{46}H_{59}N_4O_9 \cdot H_2SO_4$

Mol. wt: 909.1

---

[1] Many of the reports cited in this monograph refer to 'vinblastine' and not to the sulphate; however, since only the sulphate is produced commercially, that was assumed to be the compound under study.

1.3 Chemical and physical properties of the pure substance

From Wade (1977) or Burns (1972)

(a) *Description:* White to slightly yellow, odourless, very hygroscopic, amorphous or crystalline powder

(b) *Melting-point:* 284-285°C (monohydrate)

(c) *Optical rotation:* $[\alpha]_D^{22}$ = −28° (c = 1.01; in methanol)

(d) *Spectroscopy data:* λ_{max} 214 nm, A_1^1 = 592; 262 nm, A_1^1 = 186 (in 95% ethanol). Infra-red, mass and nuclear magnetic resonance spectra have been tabulated.

(e) *Solubility:* Soluble in water (1 in 10), ethanol (1 in 12,200), chloroform (1 in 50) and methanol; insoluble in diethyl ether

(f) *Stability:* Sensitive to hydrolysis, oxidation and heat

1.4 Technical products and impurities

Various national and international pharmacopoeias give specifications for the purity of vinblastine sulphate in pharmaceutical products. For example, it is available in the US as a USP grade measured as containing 96.0 - 101.0% active ingredient calculated on the dried basis, with 17% max. loss on drying, $[\alpha]$ = −28° to −35° (calculated on the dried basis, determined in a methanol solution containing 200 mg vinblastine sulphate in each 10 ml) and producing an aqueous solution (3 mg in 2 ml of water) with a pH of 3.5 - 5.0. Vinblastine sulphate is also available in the US, Europe and Japan as a sterile preparation of 10 mg in vials for parenteral use, measured as containing 90.0 - 110.0% of the stated amount (Wade, 1977; US Pharmacopeial Convention, Inc., 1980). In Japan, vials containing 5 mg are also available.

2. PRODUCTION, USE, OCCURRENCE AND ANALYSIS

(a) *Production*

Vinblastine is an alkaloid which was isolated independently by two research groups in 1958-1959 (Noble *et al.*, 1958; Johnson *et al.*, 1959) from the leaves, bark or stems of the plant *Vinca rosea* Linn. (now called *Catharanthus roseus* G. Don) of the family Apocynaceae (Madagascar periwinkle). The final structure elucidation of vinblastine was achieved by X-ray crystallography in 1965 (Moncrief & Lipscomb, 1965). The crude extract is obtained by aqueous or aqueous-ethanolic sulphuric acid extraction and final purification by chromatography on aluminium oxide. The sulphate is produced by reaction of the alkaloid with sulphuric acid (Harvey, 1975).

Commercial production of vinblastine sulphate in the US was first reported in 1965 (US Tariff Commission, 1967). The single US producer is believed to obtain most of the raw material for extraction of vinblastine from the Malagasy Republic and from Mozambique.

Vinblastine sulphate is believed to be produced by one company in Italy and by one in Hungary.

(b) Use

Vinblastine sulphate is used in human medicine as an antineoplastic agent, often in combination with other drugs, in the treatment of Hodgkin's disease, breast cancer, choriocarcinoma, testicular tumours, neuroblastoma (Creasey, 1975; Harvey, 1975; Wade, 1977), squamous-cell carcinoma of the head and neck (Vanhaelen *et al.*, 1979), renal carcinoma and Kaposi's sarcoma.

Therapy is usually started at a dose level of 2.5-8 mg/m^2 of body surface area, given intravenously at weekly intervals, to give 0.1 mg/kg bw. Thereafter the dose level is gradually increased by 0.05 mg/kg bw, usually weekly, until a response or toxicity is observed (Goodman & Gilman, 1975; Harvey, 1975; Wade, 1977).

2.2 Occurrence

Vinblastine is a naturally occurring alkaloid, which has been isolated from several members of the plant genus *Catharanthus* (formerly called *Vinca*), a pantropical shrub (Saxton, 1971).

2.3 Analysis

Analytical methods for the determination of vinblastine sulphate based on spectrophotometry, colorimetry and chromatography have been reviewed (Burns, 1972). Typical methods for the analysis of vinblastine sulphate in various matrices are summarized in Table 1.

Table 1. Methods for the analysis of vinblastine sulphate

Sample matrix	Sample preparation	Assay procedure[a]	Limit of detection	Reference
Formulations	Dissolve in methanol	UV	not given	US Pharmacopeial Convention, Inc. (1980)
	Dissolve in 25% aqueous methanol; spray plate with ceric ammonium sulphate solution	TLC	not given	Burns (1972)
Biological fluids	Dissolve in glycine buffer; incubate with ^{3}H-vinblastine and antiserum or normal rabbit serum	RIA	450 ng	Sethi *et al.* (1980)

[a]Abbreviations: UV, ultra-violet spectrometry; TLC, thin-layer chromatography; RIA, radioimmunoassay

3. BIOLOGICAL DATA RELEVANT TO THE EVALUATION OF CARCINOGENIC RISK TO HUMANS

3.1 Carcinogenicity studies in animals

(a) Intraperitoneal administration

Mouse: Two groups, each of 25 male and 25 female outbred Swiss-Webster-derived mice, 6 weeks old, were given i.p. injections of 0.09 or 0.18 mg/kg bw vinblastine sulphate dissolved in physiological saline 3 times a week for 6 months. Animals that survived over 100 days were observed for up to 12 further months, at which time they were killed. A control group of 101 male mice had a median survival time of 9.8 months, while that of 153 control mice was 18 months. The survival times of the treated animals were reported as percentages of that of the controls [no precise definition of the mode of calculation was given] : the survival time of treated males was reported to be 41 - 42% that of controls, and that of treated females 74 - 98%. Animals that died before day 100 on test were excluded from evaluation. The tumour incidences were 1/19 in treated males (a bladder tumour) and 4/14 in females (2 lung, 1 splenic and 1 uterine tumours). These incidences did not differ markedly from the 26% incidence seen in both male and female controls (Weisburger, 1977). [The Working Group considered that the inadequate reporting of certain items, such as survival times, the amalgation of various experimental groups and tumour types, as well as the lack of age-adjustment in the analyses precluded a complete evaluation of this study.]

Rat: Two groups, each of 25 male and 25 female Sprague-Dawley-derived Charles-River (CD) rats, 6 weeks of age, were given i.p. injections of 0.1 or 0.2 mg/kg bw vinblastine sulphate dissolved in physiological saline 3 times weekly for 6 months. Animals that survived over 100 days were observed for up to 12 further months, at which time they were killed. A control group of 179 males and 181 females had an overall survival time of over 18 months. The survival times of the treated animals were reported as percentages of that of the controls [no precise definition of the mode of calculation was given] : the survival of both treated males and females was reported to range from 18 - 100% of that of controls. Animals that died before day 100 on test were excluded from evaluation. Of the treated males, 11/21 (52%) animals examined had neoplasms, 7 of which were malignant: 2 lymphosarcomas, 2 pituitary tumours, 1 peritoneal sarcoma, 1 reticulum-cell sarcoma and 1 testicular neoplasm. Among male controls, 34% had tumours, most of which were found in endocrine tissues, including pituitary, adrenal, thyroid, testis and mammary gland. The tumour incidence in treated male rats was thus considered to be 1.5 - 2 times greater than that in controls. Of the treated female rats, 18/25 (72%) had neoplasms by 18 months, 3 of which were malignant. The principal sites of tumour development were the breast (11) and pituitary (7); tumours were seen at the same sites in controls, in which a 58% incidence of tumours occurred. Vinblastine was considered to produce only a slightly greater or the same tumour incidence as in controls (Weisburger, 1977). [The Working Group considered that the inadequate reporting of certain items, such as survival times, the amalgation of various experimental groups and tumour types, as well as the lack of age-adjustment in the analyses precluded a complete evaluation of this study.]

(b)   Intravenous administration

Rat: Two groups of male BR46 rats were injected intravenously with vinblastine sulphate: a group of 48 received 0.14 mg/kg bw once weekly for 52 weeks (total dose, 7.28 mg/kg bw), and a second group of 96 animals was given an injection of 0.33 mg/kg bw (17% of the LD_{50}) every 14 days for a total of 5 injections (total, 1.75 mg). A control group of 89 rats was maintained. In the first group, 25 (52%) rats were alive at the time of appearance of the first tumour, and only 1 rat (4%) died with a neoplasm, a benign thymoma, 18 months after start of treatment. In the second group, 31 animals were still alive at the time of appearance of the first tumour; a 3% incidence of malignant tumours and a 9% incidence of benign tumours were seen. Of the controls, 65 (73%) survived to the time of the first tumour, and 5% died with benign tumours and 6% with malignancies after a median latent period of 23 months (Schmähl & Osswald, 1970).

3.2 Other relevant biological data

(a) Experimental systems

Toxic effects

Vinblastine is more toxic in mice by i.p. injection (LD_{50} 5.6 mg/kg bw) than by i.v. or oral administration (LD_{50} 15 mg/kg bw) (Németh et al., 1970). In another series of experiments, the i.v. LD_{50} of vinblastine sulphate was found to be 10.0 mg/kg bw in mice and 2.9 mg/kg bw in rats (Todd et al., 1976). In Wistar rats the i.p. LD_{50} was 2.2 mg/kg bw (Németh et al., 1970).

In rats, the prominent signs of toxicity after a lethal dose were diarrhoea, anorexia, locomotor inactivity, diuresis, weight loss and dyspnoea (Todd et al., 1976). Deaths usually occurred 3 - 7 days after dosing; survivors improved from day 7.

A distinctive feature of the vinca alkaloids is their ability to arrest cell division in metaphase by a direct effect on the spindle apparatus. In the absence of a complete spindle, the chromosome may be dispersed through the cytoplasm or may adopt various unusual groupings. Other microtubular structures may also be affected (Creasey, 1975).

Effects on reproduction and prenatal toxicity

When inbred DBA/2J mice were given a single dose of 0.35 mg/kg bw vinblastine sulphate on day 9 of pregnancy, 69% of the fetuses were resorbed, and 35 of 74 surviving fetuses showed morphological defects such as anophthalmia, gastroschisis, umbilical hernia and twisted hindlimbs; 10 of the 74 fetuses were growth retarded. With 0.3 mg/kg bw, only 3 of 55 surviving fetuses showed malformations, but the resorption rate was still 52% (5% in controls). No malformations but an increased resorption rate were observed if up to 0.5 mg/kg bw were given on day 7, 8, 10 or 11 of pregnancy (Joneja & LeLiever, 1974).

A single i.m. dose of 0.025 mg vinblastine sulphate given to 31 female Long-Evans or 16 Holtzman rats 8 - 8.5 days after mating produced 51% and 33% resorptions in the two strains, respectively; 66 of the surviving 143 fetuses (Long-Evans) or 43 of the surviving 102 fetuses (Holtzman) showed malformations, such as anophthalmia, microphthalmia, microcephaly or micrognathia (DeMyer, 1964).

When 0.12 - 0.5 mg/kg bw vinblastine was given intraperitoneally to 94 Wistar (CR) rats from day 7 - 12 of pregnancy, embryomortality of 20% (with 0.12 mg/kg bw) to 80% (with 0.50 mg/kg bw) was found. Malformations occurred in 9.4% of the fetuses that survived the maternal dose of 0.25 mg/kg bw but in only 2.6% (2/78) of the fetuses of animals that received 0.12 mg/kg bw. The abnormalities observed included exencephaly, rachischisis and gastroschisis. When 15-day pregnant rats were given an i.v. injection of 1 mg vinblastine, the number of mitotic figures per 1000 cells after 4 hours increased 6.5-fold in maternal bone marrow and 5.7-fold in fetal cell suspensions, but only 1.7-fold in a placental cell suspension (Cohlan *et al.*, 1964; Cohlan & Kitay, 1965).

Ultrastructural changes were observed 6 hours later in the primitive neural cells of the telencephalic wall of rat fetuses exposed *in utero* by i.p. injection of 1 mg/kg bw vinblastine sulphate to pregnant MP 1 albino rats on day 14 of pregnancy. The changes included abnormal accumulation of mitotic cells in metaphase on the paraventricular surface, condensation and fragmentation of chromatin materials in some cells and decrease or complete disappearance of endoplasmic reticulum and Golgi apparatus. These changes were transient: 9 hours after the injection none could be seen, except for occasional necrotic cells (Takeuchi *et al.*, 1977).

When 10 pregnant golden hamsters were given i.v. injections of 0.25 mg/kg bw vinblastine on the 8th day of pregnancy, 58% embryomortality was seen on the 14th day of gestation, and 16% of the 56 surviving fetuses were grossly abnormal. The malformations included microphthalmia, anophthalmia, spina bifida and skeletal defects (mostly rib fusions and vertebral arch deformities). Only 3% of fetuses were abnormal after 4 pregnant hamsters were treated with 0.1 mg/kg bw on the 8th day of pregnancy, but fetomortality was still 18% (compared with 7% in controls) (Ferm, 1963).

Absorption, distribution, excretion and metabolism

Twenty-four hours after i.v. injection to rats of tritiated vinblastine (free base), radioactivity was distributed evenly throughout the body. Less than 7% of the total injected radioactivity was excreted in the urine in that time. There was evidence of biliary excretion, and 2 hours after injection lung, liver, spleen and kidney contained the highest concentrations of drug, whether it was administered intraperitoneally or intravenously (Beer & Richards, 1964; Beer *et al.*, 1964). In dogs, plasma levels of tritiated vinblastine sulphate fell in a biphasic mode, with half lives of 17 - 38 min and 3 - 5 hours, respectively. Unchanged vinblastine was a major component of bile radioactivity; over a 9-day period 12 - 17% of administered radioactivity was excreted in the urine and 30-36% in the bile (Creasey *et al.*, 1975).

Mutagenicity and other short-term tests

The genetic and related effects of vinblastine have been reviewed (Degraeve, 1978).

Vinblastine sulphate did not induce reverse mutations in *Salmonella typhimurium* tester strains TA1535, TA1537, TA98 or TA100, in the presence or absence of a liver microsomal preparation from induced rats (Heddle & Bruce, 1977; Seino *et al.*, 1978).

In Don lung cells from Chinese hamsters, vinblastine sulphate produced a dose- and time-dependent increase in various chromosomal aberrations, including chromatid breaks and sister chromatid exchanges (Segawa *et al.*, 1979).

Vinblastine also produced an increase in bone-marrow micronuclei formation and sperm abnormalities in mice (Heddle & Bruce, 1977). [Since vinblastine produces changes in mitotic spindle formation, whether these changes are related to mutagenicity is questionable.]

Vinblastine sulphate produced no preimplantation loss above control limits in mice in the dominant lethal assay (Epstein *et al.*, 1972).

(b) Humans

Toxic effects

The dominant toxic effect of vinblastine is leucopenia (Goodman & Gilman, 1975), which limits the therapeutic dose that can be given. However, high doses have the same spectrum of neurotoxic effects as vincristine: peripheral neuropathy, constipation and ileus (Creasey, 1975). Alopecia (Goodman & Gilman, 1975), inappropriate antidiuretic hormone secretion (Ginsberg *et al.*, 1977), vocal cord paralysis (Brook & Schreiber, 1971) and laryngeal nerve paralysis (Whittaker & Griffith, 1977) have also been reported. The majority of these effects are reversible when the drug is discontinued. Raynaud's phenomenon has also been reported as a possible complication of vinblastine therapy (Teutsch *et al.*, 1977; Rothberg, 1978).

Effects on reproduction and prenatal toxicity

Only case reports are available regarding the possible teratogenicity of this agent. In two reports of first-trimester exposure, the infants were considered normal. In one case the mother had received 25 mg per week or less of vinblastine throughout her entire pregnancy (Armstrong *et al.*, 1964). The other mother had received a total dose of 127 mg vinblastine sulphate between conception and the third month and between the sixth and seventh months of pregnancy; in addition, she had received a total of 5660 rads during pregnancy (Rosenzweig *et al.*, 1964).

No birth defect was observed in the infant of a woman exposed to a total dose of 48 mg vinblastine sulphate in the third trimester of pregnancy (Lacher, 1964). A normal infant was also born to a mother who received a total dose of 111 mg vinblastine sulphate between the 4th month of pregnancy and term (Lacher & Geller, 1966).

An infant whose mother received combination therapy consisting of nitrogen mustard, vinblastine sulphate and procarbazine during the first trimester had only 4 toes on each foot with syndactyly of the third and fourth right toes. The fourth metatarsal was absent in the left toe (Garrett, 1974).

Absorption, distribution, excretion and metabolism

Owellen *et al.* (1977) studied the disposition of ring-labelled tritiated vinblastine sulphate both by its radioactivity and by a radioimmunoassay which detected all the vinca alkaloid derivatives. A triphasic decay, with half-lives of 3.9, 53 and 1173 minutes, was identified. Approximately 10% of the administered radioactivity was found in the faeces and 14% in the urine, the majority remaining unaccounted for. One cytotoxic metabolite, deacetyl vinblastine, was identified by thin-layer chromatography.

Mutagenicity and chromosomal effects

No data were available to the Working Group.

3.3 Case reports and epidemiological studies of carcinogenicity in humans

There have been 17 case reports of acute nonlymphocytic leukaemia occurring after treatment for Hodgkin's disease that included vinblastine (Osta *et al.*, 1970; Swain *et al.*, 1971; Chan & McBride, 1972; Focan *et al.*, 1974; Sahakian *et al.*, 1974; Canellos, 1975; Rosner & Grünwald, 1975; Cadman *et al.*, 1977; Cavalli *et al.*, 1977; Kaye *et al.*, 1979). One patient with non-Hodgkin's lymphoma developed leukaemia after receiving treatment including vinblastine (Zarrabi, 1980).

Two of the leukaemia patients, both of whom had also received radiation, had received vinblastine as the only cytotoxic drug (Osta *et al.*, 1970; Rosner & Grünwald, 1975).

Several authors have described the occurrence of acute nonlymphocytic leukaemia in cohorts of Hodgkin's disease patients treated with varying combinations of multi-drug chemotherapy and radiation (Auclerc *et al.*, 1979; Papa *et al.* 1979). The treatment regimens typically included procarbazine, vincristine and/or vinblastine and nitrogen mustard. However, these cohorts were not described in detail, and the relative risk of acute leukaemia in treated patients was not quantified. Taken together, the reports present data on approximately 2600 patients with Hodgkin's disease in whom 17 cases of acute nonlymphocytic leukaemia were diagnosed subsequently.   Thirteen of these 17 leukaemia cases occurred in patients who had received both combination chemotherapy and radiation.   The occurrence of solid tumours was not systematically documented.

Valagussa *et al.* (1980) followed 55 patients with Hodgkin's disease treated with vinblastine in combination with adriamycin, bleomycin and dacarbazine for a median period of 43 months, without observing secondary neoplasms.   No other epidemiological study in which patients with Hodgkin's disease were followed up has specifically indicated that vinblastine was among the agents used for treatment.

4. SUMMARY OF DATA REPORTED AND EVALUATION

4.1   Experimental data

Vinblastine sulphate was tested in three studies, two by intraperitoneal injection in mice and rats, and one by intravenous injection in rats.   No evidence of carcinogenicity was found, but vinblastine sulphate has not been adequately tested at high doses.

Vinblastine sulphate can induce teratogenic effects in several animal species and embryo-lethality at doses nontoxic to the mother.   On the basis of the available data, this compound cannot be considered to be mutagenic.

4.2   Human data

Vinblastine sulphate has been widely used since the early 1960s, almost always in combination with other cytotoxic agents, in the treatment of neoplastic diseases, particularly lymphoma.

The available data are insufficient to evaluate its teratogenic effects in humans.   No data on the mutagenicity or chromosomal effects of vinblastine sulphate in humans were available.

Vinblastine sulphate, mainly in combination therapy, has been associated in case reports with the subsequent development of leukaemias.   The only epidemiological study was small and of short duration and showed no excess of subsequent neoplasms in patients treated with a regimen including vinblastine sulphate, adriamycin, bleomycin and dacarbazine.

4.3 Evaluation

There is no evidence of carcinogenicity in rats or mice on the basis of the available data. The data from studies in man are inadequate to evaluate the carcinogenicity of vinblastine sulphate in humans.

There is no evidence currently available to indicate that vinblastine sulphate is carcinogenic to humans, but the compound has not been extensively investigated.

5. REFERENCES

Armstrong, J.G., Dyke, R.W. & Fouts, P.J. (1964) Vinblastin sulfate treatment of Hodgkin's disease during pregnancy. *Science, 143,* 703

Auclerc, G., Jacquillat, C., Auclerc, M.F., Weil, M. & Bernard, J. (1979) Post-therapeutic acute leukemia. *Cancer, 44,* 2017-2025

Beer, C.T. & Richards, J.F. (1964) The metabolism of vinca alkaloids. II. The fate of tritiated vinblastine in rats. *Lloydia, 27,* 352-360

Beer, C.T., Wilson, M.L. & Bell, J. (1964) A preliminary investigation of the fate of tritiated vinblastine in rats. *Can. J. Physiol. Pharmacol., 42,* 368-373

Brook, J. & Schreiber, W. (1971) Vocal cord paralysis: a toxic reaction to vinblastine (NSC-49842) therapy. *Cancer Chemother. Rep., Part 1, 55,* 591-593

Burns, J.H. (1972) *Vinblastine sulfate.* In: Florey, K., ed., *Analytical Profiles of Drug Substances,* Vol. 1, New York, Academic Press, pp. 443-462

Cadman, E.C., Capizzi, R.L. & Bertino, J.R. (1977) Acute nonlymphocytic leukemia. A delayed complication of Hodgkin's disease therapy: analysis of 109 cases. *Cancer, 40,* 1280-1296

Canellos, G.P. (1975) Second malignancies complicating Hodgkin's disease in remission. *Lancet, i,* 1294

Cavalli, F., Gerber, A., Mosimann, W., Sonntag, R.W. & Tschopp, L. (1977) Acute myeloid leukaemia in the course of Hodgkin's disease (Ger.). *Dtsch. med. Wochenschr., 102,* 1019-1024

Chan, B.W.B. & McBride, J.A. (1972) Hodgkin's disease and leukemia. *Can. med. Assoc. J., 106,* 558-561

Cohlan, S.Q. & Kitay, D. (1965) The teratogenic effect of vincaleukoblastine in the pregnant rat. *J. Pediatr., 66,* 541-544

Cohlan, S.Q., Dancis, J. & Kitay, D. (1964) Vinblastine. *Lancet, i,* 1390

Creasey, W.A. (1975) *Vinca alkaloids and colchicine.* In: Sartorelli, A.C. & Johns, D.G., eds, *Antineoplastic and Immunosuppressive Agents,* Part II, New York, Springer, pp. 670-694

Creasey, W.A., Scott, A.I., Wei, C.-C., Kutcher, J., Schwartz, A. & Marsh, J.C. (1975) Pharmacological studies with vinblastine in the dog. *Cancer Res., 35,* 1116-1120

Degraeve, N. (1978) Genetic and related effects of *Vinca rosea* alkaloids. *Mutat. Res., 55,* 31-42

DeMyer, W. (1964) Vinblastine-induced malformations of face and nervous system in two rat strains. *Neurology, 14,* 806-808

Epstein, S.S., Arnold, E., Andrea, J., Bass, W. & Bishop, Y. (1972) Detection of chemical mutagens by the dominant lethal assay in the mouse. *Toxicol. appl. Pharmacol., 23,* 288-325

Ferm, V.H. (1963) Congenital malformations in hamster embryos after treatment with vinblastine and vincristine. *Science, 141,* 426

Focan, C., Brictieux, N., Lemaire, M. & Hugues, J. (1974) Secondary neoplasias as complications in Hodgkin's disease (Fr.). *Nouv. Presse méd., 3,* 1385

Garrett, M.J. (1974) Teratogenic effects of combination chemotherapy. *Ann. intern. Med., 80,* 667

Ginsberg, S.J., Comis, R.L. & Fitzpatrick, A.V. (1977) Vinblastine and inappropriate ADH secretion. *New Engl. J. Med., 296,* 941

Goodman, L.S. & Gilman, A., eds (1975) *The Pharmacological Basis of Therapeutics,* 5th ed., New York, Macmillan, pp. 1375-1378

Harvey, S.C. (1975) *Antineoplastic and immunosuppressive drugs.* In: Osol, A., ed., *Remington's Pharmaceutical Sciences,* 15th ed., Easton, PA, Mack Publishing Co., pp. 1085-1086

Heddle, J.A. & Bruce, W.R. (1977) *On the use of multiple assays for mutagenicity, especially the micronucleus,* Salmonella, *and sperm abnormality assays.* In: Scott, D., Bridges, B.A. & Sobels, F.H., eds, *Progress in Genetic Toxicology,* Vol. 2, Amsterdam, Elsevier/North-Holland Biomedical Press, pp. 265-274

Johnson, I.S., Wright, H.F. & Svoboda, G.H. (1959) Experimental basis for clinical evaluation of antitumour principles derived from *Vinca rosea* Linn. (Abstract no. 72). *J. Lab. clin. Med., 54,* 830

Joneja, M.G. & LeLiever, W.C. (1974) Effects of vinblastine and podophyllin on DBA mouse fetuses. *Toxicol. appl. Pharmacol., 27,* 408-414

Kaye, S.B., Juttner, C.A., Smith, I.E., Barrett, A., Austin, D.E., Peckham, M.J. & McElwain, T.J. (1979) Three years' experience with Ch1VPP (a combination of drugs of low toxicity) for the treatment of Hodgkin's disease. *Br. J. Cancer, 39,* 168-174

Lacher, M.J. (1964) Use of vinblastine sulfate to treat Hodgkin's disease during pregnancy. *Ann. intern. Med., 61,* 113-115

Lacher, M.J. & Geller, W. (1966) Cyclophosphamide and vinblastine sulfate in Hodgkin's disease during pregnancy. *J. Am. med. Assoc., 195,* 192-194

Moncrief, J.W. & Lipscomb, W.N. (1965) Structures of leurocristine (vincristine) and vincaleukoblastine. X-ray analysis of leurocristine methiodide. *J. Am. chem. Soc., 87,* 4963-4964

Németh, L., Somfai, S., Gál, F. & Kellner, B. (1970) Comparative studies concerning the tumour inhibition and the toxicology of vinblastine and vincristine. *Neoplasma, 17,* 345-347

Noble, R.L., Beer, C.T. & Cutts, J.H. (1958) Role of chance observations in chemotherapy: *Vinca rosea. Ann. N.Y. Acad. Sci., 76,* 887-894

Osta, S., Wells, M., Viamonte, M. & Harkness, D. (1970) Hodgkin's disease terminating in acute leukemia. *Cancer, 26,* 795-799

Owellen, R.J., Hartke, C.A. & Hains, F.O. (1977) Pharmacokinetics and metabolism of vinblastine in humans. *Cancer Res., 37,* 2597-2602

Papa, G., Alimena, G., Annino, L., Anselmo, A.P., Ciccone, F., De Luca, A.M., Granati, L., Petti, N. & Mandelli, F. (1979) Acute non lymphoid leukaemia following Hodgkin's disease. Clinical, biological and cytogenetic aspects of 3 cases. *Scand. J. Haematol., 23,* 339-347

Rosenzweig, A.I., Crews, Q.E., Jr & Hopwood, H.G. (1964) Vinblastine sulfate in Hodgkin's disease in pregnancy. *Ann. intern. Med., 61,* 108-112

Rosner, F. & Grünwald, H. (1975) Hodgkin's disease and acute leukemia. Report of eight cases and review of the literature. *Am. J. Med., 58,* 339-353

Rothberg, H. (1978) Raynaud's phenomenon after vinblastine-bleomycin chemotherapy. *Cancer Treat. Rep., 62,* 569-570

Sahakian, G.J., Al-Mondhiry, H., Lacher, M.J. & Connolly, H.C. (1974) Acute leukemia in Hodgkin's disease. *Cancer, 33,* 1369-1375

Saxton, J.E. (1971) *The Alkaloids,* Vol. 1, London, The Chemical Society, pp. 483-484

Schmähl, D. & Osswald, H. (1970) Experimental studies on carcinogenic effects of anticancer chemotherapeutics and immunosuppressives (Ger.). *Arzneimittel-Forsch./Drug Res., 20,* 1461-1467

Segawa, M., Nadamitsu, S., Kondo, K. & Yoshizaki, I. (1979) Chromosomal aberrations of Don lung cells of Chinese hamster after exposure to vinblastine *in vitro. Mutat. Res., 66,* 99-102

Seino, Y., Nagao, M., Yahagi, T., Hoshi, A., Kawachi, T. & Sugimura, T. (1978) Mutagenicity of several classes of antitumor agents to *Salmonella typhimurium* TA98, TA100, and TA92. *Cancer Res., 38,* 2148-2156

Sethi, V.S., Burton, S.S. & Jackson, D.V. (1980) A sensitive radioimmunoassay for vincristine and vinblastine. *Cancer Chemother. Pharmacol., 4,* 183-187

Swain, W.R., Windschitl, H.E., Doscherholmen, A., Bankole, R.O. & Bates, H.A. (1971) Chronic myelogenous leukemia in Hodgkin's disease: immunofluorescence of cells. *Cancer, 27,* 569-573

Takeuchi, I.K., Takeuchi, Y.K. & Murakami, U. (1977) Electron microscopy on the effect of vinblastine on the telencephalic wall of the rat fetus. *Br. J. exp. Pathol., 58,* 521-532

Teutsch, C., Lipton, A. & Harvey, H.A. (1977) Raynaud's phenomenon as a side effect of chemotherapy with vinblastine and bleomycin for testicular carcinoma. *Cancer Treat. Rep., 61,* 925-926

Todd, G.C., Gibson, W.R. & Morton, D.M. (1976) Toxicology of vindesine (desacetyl vinblastine amide) in mice, rats and dogs. *J. Toxicol. environ. Health, 1,* 843-850

US Pharmacopeial Convention, Inc. (1980) *The US Pharmacopeia,* 20th rev., Rockville, MD, p. 843

US Tariff Commission (1967) *Synthetic Organic Chemicals, US Production and Sales, 1965,* TC Publication 206, Washington DC, US Government Printing Office, p. 119

Valagussa, P., Santoro, A., Kenda, R., Fossati Bellani, F., Franchi, F., Banfi, A., Rilke, F. & Bonadonna, G. (1980) Second malignancies in Hodgkin's disease: a complication of certain forms of treatment. *Br. med J., i,* 216-219

Vanhaelen, C., Bertrand, M., De Jager, R. & Kenis, Y. (1979) Vinblastine, methotrexate, bleomycin, in the management of head and neck cancer. *Eur. J. Cancer, 15,* 1315-1318

Wade, A., ed. (1977) *Martindale, The Extra Pharmacopoeia,* 27th ed., London, The Pharmaceutical Press, pp. 172-173

Weisburger, E.K. (1977) Bioassay program for carcinogenic hazards of cancer chemotherapeutic agents. *Cancer, 40,* 1935-1949

Whittaker, J.A. & Griffith, I.P. (1977) Recurrent laryngeal nerve paralysis in patients receiving vincristine and vinblastine. *Br. med. J., i,* 1251-1252

Zarrabi, M.H. (1980) Association of non-Hodgkin's lymphoma (NHL) and second neoplasms. *Semin. Oncol., 7,* 340-351

VINCRISTINE SULPHATE[1]

1. CHEMICAL AND PHYSICAL DATA

1.1 Synonyms and trade names

Chem. Abstr. Services Reg. No.: 2068-78-2

Chem. Abstr. Name: Vincaleukoblastine, 22-oxo-, sulfate (1:1) (salt)

IUPAC Systematic Name: Leurocristine sulfate (1:1) (salt)

Synonyms: Des-N_a-methyl-N_a-formylvinblastine sulphate; LCR sulphate; leurocristine sulphate; leurocristine, sulphate (1:1) (salt); VCR sulphate

Trade names: NSC 67574; Oncovin; Onkovin; Vincristin; Vincrisul; 37231

1.2 Structural and molecular formulae and molecular weight

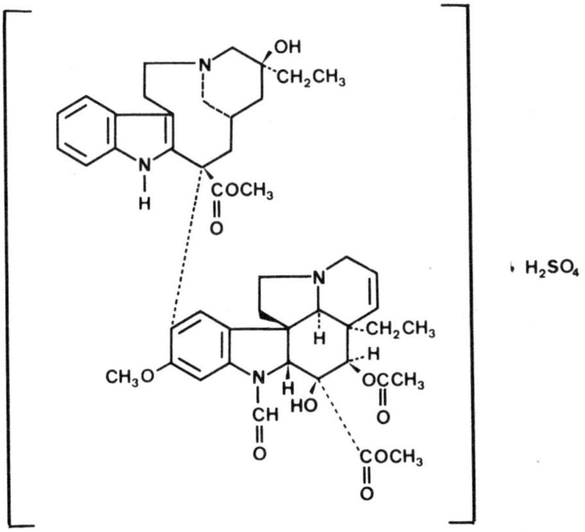

$$C_{46}H_{56}N_4O_{10} \cdot H_2SO_4$$

Mol. wt: 923.0

---

[1] Many of the reports cited in this monograph refer to 'vincristine' and not to the sulphate; however, since only the sulphate is produced commercially, that was assumed to be the compound under study.

1.3 Chemical and physical properties of the pure substance

From Wade (1977) or Burns (1972)

(a) *Description:* White to slightly yellow, odourless, very hygroscopic, amorphous or crystalline powder

(b) *Melting-point:* After recrystallization from absolute ethanol, 273-281°C

(c) *Optical rotation:* $[\alpha]_D^{25}$ = 8.5 (c = 0.8) (in methanol)

(d) *Spectroscopy data:* λ_{max} 221 nm, A_1^1 = 510; 255 nm, A_1^1 = 167; 296 nm, A_1^1 = 169 (in 95% ethanol). Infra-red, mass and nuclear magnetic resonance spectra have been tabulated.

(e) *Solubility:* Soluble in water (1 in 2), ethanol (1 in 600), chloroform (1 in 30) and methanol; insoluble in diethyl ether

(f) *Stability:* Sensitive to hydrolysis, oxidation and heat

1.4 Technical products and impurities

Various national and international pharmacopoeias give specifications for the purity of vincristine sulphate in pharmaceutical products. For example, it is available in the US as a USP grade measured as containing 90.0 - 105.0% active ingredient calculated on the dried basis, with 12% max. loss on drying and producing an aqueous solution (1 in 1000) with pH 3.5 - 4.5. Vincristine sulphate is also available in vials of 1 or 5 mg measured as containing 90.0-110.0% of the stated amount (Baker, 1980; US Pharmacopeial Convention, Inc., 1980). One company provides ampoules containing 1 mg or 5 mg vincristine sulphate plus 10 mg or 50 mg lactose, respectively, for use with 10-ml ampoules of solvent containing 0.9% sodium chloride and 0.9% benzyl alcohol (Wade, 1977).

Vincristine sulphate is available in Japan in 1 mg amounts for injection.

2. PRODUCTION, USE, OCCURRENCE AND ANALYSIS

2.1 Production and use

(a) *Production*

Vincristine is an alkaloid which was isolated independently by two research groups in 1958 - 1959 (Noble *et al.*, 1958; Johnson *et al.*, 1959) from the leaves, bark or stem of the plant *Vinca rosea* Linn. (now called *Catharanthus roseus* G. Don) of the family Apocynaceae

(Madagascar periwinkle). The final structure elucidation of vincristine was achieved by X-ray crystallography in 1965 (Moncrief & Lipscomb, 1965). The crude extract is obtained by aqueous or aqueous-ethanolic sulphuric acid extraction and final purification by chromatography on aluminium oxide (Harvey, 1975). The sulphate is produced by reaction of the alkaloid with sulphuric acid.

Commercial production of vincristine sulphate in the US was first reported in 1965 (US Tariff Commission, 1967). The single US producer is believed to obtain most of the raw material for extraction of vincristine from the Malagasy Republic and Mozambique.

Vincristine sulphate is believed to be produced by one company in Italy and by one in Hungary.

(b) Use

Vincristine sulphate is used in human medicine as an antineoplastic agent, usually in combination with other antineoplastic drugs. It is used in the induction phase of therapy for acute lymphoblastic leukaemia of childhood with prednisone and with prednisone, mercaptopurine and methotrexate in various protocols. It is combined with nitrogen mustard, procarbazine and prednisone in the MOPP regimen used for treatment of Hodgkin's disease. Vincristine sulphate is also used in the treatment of non-Hodgkin's lymphoma, blast crisis of chronic myelogenous leukaemia, neuroblastoma, Wilms' tumour, Ewing's sarcoma, embryonal rhabdomyosarcoma, soft-tissue sarcoma, osteogenic sarcoma, breast cancer, small-cell carcinoma of the lung and carcinoma of uterine cervix (Goodman & Gilman, 1975; Harvey, 1975; Wade, 1977). It has also been used in the treatment of non-malignant conditions, including refractory idiopathic thrombocytopenia (Ahn *et al.*, 1974).

Vincristine sulphate is given intravenously, usually at a dose of 1.4 mg/m^2 body surface area for adults and 2.0 mg/m^2 body surface area for children, once a week, although different amounts of the drug are used in various combination regimens (Goodman & Gilman, 1975; Harvey, 1975; Wade, 1977).

2.2 Occurrence

Vincristine is a naturally occurring alkaloid, which has been isolated from several members of the plant genus *Catharanthus* (formerly called *Vinca*), a pantropical shrub (Saxton, 1971).

2.3 Analysis

Analytical methods for the determination of vincristine sulphate based on spectrophotometry, colorimetry, thin-layer chromatography and bioassay techniques have been reviewed
(Burns, 1972). Typical methods for the analysis of vincristine sulphate in various matrices
are summarized in Table 1.

Table 1. Methods for the analysis of vincristine sulphate

Sample matrix	Sample preparation	Assay procedure[a]	Limit of detection	Reference
Formulations	Dissolve in methanol	UV	not given	US Pharmacopeial Convention, Inc. (1980)
Formulations, bile, blood serum, homogenized tissues, and urine	Extract with phosphate buffer and benzene; shake and centrifuge; add to scintillation solution	SS	not given	El Dareer et al. (1977)
Blood serum	Add known amounts of vincristine to control serum; dilute; add to KB human epidermoid cell cultures; measure protein content of cultures	BA	0.01 mg/l	Dixon et al. (1969)
	Add to human leucocyte cultures; count cells	BA	not given	Hirshaut et al. (1969)
Biological fluids	Dissolve in glycine buffer; incubate with ^{3}H-vincristine and antiserum or normal rabbit serum	RIA	460 ng	Sethi et al. (1980)

[a]Abbreviations: UV, ultra-violet spectrometry; SS, scintillation spectrometry; BA, bioassay; RIA,
radioimmunoassay

3. BIOLOGICAL DATA RELEVANT TO THE EVALUATION
OF CARCINOGENIC RISK TO HUMANS

3.1 Carcinogenicity studies in animals

(a) Intraperitoneal administration

Mouse: Two groups, each of 25 male and 25 female outbred Swiss-Webster-derived mice, 6 weeks old, were given i.p. injections of 0.075 or 0.15 mg/kg bw vincristine sulphate dissolved in physiological saline 3 times a week for 6 months. Animals that survived over 100 days were observed for up to 12 further months, at which time they were killed. A control group of 101 male mice had a median survival time of 9.8 months, while that of 153 female control mice was 18 months. The survival times of the treated animals were reported as percentages of that of the controls [no precise definition of the mode of calculation was given]: the survival of treated males given the low dose was reported to be 34 - 55% that of controls. The high dose was toxic to male mice. The survival of treated females was reported to be 97 - 100% of that of controls. Animals that died before day 100 on test were excluded from evaluation. The overall tumour incidence in treated males was 1/15 (7%) (a benign skin tumour), while that in treated females was 4/13 (31%) (3 of which were malignant; 3 lung-tumours, 1 leukaemia). These incidences were not greater than the 26% tumour incidence observed in both male and female controls (Weisburger, 1977). [The Working Group considered that the inadequate reporting of certain items, such as survival times, the amalgamation of various experimental groups and tumour types, as well as the lack of age-adjustment in the analyses precluded a complete evaluation of this study.]

Rat: Two groups, each of 25 male and 25 female Sprague-Dawley-derived Charles River (CD) rats, 6 weeks of age, were given i.p. injections of 0.06 or 0.12 mg/kg bw vincristine sulphate dissolved in physiological saline 3 times weekly for 6 months. Animals that survived over 100 days were observed for up to 12 further months, at which time they were killed. A control group of 179 males and 181 females had an overall survival time of over 18 months. The survival times of the treated animals were reported as percentages of that of the controls [no precise definition of the mode of calculation was given]: the survival of treated males was reported to be 19 - 100% that of controls, while the survival of treated females was 100% that of controls. Animals that died before day 100 on test were excluded from evaluation. Three of 16 (19%) treated male rats which survived longer than 100 days had benign neoplasms, 2 in the pituitary and 1 in the testis. The tumour incidence in control males was 34%; tumours occurred predominantly in the pituitary, but were also seen in other endocrine glands including the adrenal, thyroid and testis. Of the treated female rats, 12/22 (55%) had neoplasms by 18 months, 2 of which were malignant; the tumours occurred in the mammary gland (10), pituitary (3), and adrenal (1). In control females, there was a 58% incidence of tumours, involving the same organs as in the treated females. The tumour incidences in treated males and females were not considered to be greater than those in controls (Weisburger, 1977). [The Working Group considered that the inadequate reporting of certain items, such as survival times, the amalgamation of various experimental groups and tumour types, as well as the lack of age-adjustment in the analyses precluded a complete evaluation of this study.]

3.2   Other relevant biological data

(a)   Experimental systems

Toxic effects

The LD_{50} of vincristine in mice was 4.7 mg/kg bw by i.p. injection and 3.0 mg/kg bw by i.v. injection; in rats the i.p. LD_{50} was 1.2 mg/kg bw (Németh et al., 1970). The i.v. LD_{50} has also been reported as 2.1 mg/kg bw for mice and 1.0 mg/kg bw for rats (Todd et al., 1976). The acute i.v. LD_{50} of vincristine sulphate has also been found to be 1.33 mg/kg bw in adult female albino rats and 1.13 mg/kg bw in weanling females; and the i.p. LD_{50} in mice was 5.2 mg/kg bw (Adamson et al., 1965).

Mice given 7 mg/kg bw vincristine sulphate intraperitoneally showed muscular weakness and hind limb paralysis and died within 8 days. In rats, the prominent signs of toxicity after a lethal dose were diarrhoea, anorexia, locomotor inactivity, diuresis, loss of weight and dyspnoea. Deaths usually occurred 3 - 7 days after dosing, with survivors improving from day 7 (Adamson et al., 1965).

In a six-week study in dogs, vincristine sulphate was given as i.v. injections of 0.08, 0.04 or 0.02 mg/kg bw per week. With the highest dose, 2/4 animals died with extensive damage to gut, lymphoid hypoplasia and maturation arrest of spermatocytes. The two survivors had no drug-induced lesions at necropsy 44 and 97 days after start of treatment, respectively, but nonspecific lesions of the nervous system occurred with all dose levels. Monkeys treated with i.v. doses of 0.08, 0.16 or 0.32 mg/kg bw per week survived treatment, but showed dose-related leucopenia, anaemia and reticulocytosis. One of two monkeys given 0.64 mg/kg bw per week died; both animals had swollen neurons in the ventral horn of the spinal cord and severe damage to the intestinal mucosa. In monkeys, as in man, the nervous system was the most sensitive tissue; while in dogs, the gut was the most sensitive (Folk et al., 1974). Chickens and cats are also sensitive to the neurotoxic effects of vincristine (Todd et al., 1979).

Vincristine sulphate is one of a number of agents whose characteristic action is to arrest cells in metaphase by an effect on microtubules (Creasey, 1975).

Effects on reproduction and prenatal toxicity

When inbred C3H/HeJ or DBA/2J mice or random-bred ICR/Ha Swiss mice received a single i.p. injection of 0.25 - 0.35 mg/kg bw vincristine sulphate on day 9 of pregnancy, the rate of resorptions was 49 - 57% in the three strains as compared with up to 6% in controls; 32 - 66% of the surviving fetuses of inbred mice showed malformations. Anomalies involved the central nervous system, eyes, limbs, tail and ribs (Joneja & Ungthavorn, 1969; Ungthavorn & Joneja, 1969).

When 0.1 - 0.5 mg/kg bw vincristine was injected intravenously into golden hamsters on the 8th day of pregnancy, a high percentage of resorptions occurred (23% with 0.1 mg/kg bw; 85% with 0.5 mg/kg bw). Although up to 6% of 39 surviving fetuses were grossly abnormal (compared with 0/111 control fetuses), the effect was not clearly dose-dependent. The malformations included microphthalmia, anophthalmia and rib defects (Ferm, 1963).

Of the fetuses of 5 *Macaca mulatta* (rhesus) monkeys treated with a single i.m. injection of 0.15 - 0.20 mg/kg bw vincristine sulphate between days 27 to 34 of pregnancy, 3 were normal and 2 showed gross morphological abnormalities (one syndactyly and one encephalocele). Both abnormal monkeys were viable (Courtney & Valerio, 1968).

Absorption, distribution, excretion and metabolism

The distribution and metabolism of tritiated vincristine have been studied in a number of species. After i.p. injection into mice and rats, peak plasma levels of vincristine are attained after 15 min; it is excreted with half-lives of 60 min in mice and 60 - 100 min in rats (Castle *et al.*, 1976; El Dareer *et al.*, 1977).

In mice, metabolites in serum increase for 30 min after injection and then remain constant for 180 min. There is a marked accumulation of unchanged drug in liver, kidneys and spleen compared with the serum level; the level of unchanged drug was very low in the brain, although metabolite levels were significantly higher than in other organs. By 24 hours, the levels of radioactivity from tritiated vincristine had fallen in most tissues, except for the spleen and the large intestine, indicating biliary excretion of the drug or its metabolites. In mice, 22% of the total dose was excreted in the urine over 48 hours as vincristine and 25% as metabolites; and in the faeces, 18% of the total dose was vincristine and 19% metabolites. At that time, the carcass contained 8% of the total dose as vincristine and 9% as metabolites. Urinary excretion of radioactivity over the first few hours after injection was also low in dogs and monkeys. In both species, the drug was distributed to most tissues, but highest concentrations were found in the lung, kidney, spleen, pancreas and liver (El Dareer *et al.*, 1977). In monkeys, vincristine and its metabolites rapidly entered the cerebrospinal fluid from the plasma to form a low concentration of drug, which persisted for several days (Jackson *et al.*, 1980).

Mutagenicity and other short-term tests

Genetic and related effects of vincristine have been reviewed (Degraeve, 1978).

Vincristine sulphate was not mutagenic in *Salmonella typhimurium* tester strains TA98 and TA100 with or without rat liver microsomal activation (Seino *et al.*, 1978). In a study with the mouse lymphoma line L5178Y, using excessive concentrations (> 0.5 to 40 μg/ml), vincristine exhibited mutagenic activity (Matheson *et al.*, 1978).

No chromosomal aberration was found with the drug in CHO cells (Maier & Schmid, 1976), or in a Syrian hamster fibroblast cell line (Benedict *et al.*, 1977).

Statistically significant increases in the number of bone-marrow cells with numerical and structural aberrations were found in pregnant mice 48 hours after a single i.p. injection of 0.3 mg/kg bw vincristine sulphate when given on day 6. Increases in numerical aberrations were also found in embryonic tissues 48 hours after the same dose of vincristine on day 8 of pregnancy. No increase in chromosomal aberrations occurred in maternal cells when vincristine sulphate was injected on day 7 or 8, or in embryonic cells when the drug was injected on day 6 or 7 of pregnancy (Sieber *et al.*, 1978).

Vincristine sulphate also produced a dose-dependent increase in micronuclei formation in mouse bone-marrow cells (Maier & Schmid, 1976).

A less than two-fold increase in sister chromatid exchanges has been seen in a hamster cell line (Banerjee & Benedict, 1979). A slightly greater than two-fold increase in sister chromatid exchanges was reported in phytohaemagglutinin-stimulated human lymphocytes in culture (Raposa, 1978); however, in a more extensive study with the same test system, no increase in sister chromatid exchanges was observed (Morgan & Crossen, 1980).

No morphological transformation was induced in C3H/10T½ clone 8 cells even with highly toxic doses of vincristine (Benedict *et al.*, 1977).

(b) Humans

Toxic effects

The toxic effect of vincristine sulphate that limits the therapeutic dose that can be given is on the nervous system (Goodman & Gilman, 1975). The majority of patients experience some degree of peripheral neuropathy, with decreased tendon reflexes, paraesthesiae and weakness. Abdominal pain and constipation (related to an effect on the autonomic nervous system) are common (Creasey, 1975). Other manifestations include laryngeal nerve paralysis

(Whittaker & Griffith, 1977) and foot drop (Goodman & Gilman, 1975). Unexplained seizures occur in about 1% of patients and may be related to the drug (Dieterich, 1979). Ataxia, athetosis and coma have also been reported (Whittaker *et al.*, 1973; Carpentieri & Lockhart, 1978), although the causal role of vincristine has not been proven. Neurological effects are partially reversible on withdrawal of the drug. Although vincristine may cause myelosuppression (Goodman & Gilman, 1975), thrombocytosis is usual (Carbone *et al.*, 1963); however, platelets in vincristine-treated patients may undergo abnormal aggregation (Steinherz *et al.*, 1976).

Alopecia occurs in approximately 20% of patients (Goodman & Gilman, 1975). Other toxic effects that may follow vincristine treatment are the syndrome of inappropriate anti-diuretic hormone secretion (Slater *et al.*, 1969) and, possibly, myocardial infarction (Mandel *et al.*, 1975).

Effects on reproduction and prenatal toxicity

In a fetus of a woman given 1.5 mg vincristine sulphate and 4 mg nitrogen mustard, as single doses, and 100 mg/day procarbazine hydrochloride and 60 mg/day prednisone for 7 days during the first trimester of gestation, both kidneys were located in the pelvic inlet at the level of the bifurcation of the aorta after abortion at 3 months (Mennuti *et al.*, 1975).

In two negative case reports of use of this drug during pregnancy, exposure did not occur during the first trimester (Durie & Giles, 1977; Ortega, 1977).

Absorption, distribution, excretion and metabolism

After i.v. administration of a dose of tritiated vincristine, a triphasic plasma decay was observed, with half-lives of 0.85, 7.4 and 164 min; 69% of the radioactivity was recovered in the faeces and 12% in the urine over a 72-hour period. Approximately half of the recovered radioactivity was in the form of metabolites, whose ultra-violet spectrum suggested that the vincristine dimer was intact (Bender *et al.*, 1977). Studies of a patient with a biliary fistula showed extensive biliary excretion of the intact drug (46.5%) and of metabolites (53.5%) (Jackson *et al.*, 1978). These observations suggest that the biliary-faecal route is predominant in the excretion of vincristine and its metabolites.

Mutagenicity and chromosomal effects

No data were available to the Working Group.

3.3   Case reports and epidemiological studies of carcinogenicity in humans

There have been 15 case reports of acute nonlymphocytic leukaemia occurring following treatment of Hodgkin's disease with vincristine in combination with other drugs (Castro *et al.*, 1973; Weiden *et al.*, 1973; Focan *et al.*, 1974; Sahakian *et al.*, 1974; Rosner & Grünwald, 1975; Cadman *et al.*, 1977; Cavalli *et al.*, 1977). Other second neoplasms reported in patients with Hodgkin's disease given treatments including vincristine are: 1 squamous-cell carcinoma of the skin (Poleksic & Yeung, 1978), 1 lung cancer (O'Sullivan *et al.*, 1979) and 1 non-Hodgkin's lymphoma (Spaulding *et al.*, 1979).

Acute nonlymphocytic leukaemia has also been reported in patients treated with vincristine in combination with other therapies for the following primary neoplasms: 1 chronic lymphocytic leukaemia (Zarrabi *et al.*, 1977), 1 lymphosarcoma (Poth *et al.*, 1971), 1 Ewing's sarcoma (Smithson *et al.*, 1978) and 1 breast cancer (Portugal *et al.*, 1979). One renal medullary neuroblastoma and 1 bone fibrosarcoma were reported in patients with Ewing's sarcoma treated with vincristine and other cytotoxic drugs (Greene *et al.*, 1979); and Hodgkin's disease was reported to have occurred after vincristine and other cytotoxic drugs were given for an astrocytoma (Crafts *et al.*, 1978). In none of these cases was vincristine the only cytotoxic drug given, and many of the patients had also received radiation therapy.

Several authors have described the occurrence of acute nonlymphocytic leukaemia in cohorts of Hodgkin's disease patients treated with varying combinations of multi-drug chemotherapy and radiation (Ayoub *et al.*, 1978; Auclerc *et al.*, 1979; Papa *et al.*, 1979). The treatment regimens typically included procarbazine, vincristine and/or vinblastine sulphate and nitrogen mustard. However, these cohorts were not described in detail, and the relative risk of acute leukaemia in treated patients was not quantified. Taken together, the reports present data on approximately 2400 patients with Hodgkin's disease in whom 21 cases of acute nonlymphocytic leukaemia were diagnosed subsequently. Seventeen of these 21 leukaemia cases occurred in patients who had received both combination chemotherapy and radiation. The occurrence of solid tumours was not systematically documented.

A cohort of 452 patients with Hodgkin's disease treated at the US National Cancer Institute has been studied with reference to subsequent neoplasms (Arseneau *et al.*, 1972, 1977; Canellos *et al.*, 1974, 1975). The primary chemotherapeutic regimens employed were incompletely described but consisted primarily of procarbazine, vincristine, prednisone plus nitrogen mustard (MOPP) or cyclophosphamide (COPP). [An apparent initial excess of solid tumours, particularly in patients receiving both radiation and chemotherapy, may have been due to the inappropriate inclusion of non-melanoma skin cancers among their observations when such tumours were not included in the cancer incidence rates used to calculate the expected values.] With additional follow-up, 3 cases of acute non-lymphocytic leukaemia developed among the 65 patients treated with both combination chemotherapy (which included vincristine) and intensive radiation. This was described as a significant excess, although no expected number was given. The latent periods for development of leukaemia in these 3 patients were 12, 48 and 84 months.

A series of 1028 patients with Hodgkin's disease was reported from the Sloan-Kettering Cancer Centre, New York (Brody et al., 1977); in this cohort a significant excess of all cancers was noted among patients receiving various incompletely described regimens including combination chemotherapy (primarily procarbazine, vincristine, prednisone and nitrogen mustard - MOPP) and among patients treated with single-agent chemotherapy. Risk estimates were not provided for specific cancer types, but at least 3 cases of acute non-lymphocytic leukaemia occurred.

At Stanford University, California, 680 patients with Hodgkin's disease were followed for at least one year, for a median period of 5 years. Of these, 320 received radiation alone, 30 chemotherapy alone and 330 radiation plus chemotherapy. Chemotherapy consisted of nitrogen mustard, vincristine, prednisone and procarbazine (MOPP). Eight cases of acute nonlymphocytic leukaemia occurred among those treated with chemotherapy plus radiation, whereas none occurred in either of the other two groups. Although no expected number was calculated, the actuarial risk at 7 years was estimated to be $3.9 \pm 1.5\%$ (Coleman et al., 1977). An excess risk of non-Hodgkin's lymphoma was also observed, all 5 cases occurring in those 344 patients treated with both radiation and combination chemotherapy. The 10-year actuarial risk was estimated to be 15.2% among 579 patients with Hodgkin's disease at the same centre (Krikorian et al., 1979). The median latent period for development of leukaemia was 52 months, and that for non-Hodgkin's lymphoma was 94 months.

In Denmark, three cases of acute nonlymphocytic leukaemia were observed in a series of 201 consecutive patients with Hodgkin's disease, compared with 0.04 cases expected (Larsen & Brincker, 1977). One patient had received radiation and chemotherapy without vincristine, and the other two had received both radiation and combination chemotherapy including procarbazine, vincristine, prednisone and nitrogen mustard (MOPP). The latent period ranged from 2 - 8 years. No risk estimate for specific therapeutic subgroups was provided.

Among 232 patients with Hodgkin's disease treated in Manitoba, Canada (Neufeld et al., 1978), 2 cases of acute nonlymphocytic leukaemia developed, while 0.05 were expected. Both patients had received combination drug regimens which included procarbazine and vincristine, with radiation. The latent periods were 37 and 48 months. No risk estimate for specific therapeutic subgroups was provided.

Among 643 patients with Hodgkin's disease (Toland *et al.*, 1978) treated under the auspices of the Southwest Oncology Group in the US, 11 cases of acute nonlymphocytic leukaemia were reported, compared with 0.04 cases expected. The excess was greatest in patients treated with both radiation and combination chemotherapy (procarbazine, vincristine, prednisone and nitrogen mustard [MOPP] with or without bleomycin), among whom 8 cases of acute nonlymphocytic leukaemia were observed compared with 0.02 cases expected. A smaller excess was noted among patients treated with chemotherapy alone (3 observed, 0.012 expected). No leukaemia was observed among 106 patients who had received radiation only.

Pajak *et al.* (1979) reported in an abstract 9 cases of acute nonlymphocytic leukaemia among 802 patients with Hodgkin's disease who were in complete remission following treatment regimens consisting of procarbazine, prednisone and nitrogen mustard (MOPP) or procarbazine, vincristine, prednisone and BCNU (BOP). All patients were subsequently given maintenance therapy with chlorambucil (with or without vincristine and prednisone), and many also received radiation therapy. The median latent period for developing leukaemia was 53 months.

In a series of 764 patients with Hodgkin's disease from Milan (Valagussa *et al.*, 1980), 9 cases of acute nonlymphocytic leukaemia were noted (expected numbers were not calculated). Three combined chemotherapy regimens were employed: procarbazine, vincristine, prednisone and nitrogen mustard (MOPP); vincristine, nitrogen mustard, adriamycin, bleomycin and prednisone (MABOP); and vinblastine, adriamycin, bleomycin and dacarbazine (ABVD). Many patients received radiation therapy as well. Six cases of leukaemia developed in 350 patients who received a drug regimen containing both procarbazine and vincristine (plus radiation therapy), two developed in 87 patients who received a drug regimen containing vincristine (plus radiation therapy), and one developed in 36 patients who received a drug regimen containing vincristine (without radiation therapy). The frequency of leukaemia was greatest among the 147 patients treated with MOPP plus radiation, among whom 5 cases resulted in a 5-year actuarial risk of leukaemia of 5.4%. The median latent period for developing the leukaemia was 34 months. Patients in this study also developed 15 solid tumours (5 of which arose in an irradiated field), for which the 10-year actuarial risk was 7.3%. No specific chemotherapy regimen was implicated in these cases, and no risk estimates were presented for specific tumour types.

A cohort study specifically designed to evaluate the carcinogenicity of treatment for Hodgkin's disease was undertaken in 1553 patients diagnosed between 1940-1975 in Montreal and Boston (Boivin, 1981). Patients were classified as having received intensive chemotherapy, no intensive chemotherapy, intensive radiation or no intensive radiation therapy. No specific data were provided on the drugs used, although the 'intensive chemotherapeutic regimen' generally comprised procarbazine/vincristine, prednisone and nitrogen mustard (MOPP). Six cases of acute nonlymphocytic leukaemia (0.36 expected) and 21 other cancers (14.0 expected) were reported. In the subgroup treated with both intensive chemotherapy and intensive radiation (87 patients, 193 person years of observation), 2 cases of leukaemia were noted, compared with 0.007 cases expected. The relative risks for cancers other than leukaemia were not significantly elevated with any treatment category.

The occurrence of second malignancies was evaluated in a series of 438 patients with non-Hodgkin's lymphoma from the State University of New York at Stony Brook (Zarabbi, 1980). Three cases of acute nonlymphocytic leukaemia were observed, compared with 0.3 cases expected. All 3 patients had received both radiation and a combination regimen containing procarbazine and vincristine. Sixteen solid cancers were diagnosed, compared with 15.0 expected; no significant excess of any specific non-haematological malignancy was noted. The excess of leukaemia was not attributed to a specific therapeutic modality.

[The multiple agents, the inadequate description of methods of computation and the different formats of data presentation all preclude comparisons between studies and accurate calculation of the magnitude of risk.

[Nonetheless, the increase in risk of acute nonlymphocytic leukaemia has consistently been very large and cannot be explained by the above factors. This risk has been shown to increase over time in the same institutions (coincident with the introduction and increased use of multiple cytotoxic agents) independent of the effects of age, sex, stage of disease and interval since diagnosis (Brody et al., 1977; Boivin , 1981). The latent period for these leukaemias was consistently 3 - 5 years. Internal comparisons are consistent in implicating the combination of intensive chemotherapy and intensive radiation, and while solid tumours have tended to occur following radiation, the remaining cases of acute nonlymphocytic leukaemia have tended to occur after intensive chemotherapy alone.

[These studies do not permit distinctions to be made between alkylating agents, vincristine and procarbazine as potential causes of acute nonlymphocytic leukaemia.

[An excess of non-Hodgkin's lymphoma after combined chemotherapy for Hodgkin's disease has so far been reported from only one centre. Other centres have sufficient follow-up, and the chemotherapeutic regimen is a standard one.]

4. SUMMARY OF DATA REPORTED AND EVALUATION

4.1 Experimental data

Vincristine sulphate was tested in mice and rats by intraperitoneal injection. In these limited studies no evidence of carcinogenicity was found.

Vincristine sulphate can induce teratogenic effects in several animal species, and it induced embryolethality at doses nontoxic to the mother. There is no evidence to suggest that this compound is mutagenic.

4.2 Human data

Vincristine sulphate has been used since the early 1960s for treatment of acute leukaemia in children, often in combination with other antineoplastic agents. It is also frequently a part of combination chemotherapeutic regimens for Hodgkin's disease, non-Hodgkin's lymphoma, chronic lymphocytic leukaemia and other adult neoplasms.

The available data are insufficient to evaluate the teratogenicity of this drug in humans. No data were available on its mutagenic or chromosomal effects.

Both case reports and epidemiological studies indicate that acute nonlymphocytic leukaemia is produced in patients with Hodgkin's disease treated with combined therapeutic regimens which include vincristine sulphate, alkylating agents and procarbazine hydrochloride, often in conjunction with radiotherapy. No data were available on vincristine sulphate alone.

4.3 Evaluation

The available data in experimental animals were insufficient for evaluation. There is *sufficient evidence*[1] for the carcinogenicity in humans of intensive chemotherapeutic regimens that include alkylating agents, vincristine sulphate, procarbazine hydrochloride and prednisone. There is inadequate evidence for the carcinogenicity of vincristine sulphate itself.

On the basis of the available data, no conclusion could be drawn as to the carcinogenicity of vincristine sulphate.

---

[1]
See preamble, p. 17.

5. REFERENCES

Adamson, R.H., Dixon, R.L., Ben, M., Crews, L., Shohet, S.B. & Rall, D.P. (1965) Some pharmacologic properties of vincristine. *Arch. int. Pharmacodyn., 157,* 299-311

Ahn, Y.S., Harrington, W.J., Seelman, R.C. & Eytel, C.S. (1974) Vincristine therapy of idiopathic and secondary thrombocytopenias. *New Engl. J. Med., 291,* 376-380

Arseneau, J.C., Sponzo, R.W., Levin, D.L., Schnipper, L.E., Bonner, H., Young, R.C., Canellos, G.P., Johnson, R.E. & DeVita, V.T. (1972) Nonlymphomatous malignant tumors complicating Hodgkin's disease. Possible association with intensive therapy. *New Engl. J. Med., 287,* 1119-1122

Arseneau, J.C., Canellos, G.P., Johnson, R.C. & DeVita, V.T. (1977) Risk of new cancers in patients with Hodgkin's disease. *Cancer, 40,* 1912-1916

Auclerc, G., Jacquillat, C., Auclerc, M.F., Weil, M. & Bernard, J. (1979) Post-therapeutic acute leukemia. *Cancer, 44,* 2017-2025

Ayoub, J.I.G., Dubois, A., Cosendal, A.-M., Teitreault, L. & Pretty, H. (1978) Pre- and post-treatment second malignant neoplasms (SMN) in Hodgkin's disease (HD) (Abstract no. C-61). *Proc. Am. Soc. clin. Oncol., 19,* 322

Baker, C.E., Jr, ed. (1980) *Physicians' Desk Reference,* 34th ed., Oradell, NJ, Medical Economics Co., pp. 1068-1069

Banerjee, A. & Benedict, W.F. (1979) Production of sister chromatid exchanges by various cancer chemotherapeutic agents. *Cancer Res., 39,* 797-799

Bender, R.A., Castle, M.C., Margileth, D.A. & Oliverio, V.T. (1977) The pharmacokinetics of [^{3}H]-vincristine in man. *Clin. Pharmacol. Ther., 22,* 430-438

Benedict, W.F., Banerjee, A., Gardner, A. & Jones, P.A. (1977) Induction of morphological transformation in mouse C3H/10T½ clone 8 cells and chromosomal damage in hamster A(T$_1$)C1-3 cells by cancer chemotherapeutic agents. *Cancer Res., 37,* 2202-2208

Boivin, J.-F. (1981) *Late Side Effects of Treatment for Hodgkin's Disease.* Thesis, Boston, MA, Harvard School of Public Health, pp. 34-79

Brody, R.S., Schottenfeld, D. & Reid, A. (1977) Multiple primary cancer risk after therapy for Hodgkin's disease. *Cancer, 40,* 1917-1926

Burns, J.H. (1972) *Vincristine sulfate.* In: Florey, K., ed., *Analytical Profiles of Drug Substances,* Vol. 1, New York, Academic Press, pp. 463-480

Cadman, E.C., Capizzi, R.L. & Bertino, J.R. (1977) Acute nonlymphocytic leukemia. A delayed complication of Hodgkin's disease therapy: analysis of 109 cases. *Cancer, 40,* 1280-1296

Canellos, G.P., DeVita, V.T., Arseneau, J.C. & Johnson, R.C. (1974) Carcinogenesis by cancer chemotherapeutic agents: second malignancies complicating Hodgkin's disease in remission. *Recent Results
Cancer Res., 49,* 108-114

Canellos, G.P., DeVita, V.T., Arseneau, J.C., Whang-Peng, J. & Johnson, R.E.C. (1975) Second malignancies
complicating Hodgkin's disease in remission. *Lancet, i,* 947-949

Carbone, P.P., Bono, V., Frei, E., III & Brindley, C.O. (1963) Clinical studies with vincristine. *Blood, 21,*
640-647

Carpentieri, U. & Lockhart, L.H. (1978) Ataxia and athetosis as side effects of chemotherapy with vincristine in non-Hodgkin's lymphoma. *Cancer Treat. Rep., 62,* 561-562

Castle, M.C., Margileth, D.A. & Oliverio, V.T. (1976) Distribution and excretion of [^{3}H] vincristine in the
rat and the dog. *Cancer Res., 36,* 3684-3689

Castro, G.A.M., Church, A., Pechet, L. & Snyder, L.M. (1973) Leukemia after chemotherapy of Hodgkin's
disease. *New Engl. J. Med., 289,* 103-104

Cavalli, F., Gerber, A., Mosimann, W., Sonntag, R.W. & Tschopp, L. (1977) Acute myeloid leukaemia
in the course of Hodgkin's disease (Ger.). *Dtsch. med. Wochenschr., 102,* 1019-1024

Coleman, C.N., Williams, C.J., Flint, A., Glatstein, E.J., Rosenberg, S.A. & Kaplan, H.S. (1977) Hematologic
neoplasia in patients treated for Hodgkin's disease. *New Engl. J. Med., 297,* 1249-1252

Courtney, K.D. & Valerio, D.A. (1968) Teratology in the *Macaca mulatta. Teratology, 1,* 163-172

Crafts, D.C., Townsend, J., Wilson, C.B. & Levin, V.A. (1978) Development of Hodgkin's disease in a
patient receiving procarbazine, CCNU, and vincristine therapy for a gemistocytic astrocytoma. *Cancer
Treat. Rep., 62,* 177-178

Creasey, W.A. (1975) *Vinca alkaloids and colchicine.* In: Sartorelli, A.C. & Johns, D.G., eds, *Antineoplastic
and Immunosuppressive Agents,* Part II, New York, Springer, pp. 670-694

Degraeve, N. (1978) Genetic and related effects of *Vinca rosea* alkaloids. *Mutat. Res., 55,* 31-42

Dieterich, E. (1979) Encephalopathy due to vincristine (Ger.). *Klin. Pädiatr., 191,* 145-147

Dixon, G.J., Dulmadge, E.A., Mulligan, L.T. & Mellett, L.B. (1969) Cell culture bioassay for vincristine
sulfate in sera from mice, rats, dogs, and monkeys. *Cancer Res., 29,* 1810-1813

Durie, B.G.M. & Giles, H.R. (1977) Successful treatment of acute leukemia during pregnancy: combination
therapy in the third trimester. *Arch. intern. Med., 137,* 90-91

El Dareer, S.M., White, V.M., Chen, F.P., Mellett, L.B. & Hill, D.L. (1977) Distribution and metabolism of
vincristine in mice, rats, dogs, and monkeys. *Cancer Treat. Rep., 61,* 1269-1277

Ferm, V.H. (1963) Congenital malformations in hamster embryos after treatment with vinblastine and
vincristine. *Science, 141,* 426

Focan, C., Brictieux, N., Lemaire, M. & Hugues, J. (1974) Secondary neoplasias as complications in Hodgkin's disease (Fr.). *Nouv. Presse méd., 3,* 1385

Folk, R.M., Peters, A.C., Pavkov, K.L. & Swenberg, J.A. (1974) Vincristine (NSC-67574): a retrospective, toxicologic evaluation in monkeys and dogs using weekly intravenous injections for 6 weeks. *Cancer Chemother. Rep., Part 3, 5,* 17-23

Goodman, L.S. & Gilman, A., eds (1975) *The Pharmacological Basis of Therapeutics,* 5th ed., New York, Macmillan, pp. 1375-1379

Greene, M.H., Glaubiger, D.L., Mead, G.D. & Fraumeni, J.F., Jr (1979) Subsequent cancer in patients with Ewing's sarcoma. *Cancer Treat. Rep., 63,* 2043-2046

Harvey, S.C. (1975) *Antineoplastic and immunosuppressive drugs.* In: Osol, A., ed., *Remington's Pharmaceutical Sciences,* 15th ed., Easton, PA, Mack Publishing Company, p. 1086

Hirshaut, Y., Weiss, G. & Blackham, E. (1969) Bioassay of antileukemic drugs using human leukocytes in long-term culture (Abstract). *Clin. Res., 16,* 360

Jackson, D.V., Jr, Castle, M.C. & Bender, R.A. (1978) Biliary excretion of vincristine. *Clin. Pharmacol. Ther., 24,* 101-107

Jackson, D.V., Jr, Castle, M.C., Poplack, D.G. & Bender, R.A. (1980) Pharmacokinetics of vincristine in the cerebrospinal fluid of subhuman primates. *Cancer Res., 40,* 722-724

Johnson, I.S., Wright, H.F. & Svoboda, G.H. (1959) Experimental basis for clinical evaluation of antitumour principles derived from *Vinca rosea* Linn. (Abstract no. 72). *J. Lab. clin. Med., 54,* 830

Joneja, M. & Ungthavorn, S. (1969) Teratogenic effects of vincristine in three lines of mice. *Teratology, 2,* 235-240

Krikorian, J.G., Burke, J.S., Rosenberg, S.A. & Kaplan, H.S. (1979) Occurrence of non-Hodgkin's lymphoma after therapy for Hodgkin's disease. *New Engl. J. Med., 300,* 452-458

Larsen, J. & Brincker, H. (1977) The incidence and characteristics of acute myeloid leukaemia arising in Hodgkin's disease. *Scand J. Haematol., 18,* 197-206

Maier, P. & Schmid, W. (1976) Ten model mutagens evaluated by the micronucleus test. *Mutat. Res., 40,* 325-338

Mandel, E.M., Lewinski, U. & Djaldetti, M. (1975) Vincristine-induced myocardial infarction. *Cancer, 36,* 1979-1982

Matheson, D., Brusick, D. & Carrano, R. (1978) Comparison of the relative mutagenic activity for eight antineoplastic drugs in the Ames *Salmonella*/microsome and TK$^{+/-}$ mouse lymphoma assays. *Drug chem. Toxicol., 1,* 277-304

Mennuti, M.T., Shepard, T.H. & Mellman, W.J. (1975) Fetal renal malformation following treatment of Hodgkin's disease during pregnancy. *Obstet. Gynecol., 46,* 194-196

Moncrief, J.W. & Lipscomb, W.N. (1965) Structures of leurocristine (vincristine) and vincaleukoblastine. X-ray analysis of leurocristine methiodide. *J. Am. chem. Soc., 87,* 4963-4964

Morgan, W.F. & Crossen, P.E. (1980) Mitotic spindle inhibitors and sister-chromatid exchange in human chromosomes. *Mutat. Res., 77,* 283-286

Németh, L., Somfai, S., Gál, F. & Kellner, B. (1970) Comparative studies concerning the tumour inhibition and the toxicology of vinblastine and vincristine. *Neoplasma, 17,* 345-347

Neufeld, H., Weinerman, B.H. & Kemel, S. (1978) Secondary malignant neoplasms in patients with Hodgkin's disease. *J. Am. med. Assoc., 239,* 2470-2471

Noble, R.L., Beer, C.T. & Cutts, J.H. (1958) Role of chance observations in chemotherapy: *Vinca rosea. Ann. NY. Acad. Sci., 76,* 887-894

Ortega, J. (1977) Multiple agent chemotherapy including bleomycin of non-Hodgkin's lymphoma during pregnancy. *Cancer, 40,* 2829-2835

O'Sullivan, D.D., Raghuprasad, P. & Ezdinli, E.Z. (1979) Solid tumors complicating Hodgkin's disease. A report on two patients with immunoglobin deficiency. *Arch. intern. Med., 139,* 1131-1134

Pajak, T.F., Nissen, N.I., Stutzman, L., Hoogstraten, B., Cooper, M.R., Glowienka, L.P., Glidewell, O. & Glicksman, A. (1979) Acute myeloid leukemia occurring during complete remission in Hodgkin's disease (Abstract no. C-425). *Proc. Am. Soc. clin. Oncol., 20,* 394

Papa, G., Alimena, G., Annino, L., Anselmo, A.P., Ciccone, F., De Luca, A.M., Granati, L., Petti, N. & Mandelli, F. (1979) Acute non lymphoid leukaemia following Hodgkin's disease. Clinical, biological and cytogenetic aspects of 3 cases. *Scand. J. Haematol., 23,* 339-347

Poleksic, S. & Yeung, K.-Y. (1978) Rapid development of keratoacanthoma and accelerated transformation into squamous cell carcinoma of the skin. A mutagenic effect of polychemotherapy in a patient with Hodgkin's disease? *Cancer, 41,* 12-16

Portugal, M.A., Falkson, H.C., Stevens, K. & Falkson, G. (1979) Acute leukemia as a complication of long-term treatment of advanced breast cancer. *Cancer Treat. Rep., 63,* 177-181

Poth, J.L., George, R.P., Jr, Creger, W.P. & Schrier, S.L. (1971) Acute myelogenous leukemia following localized radiotherapy. *Arch. intern. Med., 128,* 802-805

Raposa, T. (1978) Sister chromatid exchange studies for monitoring DNA damage and repair capacity after cytostatics *in vitro* and in lymphocytes of leukaemic patients under cytostatic therapy. *Mutat. Res., 57,* 241-251

Rosner, F. & Grünwald, H. (1975) Hodgkin's disease and acute leukemia. Report of eight cases and review of the literature. *Am. J. Med., 58,* 339-353

Sahakian, G.J., Al-Mondhiry, H., Lacher, M.J. & Connolly, C.E. (1974) Acute leukemia in Hodgkin's disease. *Cancer, 33,* 1369-1375

Saxton, J.E. (1971) *The Alkaloids,* Vol. 1, London, The Chemical Society, pp. 483-484

Seino, Y., Nagao, M., Yahagi, T., Hoshi, A., Kawachi, T. & Sugimura, T. (1978) Mutagenicity of several classes of antitumor agents to *Salmonella typhimurium* TA98, TA100, and TA92. *Cancer Res., 38,* 2148-2156

Sethi, V.S., Burton, S.S. & Jackson, D.V. (1980) A sensitive radioimmunoassay for vincristine and vinblastine. *Cancer Chemother. Pharmacol., 4,* 183-187

Sieber, S.M., Whang-Peng, J., Botkin, C. & Knutsen, T. (1978) Teratogenic and cytogenetic effects of some plant-derivative antitumor agents (vincristine, colchicine, maytansine, VP-16-213 and VM-26) in mice. *Teratology, 18,* 31-48

Slater, L.M., Wainer, R.A. & Serpick, A.A. (1969) Vincristine neurotoxicity with hyponatremia. *Cancer, 23,* 122-125

Smithson, W.A., Burgert, E.O., Jr, Childs, D.S. & Hoagland, H.C. (1978) Acute myelomonocytic leukemia after irradiation and chemotherapy for Ewing's sarcoma. *Mayo Clin. Proc., 53,* 757-759

Spaulding, M.B., Mogavero, H. & Montes, M. (1979) Non-Hodgkin's lymphoma after chemotherapy for Hodgkin's disease. *New Engl. J. Med., 301,* 384-385

Steinherz, P.G., Miller, D.R., Hilgartner, M.W. & Schmalzer, E.A. (1976) Platelet dysfunction in vincristine treated patients. *Br. J. Haematol., 32,* 439-450

Todd, G.C., Gibson, W.R. & Morton, D.M. (1976) Toxicology of vindesine (desacetyl vinblastine amide) in mice, rats and dogs. *J. Toxicol. environ. Health, 1,* 843-850

Todd, G.C., Griffing, W.J., Gibson, W.R. & Morton, D.M. (1979) Animal models for the comparative assessment of neurotoxicity following repeated administration of vinca alkaloids. *Cancer Treat. Rep., 63,* 35-41

Toland, D.M., Coltman, C.A., Jr & Moon, T.E. (1978) Second malignancies complicating Hodgkin's disease - the Southwest Oncology Group experience. *Cancer clin. Trials, 1,* 27-33

Ungthavorn, S. & Joneja, M. (1969) Studies on vincristine-induced teratogenesis in mice (Abstract). *Anat. Rec., 163,* 277

US Pharmacopeial Convention, Inc. (1980) *The US Pharmacopeia,* 20th rev., Rockville, MD, p. 844

US Tariff Commission (1967) *Synthetic Organic Chemicals, US Production and Sales, 1965,* TC Publication 206, Washington DC, US Government Printing Office, p. 119

Valagussa, P., Santoro, A., Kenda, R., Fossati Bellani, F., Franchi, F., Banfi, A., Rilke, F. & Bonadonna, G. (1980) Second malignancies in Hodgkin's disease; a complication of certain forms of treatment. *Br. med. J., i,* 216-219

Wade, A., ed. (1977) *Martindale, The Extra Pharmacopoeia,* 27th ed., London, The Pharmaceutical Press, pp. 173-174

Weiden, P.L., Lerner, K.G., Gerdes, A., Heywood, J.D., Fefer, A. & Thomas, E.D. (1973) Pancytopenia and leukemia in Hodgkin's disease: report of three cases. *Blood, 42,* 571-577

Weisburger, E.K. (1977) Bioassay program for carcinogenic hazards of cancer chemotherapeutic agents. *Cancer, 40,* 1935-1949

Whittaker, J.A. & Griffith, I.P. (1977) Recurrent laryngeal nerve paralysis in patients receiving vincristine and vinblastine. *Br. med. J., i,* 1251-1252

Whittaker, J.A., Parry, D.H., Bunch, C. & Weatherall, D.J. (1973) Coma associated with vincristine therapy. *Br. med. J., iv,* 335-337

Zarrabi, M.H. (1980) Association of non-Hodgkin's lymphoma (NHL) and second neoplasms. *Semin. Oncol., 7,* 340-351

Zarrabi, M.H., Grünwald, H.W. & Rosner, F. (1977) Chronic lymphocytic leukemia terminating in acute leukemia. *Arch. intern. Med., 137,* 1059-1064

SUPPLEMENTARY CORRIGENDA TO VOLUMES 1 - 25

Corrigenda covering Volumes 1 - 6 appeared in Volume 7; others appeared in Volumes 8, 10 - 13, 15 - 25.

Volume 11

p. 133	para 5, line 3	*replace* 19 mg/m^3 (15 ppm) *by* 19 mg/m^3 (5 ppm)

Volume 24

p. 222	para 2, line 2	*add* although there was an association with microcephaly (7 cases; relative risk, 8).
p. 223	para, 3, line 1	*replace* eliminated *by* stimulated
p. 237	Heinonen *et al.* (1977)	*add p. no.* 495

CUMULATIVE INDEX TO IARC MONOGRAPHS ON THE EVALUATION
OF THE CARCINOGENIC RISK OF CHEMICALS TO HUMANS

Numbers in bold indicate volume, and other numbers indicate page. References to corrigenda are given in parentheses. Compounds marked with an asterisk (*) were considered by the Working Groups, but monographs were not prepared because adequate data on their carcinogenicity were not available.

4-Amino-2-nitrophenol   **16,**   43
2-Amino-4-nitrophenol*
2-Amino-5-nitrophenol*
6-Amino penicillanic acid*
Amitrole   **7,**   31
Amobarbital sodium*
Anaesthetics, volatile   **11,**   285
Aniline   **4,**   27   (corr. **7**, 320)
Anthranilic acid   **16,**   265
Apholate   **9,**   31
Aramite®   **5,**   39
Arsenic and arsenic compounds   **1,**   41
                                                   2,   48
                                                   23,   39

     Arsanilic acid
     Arsenic pentoxide
     Arsenic sulphide
     Arsenic trioxide
     Arsine
     Calcium arsenate
     Dimethylarsinic acid
     Lead arsenate
     Methanearsonic acid, disodium salt
     Methanearsonic acid, monosodium salt
     Potassium arsenate
     Potassium arsenite
     Sodium arsenate
     Sodium arsenite
     Sodium cacodylate

Asbestos   **2,**   17   (corr. **7**, 319)
                                                   14   (corr. **15**, 341)
                                                                    (corr. **17**, 351)

Beryllium carbonate

Beryllium chloride

Beryllium-copper alloy

Beryllium-copper-cobalt alloy

Beryllium fluoride

Beryllium hydroxide

Beryllium-nickel alloy

Beryllium oxide

Beryllium phosphate

Beryllium silicate

Beryllium sulphate and its tetrahydrate

Beryl ore

Zinc beryllium silicate

C

Methoxyflurane*

Methyl acrylate	**19,** 52	
2-Methylaziridine	**9,** 61	
Methylazoxymethanol	**10,** 121	
Methylazoxymethanol acetate	**1,** 164	
	10, 131	

Methyl bromide*

Methyl carbamate	**12,** 151	
N-Methyl-N,4-dinitrosoaniline	**1,** 141	
4,4'-Methylene bis(2-chloroaniline)	**4,** 65	(corr. **7,**320)
4,4'-Methylene bis(2-methylaniline)	**4,** 73	
4,4'-Methylenedianiline	**4,** 79	(corr. **7,** 320)
4,4'-Methylenediphenyl diisocyanate	**19,** 314	
Methyl iodide	**15,** 245	
Methyl methacrylate	**19,** 187	
Methyl methanesulphonate	**7,** 253	
N-Methyl-N'-nitro-N-nitrosoguanidine	**4,** 183	

Methyl protoanemonin*

Methyl red	**8,** 161	
Methyl selenac	**12,** 161	
Methylthiouracil	**7,** 53	
Metronidazole	**13,** 113	
Mirex	**5,** 203	
	20, 283	
Mitomycin C	**10,** 171	
Modacrylic fibres	**19,** 86	
Monocrotaline	**10,** 291	
Monuron	**12,** 167	
5-(Morpholinomethyl)-3-[(5-nitrofurfurylidene)- amino]-2-oxazolidinone	**7,** 161	
Mustard gas	**9,** 181	(corr. **13,** 243)

Resorcinol	**15**, 155	
Retrorsine	**10**, 303	
Rhodamine B	**16**, 221	
Rhodamine 6G	**16**, 233	
Riddelliine	**10**, 313	
Rifampicin	**24**, 243	

S

Saccharated iron oxide	**2**, 161	
Saccharin	**22**, 111	(corr. **25**, 391)
Safrole	**1**, 169	
	10, 231	
Scarlet red	**8**, 217	
Selenium and selenium compounds	**9**, 245	(corr. **12**,271)
Semicarbazide hydrochloride	**12**, 209	(corr. **16**,387)
Seneciphylline	**10**, 319	
Senkirkine	**10**, 327	
Sodium cyclamate	**22**, 56	(corr. **25**, 391)
Sodium diethyldithiocarbamate	**12**, 217	
Sodium equilin sulphate	**21**, 148	
Sodium oestrone sulphate	**21**, 147	
Sodium saccharin	**22**, 113	(corr. **25**, 391)
Soot, tars and shale oils	**3**, 22	
Spironolactone	**24**, 259	
Sterigmatocystin	**1**, 175	
	10, 245	
Streptozotocin	**4**, 221	
	17, 337	
Styrene	**19**, 231	
Styrene-acrylonitrile copolymers	**19**, 97	
Styrene-butadiene copolymers	**19**, 252	
Styrene oxide	**11**, 201	
	19, 275	

IARC MONOGRAPHS ON THE EVALUATION
OF THE CARCINOGENIC RISK OF CHEMICALS TO HUMANS

IARC SCIENTIFIC PUBLICATIONS

NON-SERIAL PUBLICATIONS:

WHO/IARC publications may be obtained, direct or through booksellers, from:

ALGERIA: Société Nationale d'Edition et de Diffusion, 3 bd Zirout Youcef, ALGIERS

ARGENTINA: Carlos Hirsch SRL, Florida 165, Galerias Güemes, Escritorio 453/465, BUENOS AIRES

AUSTRALIA: *Mail Order Sales:* Australian Government Publishing Service, P.O. Box 84, CANBERRA A.C.T. 2600; *or over the counter from* Australian Government Publishing Service Bookshops *at:* 70 Alinga Street, CANBERRA CITY A.C.T. 2600; 294 Adelaide Street, BRISBANE, Queensland 4000; 347 Swanston Street, MELBOURNE, VIC 3000; 309 Pitt Street, SYDNEY, N.S.W. 2000; Mt Newman House, 200 St. George's Terrace, PERTH, WA 6000; Industry House, 12 Pirie Street, ADELAIDE, SA 5000; 156–162 Macquarie Street, HOBART, TAS 7000 — Hunter Publications, 58A Gipps Street, COLLINGWOOD, VIC 3066 — R. Hill & Son Ltd, 608 St. Kilda Road, MELBOURNE, VIC 3004; Lawson House, 10–12 Clark Street, CROW'S NEST, NSW 2065

AUSTRIA: Gerold & Co., Graben 31, 1011 VIENNA I

BANGLADESH: The WHO Programme Coordinator, G.P.O. Box 250, DACCA 5 — The Association of Voluntary Agencies, P.O. Box 5045, DACCA 5

BELGIUM: Office international de Librairie, 30 avenue Marnix, 1050 BRUSSELS — *Subscriptions to World Health only:* Jean de Lannoy, 202 avenue du Roi, 1060 BRUSSELS

BRAZIL: Biblioteca Regional de Medicina OMS/OPS, Unidade de Venda de Publicações, Caixa Postal 20.381, Vila Clementino, 04023 SÃO PAULO, S.P.

BURMA: *see* India, WHO Regional Office

CANADA: *Single and bulk copies of individual publications (not subscriptions):* Canadian Public Health Association, 1335 Carling Avenue, Suite 210, OTTAWA, Ont. K1Z 8N8. *Subscriptions: Subscription orders, accompanied by cheque made out to the* Royal Bank of Canada, OTTAWA, Account World Health Organization, *should be sent to the* World Health Organization, P.O. Box 1800, Postal Station B, OTTAWA, Ont. K1P 5R5. *Correspondence concerning subscriptions should be addressed to the* World Health Organization, Distribution and Sales, 1211 GENEVA 27, Switzerland

CHINA: China National Publications Import Corporation, P.O. Box 88, BEIJING (PEKING)

COLOMBIA: Distrilibros Ltd, Pio Alfonso Garcia, Carrera 4a, Nos 36–119, CARTAGENA

CYPRUS: Publishers' Distributors Cyprus, 30 Democratias Ave Ayios Dhometios, P.O. Box 4165, NICOSIA

CZECHOSLOVAKIA: Artia, Ve Smeckach 30, 111 27 PRAGUE I

DENMARK: Munksgaard Export and Subscription Service, Nørre Søgade 35, 1370 COPENHAGEN K

ECUADOR: Libreria Cientifica S.A., P.O. Box 362, Luque 223, GUAYAQUIL

EGYPT: Osiris Office for Books and Reviews, 50 Kasr El Nil Street, CAIRO

EL SALVADOR: Libreria Estudiantil, Edificio Comercial B No 3, Avenida Libertad, SAN SALVADOR

FIJI: The WHO Programme Coordinator, P.O. Box 113, SUVA

FINLAND: Akateeminen Kirjakauppa, Keskuskatu 2, 00101 HELSINKI 10

FRANCE: Librairie Arnette, 2 rue Casimir-Delavigne, 75006 PARIS

GERMAN DEMOCRATIC REPUBLIC: Buchhaus Leipzig, Postfach 140, 701 LEIPZIG

GERMANY, FEDERAL REPUBLIC OF: Govi-Verlag GmbH, Ginnheimerstrasse 20, Postfach 5360, 6236 ESCHBORN — W. E. Saarbach, Postfach 101610, Follerstrasse 2, 5000 KÖLN I — Alex. Horn, Spiegelgasse 9, Postfach 3340, 6200 WIESBADEN

GHANA: Fides Enterprises, P.O. Box 1628, ACCRA

GREECE: G. C. Eleftheroudakis S.A., Librairie internationale, rue Nikis 4, ATHENS (T. 126)

HAITI: Max Bouchereau, Librairie "A la Caravelle", Boîte postale 111-B, PORT-AU-PRINCE

HONG KONG: Hong Kong Government Information Services, Beaconsfield House, 6th Floor, Queen's Road, Central, VICTORIA

HUNGARY: Kultura, P.O.B. 149, BUDAPEST 62 — Akadémiai Könyvesbolt, Váci utca 22, BUDAPEST V

ICELAND: Snaebjørn Jonsson & Co., P.O. Box 1131, Hafnarstraeti 9, REYKJAVIK

INDIA: WHO Regional Office for South-East Asia, World Health House, Indraprastha Estate, Ring Road, NEW DELHI 110002 — Oxford Book & Stationery Co., Scindia House, NEW DELHI 110001; 17 Park Street, CALCUTTA 700016 (*Sub-agent*)

INDONESIA: M/s Kalaman Book Service Ltd, Kwitang Raya No. 11, P.O. Box 3105/Jkt., JAKARTA

IRAN: Iranian Amalgamated Distribution Agency, 151 Khiaban Soraya, TEHERAN

IRAQ: Ministry of Information, National House for Publishing, Distributing and Advertising, BAGHDAD

IRELAND: The Stationery Office, DUBLIN 4

ISRAEL: Heiliger & Co., 3 Nathan Strauss Street, JERUSALEM

ITALY: Edizioni Minerva Medica, Corso Bramante 83–85, 10126 TURIN; Via Lamarmora 3, 20100 MILAN

JAPAN: Maruzen Co. Ltd, P.O. Box 5050, TOKYO International, 100–31

KOREA, REPUBLIC OF: The WHO Programme Coordinator, Central P.O. Box 540, SEOUL

KUWAIT: The Kuwait Bookshops Co. Ltd, Thunayan Al-Ghanem Bldg, P.O. Box 2942, KUWAIT

LAO PEOPLE'S DEMOCRATIC REPUBLIC: The WHO Programme Coordinator, P.O. Box 343, VIENTIANE

LEBANON: The Levant Distributors Co. S.A.R.L., Box 1181, Makdassi Street, Hanna Bldg, BEIRUT

LUXEMBOURG: Librairie du Centre, 49 bd Royal, LUXEMBOURG

MALAWI: Malawi Book Service, P.O. Box 30044, Chichiti, BLANTYRE 3

MALAYSIA: The WHO Programme Coordinator, Room 1004, Fitzpatrick Building, Jalan Raja Chulan, KUALA LUMPUR 05–02 — Jubilee (Book) Store Ltd, 97 Jalan Tuanku Abdul Rahman, P.O. Box 629, KUALA LUMPUR 01–08 — Parry's Book Center, K. L. Hilton Hotel, Jln. Treacher, P.O. Box 960, KUALA LUMPUR

MEXICO: La Prensa Médica Mexicana, Ediciónes Cientificas, Paseo de las Facultades 26, Apt. Postal 20–413, MEXICO CITY 20, D.F.

MONGOLIA: *see* India, WHO Regional Office

MOROCCO: Editions La Porte, 281 avenue Mohammed V, RABAT

MOZAMBIQUE: INLD, Caixa Postal 4030, MAPUTO

NEPAL: *see* India, WHO Regional Office

NETHERLANDS: Medical Books Europe BV, Noorderwal 38, 7241 BL LOCHEM

NEW ZEALAND: Government Printing Office, Publications Section, Mulgrave Street, Private Bag, WELLINGTON I; Walter Street, WELLINGTON; World Trade Building, Cubacade, Cuba Street, WELLINGTON. *Government Bookshops en:* Hannaford Burton Building, Rutland Street, Private Bag, AUCKLAND; 159 Hereford Street, Private Bag, CHRISTCHURCH; Alexandra Street, P.O. Box 857, HAMILTON; T & G Building, Princes Street, P.O. Box 1104, DUNEDIN — R. Hill & Son Ltd., Ideal House, Cnr Gillies Avenue & Eden St., Newmarket, AUCKLAND I

NIGERIA: University Bookshop Nigeria Ltd, University of Ibadan, IBADAN

NORWAY: J. G. Tanum A/S, P.O. Box 1177 Sentrum, OSLO I

PAKISTAN: Mirza Book Agency, 65 Shahrah–E–Quaid–E–Azam, P.O. Box 729, LAHORE 3

PAPUA NEW GUINEA: The WHO Programme Coordinator, P.O. Box 5896, BOROKO

PHILIPPINES: World Health Organization, Regional Office for the Western Pacific, P.O. Box 2932, MANILA — The Modern Book Company Inc., P.O. Box 632, 922 Rizal Avenue, MANILA 2800

POLAND: Składnica Księgarska, ul Mazowiecka 9, 00052 WARSAW (*except periodicals*) — BKWZ Ruch, ul Wronia 23, 00840 WARSAW (*periodicals only*)

PORTUGAL: Livraria Rodrigues, 186 Rua do Ouro, LISBON 2

SIERRA LEONE: Njala University College Bookshop (University of Sierra Leone), Private Mail Bag, FREETOWN

SINGAPORE: The WHO Programme Coordinator, 144 Moulmein Road, G.P.O. Box 3457, SINGAPORE I — Select Books (Pte) Ltd, 215 Tanglin Shopping Centre, 2/F, 19 Tanglin Road, SINGAPORE 10

SOUTH AFRICA: Van Schaik's Bookstore (Pty) Ltd, P.O. Box 724, 268 Church Street, PRETORIA 0001

SPAIN: Comercial Atheneum S.A., Consejo de Ciento 130–136, BARCELONA 15; General Moscardó 29, MADRID 20 — Libreria Diaz de Santos, Lagasca 95 y Maldonado 6, MADRID 6; Balmes 417 y 419, BARCELONA 22

SRI LANKA: *see* India, WHO Regional Office

SWEDEN: Aktiebolaget C.E. Fritzes Kungl. Hovbokhandel, Regeringsgatan 12, 10327 STOCKHOLM

SWITZERLAND: Medizinischer Verlag Hans Huber, Länggass Strasse 76, 3012 BERN 9

SYRIAN ARAB REPUBLIC: M. Farras Kekhia, P.O. Box No. 5221, ALEPPO

THAILAND: *see* India, WHO Regional Office

TUNISIA: Société Tunisienne de Diffusion, 5 avenue de Carthage, TUNIS

TURKEY: Haset Kitapevi, 469 Istiklal Caddesi, Beyoglu, ISTANBUL

UNITED KINGDOM: H.M. Stationery Office: 49 High Holborn, LONDON WC1V 6HB; 13a Castle Street, EDINBURGH EH2 3AR; 41 The Hayes, CARDIFF CF1 1JW; 80 Chichester Street, BELFAST BT1 4JY; Brazennose Street, MANCHESTER M60 8AS; 258 Broad Street, BIRMINGHAM B1 2HE; Southey House, Wine Street, BRISTOL BS1 2BQ. *All mail orders should be sent to* P.O. Box 569, LONDON SE1 9NH

UNITED STATES OF AMERICA: *Single and bulk copies of individual publications (not subscriptions):* WHO Publications Centre USA, 49 Sheridan Avenue, ALBANY, N.Y. 12210. *Subscriptions: Subscription orders, accompanied by check made out to the* Chemical Bank, New York, Account World Health Organization, *should be sent to the* World Health Organization, P.O. Box 5284, Church Street Station, NEW YORK, N.Y. 10249. *Correspondence concerning subscriptions should be addressed to the* World Health Organization, Distribution and Sales, 1211 GENEVA 27, Switzerland. *Publications are also available from the* United Nations Bookshop, NEW YORK, N.Y. 10017 (*retail only*)

USSR: *For readers in the USSR requiring Russian editions:* Komsomolskij prospekt 18, Medicinskaja Kniga, MOSCOW — *For readers outside the USSR requiring Russian editions:* Kuzneckij most 18, Meždunarodnaja Kniga, MOSCOW G-200

VENEZUELA: Editorial Interamericana de Venezuela C.A., Apartado 50.785, CARACAS 105 — Libreria del Este, Apartado 60.337, CARACAS 106 — Libreria Médica Paris, Apartado 60.681, CARACAS 106

YUGOSLAVIA: Jugoslovenska Knjiga, Terazije 27/II, 11000 BELGRADE

ZAIRE: Librairie universitaire, avenue de la Paix Nº 167, B.P. 1682, KINSHASA I

Special terms for developing countries are obtainable on application to the WHO Programme Coordinators or WHO Regional Offices listed above or to the World Health Organization, Distribution and Sales Service, 1211 Geneva 27, Switzerland. Orders from countries where sales agents have not yet been appointed may also be sent to the Geneva address, but must be paid for in pounds sterling, US dollars, or Swiss francs.

Price: Sw. fr. 62.– US $ 30.00   Prices are subject to change without notice.   IARC/1/81